W9-BMI-207

Vowel Disorders

Vowel Disorders

Martin J. Ball, Ph.D.

*Hawthorne-BoRSF Distinguished Professor of
Communicative Disorders, University of Louisiana
at Lafayette*

Fiona E. Gibbon, Ph.D.

*Senior Lecturer and Director of Research, Department
of Speech and Language Sciences, Queen Margaret
University College, Edinburgh, Scotland*

Foreword by WITHDRAWN

Raymond D. Kent, Ph.D.

*Professor of Communicative Disorders, University
of Wisconson, Madison*

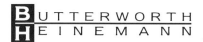

BUTTERWORTH
HEINEMANN

Boston Oxford Auckland Johannesburg Melbourne New Delhi

MW

Library of Congress Cataloging-in-Publication Data

Ball, Martin J. (Martin John)
   Vowel disorders / Martin J. Ball, Fiona Gibbon; foreword by Raymond D. Kent.
     p. cm.
   Includes bibliographical references and index.
   ISBN 0-7506-7249-8
     1. Articulation disorders in children. 2. Communicative disorders in children. 3. Tone
(Phonetics) 4. Vowels.   I. Gibbon, Fiona.   II. Title.

   RJ496.S7 B33 2001
   618.92'855--dc21

                                                                2001043714

British Library Cataloguing-in-Publication Data
A catalogue record for this book is available from the British Library.

The publisher offers special discounts on bulk orders of this book.
For information, please contact:

Manager of Special Sales
Butterworth–Heinemann
225 Wildwood Avenue
Woburn, MA 01801-2041
Tel: 781-904-2500
Fax: 781-904-2620

For information on all Butterworth–Heinemann publications available, contact our World Wide Web home page at: http://www.bh.com

10 9 8 7 6 5 4 3 2 1

Printed in the United States of America

9/14/04

Contents

Contributing Authors

Martin J. Ball, Ph.D., Hawthorne-BoRSF Distinguished Professor of Communicative Disorders, University of Louisiana at Lafayette

Sally A. R. Bates, Ph.D., Speech and Language Therapist, Department of Children's Speech and Language Service, Plymouth National Health Service Primary Care Trust, Plymouth, England

Janet Mackenzie Beck, Ph.D., Lecturer in Speech and Language Sciences, Queen Margaret University College, Edinburgh, Scotland

Patricia Donegan, Ph.D., Associate Professor of Linguistics, University of Hawaii at Mānoa, Honolulu

Fiona E. Gibbon, Ph.D., Senior Lecturer and Director of Research, Department of Speech and Language Sciences, Queen Margaret University College, Edinburgh, Scotland

Barry Heselwood, Ph.D., Lecturer in Phonetics, Department of Linguistics and Phonetics, University of Leeds, England

Sara J. Howard, Ph.D., Senior Lecturer in Human Communication Sciences, University of Sheffield, England

Karen E. Pollock, Ph.D., Associate Professor of Audiology and Speech-Language Pathology, The University of Memphis, Tennessee

Joseph Reynolds, Ph.D., Manager, Department of Speech and Language Therapy, Leeds Community and Mental Health National Health Service Trust, England

James M. Scobbie, Ph.D., Senior Research Fellow of Speech and Language Sciences, Queen Margaret University College, Edinburgh, Scotland

Jocelynne M. M. Watson, Ph.D., Lecturer in Speech and Language Sciences, Queen Margaret University College, Edinburgh, Scotland

Foreword

Vowel development in children is sometimes taken for granted, and clinical concern for vowel disorders frequently has been eclipsed by a greater concern for consonant disorders.

Historically, vowels have been rather neglected both in research on typical speech development and in research on articulatory and phonological disorders in children. Recent studies, however, have made it clear that vowels deserve far more attention than they have received. Some readers may even be surprised that there is enough to be said about vowel disorders to fill a book. The authors who contributed the seven chapters in *Vowel Disorders* succeed in showing that a book-length treatment is most certainly warranted, and that a fresh understanding of vowels is on the horizon. *Vowel Disorders* satisfies two major goals of scholarship: first, reviewing and interpreting the available information, and second, charting the way for a deeper understanding. This book stands as a unique and important milestone in speech-language pathology.

The chapters provide a cohesive and highly informative examination of children's vowel development and vowel disorders. Drawing on a variety of empirical and theoretical approaches, the authors demonstrate that vowel disorders are important and that several methods are available to describe and analyze these disorders. In a lucid and systematic way, this book discusses normal vowel development, clinical phonetics and phonology, the description and analysis of vowel errors, and therapy for children with vowel errors. This breadth of coverage is achieved without sacrificing depth. Readers will discover that each chapter provides a wealth of detail and thoughtful analysis.

Vowel Disorders is a welcome addition to the literature on clinical phonetics and phonology. Not only does it remedy a serious deficiency in this field, but it also shows the kind of synergy that can be accomplished by drawing on the expertise of carefully selected authors. Readers from novice to specialist will gain much from this book.

Raymond D. Kent, Ph.D.

Preface

Vowels have long been the poor relations of consonants. In descriptive phonetics, vowels have not proved as easily reducible to articulatory labels as have consonants. Often phoneticians have adopted an auditory classification scheme for vowels, while at the same time using a consonant classification based on place and manner of articulation. Similarly, studies of first-language phonological acquisition have devoted far more space to a chronology of consonant development and sets of normal consonant substitution patterns than to vowels (or, indeed, prosodic features). Finally, until recently, work in speech-language pathology and clinical linguistics also seems to have ignored vowels. The implicit assumption appears to have been that vowels are acquired very early, and examples of disordered vowel systems are so rare as to be unworthy of consideration. Even recently published phonological assessments for disordered speech have nowhere to enter vowel realizations.

We increasingly find, however, that vowels can be tackled by the phonetician and are not so unimportant to the developmental and clinical linguists as was once thought (phonologists, of course, had always found them fascinating). In the opening contribution to this collection, Patricia Donegan reviews research on vowel acquisition in normal phonological development. She then describes a universal set of phonological processes, grounded in articulatory and perceptual motivations, that restrict vowel systems. These restrictions operate cross-linguistically to shape the vowel systems of particular languages, but they can also be manifested by the patterns of vowel usage found in normal and delayed phonological acquisition, as well as in language change over time, and in second-language learning data. Donegan argues for a phonetic-based phonology, and she describes sets of vowel features, both context-free and context-sensitive processes, and the implicational hierarchies holding between them. Her analysis is supported with data from a wide range of languages.

Sara Howard and Barry Heselwood's chapter is concerned with how phoneticians actually describe vowel sounds. They begin with the problem of definitions: Phoneticians and phonologists have often disagreed over how to distinguish vowels from consonants. Whereas phoneticians rely on a definition giving primacy to characteristics of the vocal tract, phonologists have relied on a functional categorization of how sounds operate within the syllable. The authors' solution in this case is to deal only with segments that meet both definitions of vowel. In their chapter, they look at articulatory, acoustic, and auditory approaches to vowel description, covering both instrumental and impressionistic approaches to vowel classification. They also devote some time to the Cardinal Vowel system, which is still widely used for the representation of vowels despite developments in acoustic analysis of speech. They look at issues of transcription, both of normal and disordered speech, and finally, they examine the interaction of vocalic segments with stress. The examination of transcription practices is important: The authors note that vowel transcriptions should be thought of as representing a listener's auditory perception and not necessarily one particular setting of the articulators.

Karen Pollock's chapter is based on her work with a large-scale study of vowel disorders in the speech of children in the Memphis area, including phonologically normal, phonologically delayed, and deviant subjects. She describes many of the methodological issues that have to be dealt with in such a study. These include matters relating to differing target dialects within the subject group; how to categorize the vowel systems of the target varieties (in this case, a four-way division into nonrhotic monophthongs, nonrhotic diphthongs, rhotic monophthongs, and rhotic diphthongs); and how to label individual vowels (that is, height, frontness, tenseness, rounding). The methodology of the study is described in detail (the data collection protocol and how to decide on correct versus incorrect responses), and then preliminary findings are outlined. These include both data on the incidence of vowel disorders in the populations investigated and types of errors discovered in the speech samples.

Joe Reynolds presents a series of cases illustrating patterns of vowel error in children with phonological disorder. His chapter is based on previous work pertaining to children with phonological disorder who lived in the West Yorkshire area of the United Kingdom. Reynolds considers examples of context-free vowel error patterns, including lowering, fronting, diphthong reduction, and central vowel avoidance. He discusses possible explanatory frameworks, including perceptual salience, articulatory ease, and the application of different analytic frameworks such as natural process approaches and nonlinear phonology to vowel error patterns. Three child cases with idiosyncratic systems are presented. Reynolds notes that these abnormal vowel systems are structured differently from adult systems; in other words, they are not purely reduced and simplified versions. He refers to these interesting cases as instances where a child has moved up a phonological blind alley to create a different vowel system. He then considers the important influence of nonsegmental and suprasegmental features on some complex vowel error patterns. Finally, Reynolds discusses variability of vowel errors and presents evidence from studies of children that shows that variability does not assist development over time in all cases.

Sally Bates, Jocelynne Watson, and James Scobbie consider consonant-vowel interactions in the emerging speech of typically developing children and in the speech of children with developmental phonological disorder. These authors adopt a biological perspective that views immature productions as a reflection of organic constraints imposed by developing perceptual and motor systems. The finding that emerges from a literature review on context-conditioned error patterns in normally developing systems is the strong association of place of articulation in consonants and vowels, namely alveolar consonants with front vowels, labials with round vowels, and velars with back vowels. Illustrative examples of consonant-vowel interactions in children with phonological disorder are presented. These examples, which are drawn from a variety of English accents, show how vowels can condition consonant error patterns in some cases, and how consonants can condition vowel error types in others. The authors explain error patterns as reflecting difficulty in the timing and coordination of articulatory gestures and the compatibility of adjacent gestures.

The clinical phonology of vowels is dealt with in the chapter by Martin Ball. He discusses five different phonological approaches current in the literature and demonstrates how each of these could be applied to a commonly described characteristic of disordered vowel systems: the collapse of vowel systems to the three corner vowels of [i], [a], and [u]. The approaches described are classical rule-based generative phonology, process-based natural phonology, constraint-based optimality theory, the unary element-based government phonology, and gestural articulatory phonology. Vowel cornering is described in each of these approaches, and it is seen that while most of them have difficulty unifying different vowel simplification patterns (such as raising, lowering) into the single cornering one required, it is dealt with straightforwardly by government phonology. Furthermore, with government phonology, the mechanism required to restrict vowel systems to just the corner vowels is at the most basic level of phonological description: where governing relations between phonological elements are established. In other words, we do not require complexes of rules operating on derivations or hierarchies of constraints operating on segments or strings of segments. In government phonology, unlawful segments simply cannot be formed once the unary elements cannot enter governing relations. It is claimed that this approach has more clinical relevance than those that allow segments and then simplify them away.

The chapter by Fiona Gibbon and Janet Mackenzie Beck covers an under-researched area of speech pathology, namely therapy for abnormal vowels in children with phonological impairment. In the beginning of the chapter, the authors critically evaluate the findings of a few existing studies, and later discuss a range of possible therapy options for increasing vowel production accuracy. Gibbon and Beck conclude from their review that, despite limitations of current studies, there is evidence that direct therapy for vowel errors can have a positive effect on children's speech, with improvements in vowel production occurring over and above that expected from spontaneous development. A range of therapy approaches designed originally for consonant errors are presented and discussed, with examples illustrating ways in which clinicians could adapt these different approaches for vowel errors. A section describes new technology and computer-assisted techniques for improving children's auditory and production skills through the provision of real-time visual feedback of speech features. The authors present information that aims to be of interest and relevance to speech clinicians responsible for the management of children with phonological impairment. These clinicians are likely to have on their caseloads at least some children whose speech contains mild-to-moderate, if not severe, vowel errors.

This collection reflects the growth of interest in vowels and vowel disorders over the last decade or so. Our intention is to concentrate on those areas most underrepresented in the literature. We have restricted our discussion, therefore, to studies of disorder in the first-language acquisition of vowels; other work in vowel problems, such as in hearing impairment, is well represented elsewhere. Further, we are concerned solely with speech production. Studies of the perception of disordered vowels are certainly of interest, but these perhaps will constitute the next step in this area. Finally, we still need more data before we can describe possible typologies of vowel errors. It may well turn out that a pattern of gross simplification of vowels (such as vowel cornering) is found with some speakers, while a pattern of rearrangement of contrasts is found with others. It will take further studies of the type reported in this book before we can be sure of this.

Martin J. Ball
Fiona E. Gibbon

1

Normal Vowel Development

Patricia Donegan

The acquisition of vowels by normally developing children is an area that remains largely undocumented. Looking at vowel inventories in the languages of the world, we find great variety but certain clear patterns, and looking at adult substitutions,[1] we again find that the range of normal substitutions is very wide, but clear. There is every reason to believe that we should find at least that same range in normal children. Existing descriptions of children's speech, however, show only a very small sample of the systems and substitutions that could occur, and little effort has been made to determine whether children's limitations and substitutions are coextensive with those of adult languages.[2]

In this chapter, I briefly review some of the literature on vowel acquisition. Then I describe known adult limitations and substitutions in terms of a universal set of articulatorily and perceptually motivated phonological processes governing speech production. Although the processes are universal, their effects may be limited by learning, subject to implicational conditions, which reflect the phonetic motivations of the processes. (It may be possible to express these processes as constraints or families of constraints, but that is not an issue here.) As shown in the phonological acquisition model presented in the text, these processes constrain vowel inventories in adult and child language and account for substitutions in language histories, variation, and alternation; in second-language phonology; and in normal and disordered speech development. The implicational conditions on process application are responsible for the typical shapes of vowel inventories in child and adult speech.

Because vowel errors occur primarily at ages when children's natural speech may be difficult for outside observers to elicit, many phonological studies of vowel development focus on errors in the speech of children with speech delays (Bernhardt and Stemberger, 1998). The vowel substitutions described in studies of normally developing children and those in children with delayed development appear to be quite parallel (Pollock and Keiser, 1990; Stoel-Gammon and Dunn, 1985, contributions to this volume). The scarcity of data on normal children might leave this parallel open to question, but if we compare children's vowel errors with vowel alternation, variation, and change, we find that developmental errors can usually be attributed to processes (or constraints) like those of adult languages. This is not surprising if there is a common phonetic basis for both sets of phenomena, and one would expect normal development to follow the same pattern.

The Literature on Vowel Development

The literature on vowel development suggests that vowels are acquired early, both in production and perception. There is considerable variability in their production, but most studies suggest that vowel production is reasonably accurate by age 3, although some studies call this into question.

Studies of Children's Production

Among the studies of children's production, there have been several influential cross-sectional studies. Templin (1957) studied 480 children from 3 to 8 years old. The study elicited only single-word productions for each phoneme, but it established normative ages for the acquisition of consonant production. The mean percentage of correct vowel productions was already 93.3% for the youngest age group, and there was no significant increase in production accuracy over the age range studied. This result implies that most vowel development takes place before age 3.

Irwin and Wong (1983) coordinated and analyzed a set of studies of phonological development in children aged 18 to 72 months. The studies were administered by different investigators; each study investigated both vowel and consonant development in twenty subjects. The studies of children at 18 months (Paschall, 1983) and 2 years (Hare, 1983) are most revealing with respect to vowels, because the greater numbers of inaccurate productions at these early ages may indicate where vowel difficulties lie. The studies of 3- and 4-year-olds (Bassi, 1983; Larkins, 1983) serve mainly to establish the rarity of errors at age 3 and beyond. Studies such as these may be useful in providing criteria to identify vowel development delays, but they reveal little about the pronunciation systems of individual children who are or are not subject to such delays.

Instrumental studies of infant vocalization (Buhr, 1980; de Boysson-Bardies, Sagart, and Durand, 1984; Lieberman, 1980), and of early word production (Bond, Petrosino, and Dean, 1982) show that vowel production during the first year favors low, nonrounded vowels. Front-back vowel differences appear later than height differences, which can apparently be achieved by jaw opening alone. This suggests that in early vocalization and first words, the child does not exert much control of the tongue musculature, and does not coordinate lip with jaw movements for vowel articulation.

In these studies, the initial classification or identification of vowels by the researcher was auditory. It seems that the adult listeners who identified the vowels were using information other than vowel formant heights for identification, because some vowels that were distinguished by ear remained indistinguishable on the formant charts. One must conclude that, despite the difficulties involved in learning to transcribe vowels (especially children's vowels), the auditory identification of vowels is an irreplaceable tool in the analysis of vowel substitutions and vowel development.

There are also longitudinal studies, usually limited to individual children. Although these are narrowly focused, they often include crucial information that reveals how children's systems develop. The early studies of Velten (1943) and Leopold (1939–1949), followed by those of Smith (1973), Menn (1978), and Major (1977), describe in detail the phonological development of individual English-learning children.

Smith (1973, 37–40) describes the acquisition of English Standard Pronunciation by his son Amahl, but he has relatively little to say about Amahl's acquisition of vowels. At the start of the study, (2 years, 2 months), Amahl had acquired adultlike pronunciations of most English vowels, except for /æ, oṵ, oi̯/ (*man, soap, noisy*), and some vowels affected by following /r/. By the time Amahl was three years old, he had acquired adultlike vowels, even those affected by a following /r/. His few remaining vowel errors are attributable to contextual factors.

Major's 1977 study describes the phonological development, beginning at 1 year, 7 months, of his daughter Sylvia, who was learning both English and Brazilian Portuguese. Unlike Smith, Major gives special attention to vowel substitutions, and because Sylvia was becoming bilingual, he also emphasizes the progressive differentiation of her two developing phonologies.

Menn (1978) offers a study of the earliest stages of one American boy's phonology. Jacob (1 year, 2 months to 1 year, 9 months) shows much less regularity in vowel and consonant substitutions than the above-mentioned children, but he was considerably younger than they were at the time of the respective studies. Examination of Menn's data on Jacob at 1 year, 8 months and beyond indicates that the vowels of stressed syllables (when not influenced by adjacent liquids or glides) were beginning to stabilize but were by no means regular.

Lohuis-Weber and Zonneveld (1996) describe the prosodic development of a Dutch learner, a boy, from age 1 year, 8 months to 2 years, 11 months. They include many examples, which illustrate the child's pronunciation of a wide variety of vowels. Unstressed syllables are deleted at first, but the vowels of stressed syllables are usually correct, even including the Dutch labiopalatal vowels. (The focus of the study was not the child's segmental phonology, and the vowel transcriptions may have been normalized, but no notation to this effect was made.)

Macken (1979) describes the acquisition of Mexican Spanish by Si, a girl age 1 year, 7 months to 2 years, 1 month. Macken focuses on consonant acquisition, but her examples reveal mainly correct vowel qualities in accented syllables, even in Si's earliest words. Variation between [ə] and [ɑ] or between [i] and [ɪ] does occur.

Otomo and Stoel-Gammon (1992) describe the acquisition of American English /i, ɪ, e, ɛ, æ, ɑ/ by six normally developing children at 22, 26, and 30 months of age. /i/ and /ɑ/ were mastered early; /ɪ/ and /ɛ/ were least accurate throughout the study. Variability decreased as the subjects matured. Otomo and Stoel-Gammon noted some context-sensitive vowel substitution patterns that are discussed later in this chapter.

Contributions describing particular vowel substitutions in individual children, like that of Bleile (1989), and new data included in general discussions of phonological development (as in Bernhardt and Stemberger, 1998, and the contributions to this volume) add to what we can expect.

Production Studies Show Initial Variability and Early Accuracy

Stoel-Gammon and Dunn (1985) and Vihman (1996, Appendix C) show further examples where vowels, like consonants, are at first highly variable. In a given word, an accurate production may vary with a number of substitutes. The initial variability of vowels is not surprising when we consider the difficulty of controlling the shape of the tongue, which is a complex three-dimensional network of intrinsic longitudinal, vertical, and transverse fibers (Kent, 1992). Initial variability in consonants may resolve early into consistent substitutions, because consistency allows caregivers to interpret the child's speech. By the time children settle on consistent substitutions, however, most of the vowels in their speech may be reasonably accurate. The high percentages of accuracy at ages 2 years and above reported in Irwin and Wong (1983) confirm that many children achieve quite acceptable vowel quality before age 3 in all but the rhotic vowels. This may be because vowels can be produced satisfactorily with control of fewer and more widely used features than consonants require.

Even in languages with very rich vowel systems, the principal features that determine vowel quality are tongue/jaw height, palatality or tongue advancement, labiality, and tenseness (degree of palatality or labiality). Backness is rarely (if ever) distinguished from nonpalatality. In some languages, features

Table 1-1　Vowel Symbols and Features

	Palatal		Nonpalatal			Palatal	
	Nonlabial			Labial			
	Tense	Lax		Tense		Lax	
High	i	ɪ	ɨ	ʊ	u	y	ʏ
Mid	e	ɛ	ə	ɔ	o	ø	œ
Low	æ	a	ɑ		ɒ	ɶ	

In this framework, only three degrees of vowel height are phonologically relevant. Apparent four-height systems involve differences in tenseness (intensity of palatality or labiality for a given height). Nonpalatal nonlabial vowels are lax. I have not differentiated between the central and back nonpalatal nonlabials, that is, between mid [ə] and [ʌ], or high [ɨ] and [ɯ]. Labiopalatal vowels may be tense or lax. The current International Phonetic Alphabet includes no symbols for low, lax, labial vowels.

such as nasalization, tongue-root advancement or retraction (pharyngealization), rhoticity, and voice quality may also play a role. But many complex vowel systems, from the Germanic languages to those of Southeast Asia, result from the presence of diphthongs, which require sequential articulations but are composed of the same basic features as monophthongs (Table 1-1).

Consonant systems, on the other hand, require a comparative multiplicity of simultaneous features: Articulators usually include the lips, tongue tip, tongue dorsum, and often the tongue blade; places where constriction occurs may include bilabial, labiodental, dental, alveolar, velar, and others. Degrees of closure (stop, fricative, approximant), manner features (such as laterality, nasality, sibilance, affrication, trill, tap, and so on), and laryngeal features (voicing, aspiration, glottalization, and so on) often function in consonant systems. Even with an ordinary-sized consonant inventory, many features must be controlled in order to pronounce consonants. Vowels seem to make fewer demands.

Studies of Perceptual Development

Beginning with the work of Eimas, Siqueland, Jusczyk, and Vigorito (1971), it has been shown that very young infants (under 6 months) are able to perceive most of the phonetic differences that are used to distinguish sounds in any language (Aslin, Pisoni, Hennessy, and Perey, 1981; Best, McRoberts, and Sithole 1988; Eimas, 1975; Jusczyk and Thompson, 1978; Kuhl, 1983; Kuhl and Miller, 1982; Trehub, 1976; and others). (Eilers, Gavin, and Oller, 1982 and Eilers, Wilson, and Moore, 1979 offer some contradictory findings.) This does not mean that all distinctions are equally easy to perceive consistently, but it does mean that infants are unbiased with respect to the categories of the language they will learn. In contrast, the remarkable studies of Janet Werker and her colleagues (Werker, Gilbert, Humphrey, and Tees, 1981; Werker and Lalonde, 1988; Werker and Tees, 1984) offer considerable evidence that infants' perceptual categories for consonants, by the age of 12 months, have begun to correspond to the linguistically significant categories for the ambient language.

Perception of language-specific categories involves a narrowing of the range of distinctions perceived to something approaching phonemic perception. Werker and Pegg (1992, 298) point to various kinds of "strong evidence that infants are influenced by native-language phonological regularities before 10 months of age," but they describe the infants' categorizations as "language-specific phonetic perception" rather than "phonemic perception" (304). They say phonemic perception would imply the ability to distinguish lexical items, which they believe is not established at this early age. This objection does not seem entirely valid, however, since the phoneme, as originally conceived by Baudouin de Courtenay in 1895, is a perceived, remembered, and intended speech sound. Baudouin speaks of phonemes as "the psychological equivalent of a speec h sound," and as "representations, or images of the memory" (Baudouin, 1895, 152–158). The notion of a phoneme as a contrastive unit, a unit defined entirely in terms of the distribution of its allophones or member-sounds, originated later with the structuralists, and it is not essential to the construct.

These observations, however, are based largely on consonant acquisition. Vowel perception could be less categorical than consonant perception because of the continuously varying nature of vowel quality, as opposed to the seemingly discrete differences that characterize consonants, but there is little to support this supposition. Instead, the relatively early accuracy of vowel production seems to go hand in hand with relatively early categorization in vowel perception. Polka and Werker (1994) found that English-learning infants younger than 6 months could discriminate two German vowel contrasts that their 6-month-old counterparts could not distinguish. This indicates that the shift from a language-general toward a language-particular phonological pattern in perception takes place even earlier for vowels than for consonants.

Lieberman (1980, 137) posited "an innate, species-specific neural mechanism" that allows perceptual normalization of vowels in terms of the speaker's presumed supralaryngeal vocal-tract length, and which allows an infant to know when it has produced the perceptual equivalent of an adult vowel. Kuhl (1980, 1983; Kuhl and Miller, 1982) provides evidence for "perceptual constancy"—the ability of infants to generalize responses to speech sounds produced on different pitches and by different speakers—and thus, perhaps for such a normalization system. Kuhl also suggests (1991) that "perceptual magnet effects" show that speech sound categories are structured around prototypes: Adults rated vowels as good or poor exemplars of a phonetic category, such as /i/, and then adults and infants were tested on discrimination. If a prototypical exemplar was presented, both adult and 6-month-old infant subjects more readily accepted a poor exemplar as the same (the prototype acted as a perceptual magnet); a poor exemplar as the referent generalized less readily.

We might expect, then, that if the child forms language-specific prototypes or categories for perception, these same prototypes or categories would be used for the long-term mental representation of vowels when the child begins to imitate and use words. The function of phonemic categorization in adult speech seems to be representational as well as perceptual, and the categories may serve both functions for children as well.

Evidence Regarding Children's Representations

Evidence that children are able to categorize speech sounds accurately, however, does not allow us to conclude that children's lexical representations are always entirely accurate. The claim that children's errors, like adult alternation and variation, involve substitutions requires the implicit assumption that the child's mental representations of words are relatively accurate or adultlike. Stampe (1969) claimed that even the child's earliest phonological representations were in large part like the phonemic representations of adult speakers. Smith (1973) drew a similar conclusion. Stampe and Smith both concluded that early phonological representations are generally accurate, for three reasons: 1) the children were able to perceive differences they did not produce; 2) upon acquisition of a new pronunciation ability, they often corrected words that had undergone a substitution without rehearing them; 3) the children made substitutions that could only be explained with adultlike phonological representations.

Menn adduced another kind of evidence for early perceptual and representational accuracy, often evident in the child's earliest productions: avoidance. Menn noted that avoidance of a sound or class of sounds "implies the ability to discriminate it from sounds one does attempt to say" (1978, 71), and because avoided words are often in the child's receptive vocabulary, they must have phonological representations that include the avoided feature. In addition, instrumental phonetic studies of children's productions (Kornfeld, 1971; Macken and Barton, 1980) indicate that children may produce systematic differences, often imperceptible to adults, between sounds that are different in the adult language. While this result has been subject to a variety of interpretations, it confirms that perception of adult contrasts and the representation of contrastive features in long-term memory both proceed well in advance of adultlike production.

The coincidence of accurate children's perceptual categories with the phonemic categories of the ambient language at the onset of speech argues for adultlike representations, but it means that constraints on admissibility of lexical representations must also exist for children. Stampe's proposal that children's representations are like adult *phonemic* representations already assumed that allophonic details are not part of these representations. Limitations on both production and perception exist both in adult and child phonology: Adults often have considerable difficulty perceiving or producing distinctions that do not occur in their first language, and these difficulties are comparable to the difficulties of children.

We know that production difficulties exist for children, and it is possible that children's perceptions and representations may be more limited than those of adults. For example, because children often fail to distinguish final consonants in production, one might claim that a constraint forbidding final consonants applies to the child's perceptions and representations (Dinnsen, 1984), but we would then expect the child to be unable to distinguish receptively among sets like *tap/tack/tab/tag,* or *cat/cap/cash/calf/.* Instead, perception and memory of a distinction often can be established well in advance of the child's ability to produce it.

Part of the difficulty in deciding where the child's errors lie is that both perceptual and production limitations may be characterized with the same set of phonological processes or constraints. A process (or constraint) that specifies that all nonlow vowels must be high, or that all back vowels must be labial may affect perception or production or both. For the speaker of a language with no mid vowels or no back nonlabial vowels, the process may affect both perception and production. If this speaker attempts to learn a language with mid vowels, the constraint is ordinarily overcome in perception before it is mastered in production (although articulatory instruction can sometimes reverse this order in adults). A child learning a language with mid vowels, who produces only high vowels, may be subject to the limitation in perception and representation, or may perceive and remember the difference, but be unable to achieve nonhigh, nonlow vowel articulation. The evidence from perception favors the latter view.

Representations, particularly of longer or more complicated words, may be incomplete or inaccurate in some respects. Macken (1980) offered evidence that a child's own incorrect pronunciations may influence his mental representations of individual words. Aitcheson and Chiat (1981) proposed that many developmental phonological errors were the results of difficulties in lexical storage and retrieval, rather than results of production difficulties. However, aiming to provide a control group for the Aitcheson and Chiat study, Smith, Macaluso, and Brown-Sweeney (1991, 296) studied new-word learning in adults. They found that adults encountered difficulties with storage and recall that were similar to those of children, but that the error patterns of adults and older children were unlike the "reasonably consistent, unidirectional substitution patterns common in phonological processes among different children and even across languages."

Phonological Systems

In considering how a child learns to perceive and pronounce vowels, we must consider how a child progresses from the newborn state to the phonological system of an adult language. The conservative assumption would be that development involves no gross discontinuities, and available data support this, suggesting that paths of normal vowel development are based on the same features and processes that appear in vowel phonologies in adult languages (Stampe, 1973).

A note of explanation is required regarding my use of the terms *phonological system* and *phonology*. In this discussion, phonology simply means the mental system which underlies the perception and production of speech (Donegan and Stampe, 1979). The phonological system of a language is responsible for the perceptual and articulatory limitations and abilities of the adult native speaker—and for his or her accent. Phonology, so viewed, arises in phonetic realities and is based on phonetic causalities; these are universal, but their language-specific implementation must, of course, be learned. True phonological regularities can be stated in phonetic and prosodic terms; they do not refer to morphological information, as the rules of morphophonology (lexical phonology) do.

Some authors, in fact, would regard the system I am describing as phonetics, not phonology. The limitations and abilities this natural phonological system governs, however, involve categorization of sounds and selection of substitutions that are unquestionably language-specific. The elements of this system cannot, therefore, be necessary results of human perceptual and articulatory abilities, but only options, which can be controlled. They are subject to learning, in that control over the options is learned. They involve categorical conditions as well as gradients (which are subject to variable cut-off points). They are the regularities that have traditionally been called automatic phonology.

Much of modern generative and postgenerative phonology is concerned with relationships among the forms of lexical items (lexical phonology), and with alternations that are conditioned by morphological classes or boundaries. Myers (1997, 125), gives a clear statement of the position that *only* alternations that are obligatory, categorical (phonemic), independent of rate, and restricted to particular morphological categories are phonological. Such alternations are conventionalized and in most cases (*pace* Myers) they no longer retain their historic phonetic motivation. These alternations seem only marginally relevant to the problem of vowel (and consonant) acquisition, and their acquisition may be based on quite different principles (Stampe, 1987).

Features and Segments

With a phonetics-based phonology, we can reconsider some basic ideas about features and segments, as well as phonological processes, in child and adult speech. The evidence about perception noted previously suggests that children's perception of speech at the onset of word production is relatively accurate and, perhaps surprisingly, language specific. The next question, then, is how these perceptions are represented in the child's memory: Are the child's initial phonological representations whole words, or are they composed of features, or segments, or some other units?

When phonology is based on phonetics, its elements, the phonological features, must be phonetic. Phonological features can be viewed, not as abstract categories, but as the links of motor and proprioceptive aspects of production, on the one hand, to perceptual properties (auditory, acoustic, or in acquisition, sometimes visual) on the other. Such connections may be part of an inborn, prewired mechanism like that which appears to link the visual stimuli of adult facial expressions to production of facial gestures by infants. (Meltzoff and Moore [1977], for example, document imitation of adult facial gestures by young infants, who have never, of course, observed their own facial expressions.)

Alternatively, these connections may develop, or be discovered by the child, during the first year, in vocalization, crying, oral play, noisy eating or drinking, and babbling. During these activities, the child creates a map of the articulatory apparatus, noting the auditory effects of different laryngeal adjustments, of constrictions at different points of articulation, of different degrees and durations of closure, different cavity shapes, different velar positions, and so on. Whether innate or developed through experience, these connections are part of the child's natural language endowment.

If phonological features are acquired, children must acquire them by mapping articulatory gestures (such as oral closure, or tongue advancement or retraction, or lip rounding, or jaw lowering) or components of gestures (such as places of articulation, or degrees of closure) to their auditory effects. Thus, for example, the auditory effects of phonation are associated with particular laryngeal and respiratory gestures, and different pitches with different gestures. An oral closure and release during phonation are connected with a sudden drop and subsequent rise in intensity, and the place of closure is connected with a particular auditory pattern based on formant transitions and the pitch range of the release burst. Similarly, tongue advancement during phonation is associated with raising of the second vowel formant, tongue and jaw raising with the lowering of the first formant, and so on. This mapping of the vocal apparatus to its acoustic-auditory capabilities may begin with the infant's earliest vocalizations, and it is surely an important function of babbling. The resulting connections of gestural elements with their auditory effects are the foundation of the child's (and the adult's) ability to imitate, and they function as features in the child's (and the adult's) phonology.

Early function need not imply simplicity. If a feature is a gestural component linked to an auditory effect, that does not require that both the gesture and the effect are simple. A feature may involve a rather complex oral gesture connected with a simple, easily identifiable acoustic effect (for example, tongue advancement and F2 raising), or a fairly simple gesture linked to a complex auditory effect (such as lip rounding and its associated complex of formant lowering). A feature also may be present in varying degrees, depending on the other features with which it simultaneously co-occurs: For example, lip rounding may be present in high or low vowels, but (other things being equal) it is necessarily weaker in low vowels, where it conflicts with jaw opening.

Comparison of phonological processing in many languages is necessary in order to discover all the "natural classes" that are referred to in phonological substitutions (sets of sounds that undergo the same substitution, sets of sounds that condition a substitution, sets of sounds substituted, and so on). By this method, we can identify a universal set of features that are relevant in substitutions, and thus, presumably, in perception and production. The set will undoubtedly be larger than the sets of "distinctive features" most phonological theories currently subscribe to, but we can identify a basic set for vowels to be discussed here.

Vowel Features

Vowels consist of simultaneous features which conflict with each other. The principal vowel features (see discussion in Donegan, 1978 and Table 1-1) are palatality (frontness), labiality (usually manifested as roundness) and sonority (intrinsic intensity), which is correlated inversely with vowel height ([+low] vowels are most sonorant, [+high] vowels least). Palatality, labiality and the height features are both binary and gradient. They are binary, in the sense that they are either present or absent in a vowel: For example, [i] is palatal and [ɨ] is nonpalatal, [u] is labial and [ɨ] is nonlabial, [i] is high and [e] is nonhigh. Either the presence of these features or their absence can be referred to in phonological processing, but if present, each feature may be present to a greater or lesser degree, depending on the other features with which it simultaneously combines (see further discussion in Chapter 6).

The phonetic aspects of this claim would seem to be obvious. The more palatal a vowel is, the less open (and thus, the less sonorant) it can be. Tongue-fronting and raising decrease the size of the forward resonating cavity, raise the second formant, and thus create the palatal quality, but these gestures and their effects are attenuated by jaw or tongue lowering. Conversely, the gestures associated with palatality attenuate sonority, in that they decrease the size of the oral cavity and enlarge the pharyngeal (or back) cavity, lowering the first formant and decreasing the intrinsic intensity of the vowel. Labiality and sonority conflict in a similar way, both articulatorily and acoustically: The more open the jaw, the less rounding the lips can achieve; conversely, lip protrusion and compression lower the first formant and decrease intrinsic intensity. So, the optimal palatal vowel is [i], the optimal labial vowel is [u], and the optimal sonorant is non-palatal, nonlabial [a].

Palatality and labiality also conflict, attenuating each other's effects: Palatality raises the second formant and labiality lowers it, so pure labials such as [u] and pure palatals such as [i] are favored among the world's languages over labiopalatals such as [y]. Palatality or labiality (grouped terminologically as vowel colors) can make height differences more audible, so achromatic vowel systems such as /i, ə, ɑ/ are rare among the world's languages, and triangular systems such as /i, ɑ, u/ or /i, e, ɑ, o, u/ are common. Tenseness may be regarded as intensity of color (palatality or labiality) for a given degree of height, so that [i] is more palatal and less sonorant than [ɪ], and [e] is more palatal and less sonorant than [ɛ]. The noncolored vowels [ɨ, ə, ɑ] cannot be tense on this definition; see Donegan, 1986 for detailed arguments.

The implicational conditions on the application of phonological processes confirm this claim of features gradience. These features and their varying strengths are manifested in the susceptibility of vowels to different phonological substitutions. As shown below, features that are weakly present are most susceptible to loss, and those that are strongly present are most subject to enhancement or optimization.

Excursus on Representational Units: Words, Syllables, Segments, Features

Having proposed an interpretation of what features are, and a basic set of vowel features, it seems important to consider the child's representations and processing, and why features are part of these from the start.

Some researchers claim (Ferguson and Farwell 1975; Menyuk, Menn, and Silber 1986) that children represent their first words as unanalyzed wholes. Words may be acquired first as passive vocabulary, which the child recognizes but does not produce. At this point, they may indeed be recognized as unanalyzed wholes, or as general gestalts—as we assume a dog recognizes *Sit!* or a horse recognizes *Whoa!* But when a child first attempts to produce words, the words must undergo analysis into features (in the sense used here), because an attempt at imitation requires this:

1. The imitator must identify a set of simultaneous auditory properties: For example, for a single segment, such as [m̩], this would include the combined auditory effects of voicing, nasality, oral closure, and labiality. More likely (to

produce a word an adult will recognize), the child identifies a series of such sets of simultaneous properties; so for a series of segments, such as [mama], the above features are heard to alternate with the effects of oral openness, jaw lowering, nonlabiality, and so on.

2. The imitator must then connect those auditory/acoustic effects with articulatory gestures. This can be done only if the imitator has some knowledge of which effects are the results of which gestures. So auditory-articulatory links—or features—must be available. The success of the attempt to imitate depends, in part, on the established links between sound and gesture; these may be incomplete.

3. The imitator then must attempt to produce an appropriately timed sequence of gestures. The difficulties of this part of the imitation process are generally recognized.

Lindblom (1992) suggests that first words, usually consonant-vowel syllables, are stored as "trajectories." This implies storage as whole syllables, rather than segments, but the essential points of a trajectory are the beginning and ending points. For a word like [mã] (or reduplicated [mãmã]) the articulatory aspects that must be represented are a simultaneous combination of voicing, nasality, oral closure, and labial place of closure, and a simultaneous combination of oral openness, jaw lowering, and nonrounding. The point at which these simultaneous configurations are identified as units, or segments, may be difficult to establish. But when imitation begins, the child's analysis of speech must have proceeded far enough that these simultaneous configurations of features are part of his or her mental representations. This would include the self-imitation that occurs in babbling (Locke and Pearson, 1992) and the unsuccessful imitations that may occur before the adults in the family recognize a first word. Feature analysis is not, then, based on distribution or contrast; it is part of figuring out (or knowing) how to imitate.

Vowel Processes

Phonological processes are not limited to children's speech. They are responsible for constraints on adult phonological representations, and they underlie phonological substitutions (alternation and variation) in adult speech and phonological change in languages. Phonological processes express phonetic desiderata and eliminate phonetic difficulties. Some processes resolve difficulties in the production or perception of segments, optimizing simultaneous feature combinations; others resolve difficulties that result from the sequencing of segments.

Recent phonological theory expresses the content of phonological processes as universal constraints or families of constraints, and uses ranking rather than application or nonapplication to differentiate the phonologies of individual languages (Prince and Smolensky, 1993). The substance of a universal set of phonetic processes and that of a universal set of phonetic constraints may prove to be a matter of translation (see, for example, Lassettre, 1995). The choice of expressing phonetic limitations on the speech capacity as processes versus constraints does not directly affect this discussion. I am referring to phonological processes. Should constraints and their ranking prove adequate to describe the regularities of phonological production and perception, conversion to constraints would be possible.

If children and adults have phonetic capacities that are essentially the same, then we might expect some children to happen upon any of the substitutions we observe in alternation or variation, or in sound changes in the languages of the world. Or perhaps children only make some subset of these changes; this remains to be seen.

It is important to note that while processes create regularities in children's speech, these regularities are by no means perfect. Much has been made of the messiness of child data, and children's data may perhaps be more variable and idiosyncratic than adult data, but far too little has been noted of the comparable variability and apparent irregularity of adult data. It would be a mistake to ignore variation and irregularity wherever we find them, but it is important to remember that the regularities create the system and provide the keys to its explanation.

Phonological processes not only underlie substitutions in adult and child speech production, they also govern perception and thereby constrain the phonological inventory. Fortitive processes limit the inventory by ruling out certain simultaneous combinations of features (such as nasalized vowels), while lenitive processes allow speakers to discount certain actually occurring proscribed segments by attributing them to the application of sequence-optimizing substitutions (such as context-sensitive vowel nasalization). Stampe (1987) and Donegan (1995) offer a more complete discussion of how processes constrain phonological representations in adults.

If processes constrain perception, then why are children at first able to perceive virtually all occurring phonetic distinctions and why do these abilities become more language-specific during the first year? One important difference between the 6 month old, who can discriminate nonnative distinctions, and the 1 year old, who cannot, is the child's degree of experience of vocalization and babbling. It seems that without this experience, the child's perceptions are unconstrained by any limitations on his or her production abilities. As these production limitations are discovered, the child finds that certain feature combinations are less difficult or more perceptually satisfactory than others. The child thus discovers reasons to limit perceptual categories to the more-optimal feature configurations, insofar as this turns out to be possible in the target language. (See Donegan, 1995 for further discussion.)

In the following sections, I present examples of vowel processes that apply in the speech of children and follow these with examples of similar process applications in various languages of the world. I show that these processes are common to child speech and adult alternation, variation, and change, and that processes in child and adult speech are subject to the same implicational constraints on their application, which manifest the phonetic motivations of the processes. Further discussion of vowel processes is found in Chapters 3 and 4.

Context-Sensitive Substitutions:
Vowel-Consonant Assimilation

Certainly there are many regular vowel changes, common or rare, that we observe both in children and in adult languages. Vowel quality seems to influence adjacent consonant quality in very early speech, with high front vowels exerting the greatest influence, and labial vowels the least (Gierut, Cho, and Dinnsen, 1993; Wolfe and Blocker, 1990): Children may make labial and sometimes velar consonants alveolar before front vowels, and some make consonants velar before back vowels. Conversely, consonant quality may sometimes influence vowels: For example, So and Dodd (1995) report vowel errors only in the youngest group of Cantonese speakers they studied. They remark that errors were few, and the only consistent pattern they noted was that of vowel-to-consonant assimilation. Assimilation of vowels to adjacent consonants is less common in child speech than one might expect, but acquisition of languages like Marshallese or Kosraean or Kabardian, which have series of palatalized and labialized consonants, should receive further attention. Labialization of vowels adjacent to labial consonants (or labialized consonants, such as English [w, r, ʃ]), and palatalization of vowels adjacent to palatal or coronal consonants may occur (compare [dada] with front [a] and [mɑmɑ] with nonfront [ɑ] in many children).

Depalatalization of vowels adjacent to nonpalatal sonorants is reported, even when the liquid is replaced or deleted: for example, *bread, dress* as [bwəd], [dəs] (Otomo and Stoel-Gammon, 1992). In analyzing such substitutions, it is important to note the quality of the liquids in the child's speech. In a child who backs vowels after /r/, it is important to know if /r/ is pronounced elsewhere in the child's speech as [w], or as [j], or as some other alternative.

Assimilation to a consonant may affect the entire vowel, or it may appear in the form of diphthongization, where the beginning or the end of the vowel is assimilated to the adjacent consonant, creating an onglide or an offglide. Long vowels, or vowels in lengthening environments (open syllables, monosyllabic words, stressed syllables, and so on) are particularly susceptible to such diphthongization. For example, in English words such as *mash*, *sash*, a palatal glide may develop before the [ʃ], giving [mæiʃ,sæiʃ], as in various Southern U.S. dialects. Similar assimilative diphthongization in children's speech is not surprising.

Possible contexts for such assimilative diphthongizations should be considered carefully, because they may be subtle and sometimes surprising. One might not expect a "front" glide before a following velar consonant, but velar consonants are often palatalized after palatal vowels, and development of a palatal glide before a following palatalized velar is not surprising—in fact, pronunciations such as [bæig], [leig], [kɪiŋ] for *bag*, *leg*, and *king* are common among American adults, as well as in the speech of children. (One does not ordinarily find this diphthongization before [k] in adult speech because a following voiceless stop keeps the vowel short enough to prevent diphthongization.)

One also might not expect a palatal glide before [s], but this diphthongization is assimilative (because both [s] and palatals are coronal, and vowel assimilation favors continuants over stops such as [t, d, n]). It is fairly common among Southeast Asian languages; vowels acquire palatal offglides before palatal consonants and [s] in Temiar (Benjamin, 1976, 137–139) and Pacoh (Alves, 2000, 25–26) and before palatals in Khmer (personal observation), and in varieties of Mon (Huffman, 1990, 42) and Wa (Diffloth, 1980, 44). Consider also, that in Italian, word-final Latin /s/ has become /i/: *noi, voi, poi, sei* from *nos, vos, pos, sex*.

In view of these changes, the development of palatal glides between a front vowel and a velar, reported as common by Otomo and Stoel-Gammon (1992), is not surprising, and a child's pronunciations of *bus* as [bʌis], *bag* as [baig] and *bang* as [baiŋ] (Menn, 1978) need not arise from an idiosyncratic "word recipe," but may instead be a phonetically motivated assimilation.

Diphthongs that arise from assimilation are easily interpreted as "wrong" vowels: *mash* [mæiʃ] can be heard as /maiʃ/; *peg* [pɛig] is ordinarily heard as (British) /peig/ or (American) /pɛig/, and *big* [bɪig] is heard as /big/. This last effect can make it impossible for a child to distinguish pairs such as *seek* versus *sick*, or even *king* versus *keen*. And of course, the [ɪi] (from /ɪ/ plus offglide [i]) may monophthongize to [i], so it is not surprising that Otomo and Stoel-Gammon found [ɪ] > [i] before velars to be a common substitution.

Otomo and Stoel-Gammon report that vowels often become back before velar consonants, including velarized [ɫ]. This illustrates the fact that we may find quite opposite solutions to the problem of producing a front-vowel-velar-consonant sequence: The velar may be fronted, with assimilation of part of the vowel to the fronted velar, as in the [bæig] example above, or the vowel may be backed to match the backness of the velar. Such an assimilation happened in early Latin, where front vowels became back before a velarized /l/: *uelim, familia* with clear [l] remained unchanged, beside *uoltis, famulus*, where the /l/ was "dark" (Allen, 1970, 34).

The Similarity Principle (noted first in Hutcheson, 1974) asserts that segments that are similar are implicationally favored for further assimilation: For example, *nt > nn* implies *nd > nn*, but not the reverse. Therefore, we may find that palatal vowels assimilate to palatals and back vowels do not: thus [fɪiʃ] *fish* but not *[puiʃ] *push*. We may also find that vowels assimilate to the point of articulation of approximants such as /r, l/ in cases where they do not assimilate to obstruents or nasals, or that they assimilate to continuants such as /s/ but not to stops such as /t, d, n/, or that (as vocoids) they assimilate to vocoids but not to nonvocoids (Southern U.S. *high* [hɑẹ] > [hæẹ], but *gosh* [gɑʃ] does not become *[gaʃ]).

Context-Free Substitutions

Context-free phonological processes are typically fortitive—that is, they apply to enhance (optimize or maximize) a particular phonetic feature of an individual segment (see also Stevens and Keyser, 1989, regarding enhancement in consonants). Because fortitions optimize individual segments, they may have perceptual as well as articulatory motivation, they often apply context-free, and they may also apply dissimilatively. (Some examples of fortitions that affect consonants include devoicing and aspiration of obstruents, pre- or postnasalization of voiced stops, voicing of sonorants, and changes of glides into obstruents.) Lenitions, on the other hand, are concerned with sequences of segments; they have articulatory motivation only, they are reductive or assimilative, and their application often obscures the features of the individual segments.

Lowering, laxing, depalatalization and delabialization are vowel fortitions; all increase sonority. Raising and tensing increase palatality or labiality. Palatalization and labialization also increase palatality and labiality, of course—and in conferring these properties they make weaker degrees of sonority (in mid or high vowels) more audible. These conflicting motivations and opposite changes may make it seem that "anything is possible"—and indeed, all of these changes are found in children's substitutions as well as in the world's languages. But each process is strictly constrained by hierarchical conditions on the potential classes of input for a given substitution (Donegan, 1985). For example, other things being equal, a lower vowel is more susceptible to depalatalization than a higher vowel of the same series, so if [e] depalatalizes, [æ] must also depalatalize, and if [i] depalatalizes, then [e] and [æ] must depalatalize as well. These implicational conditions can be summarized roughly with the principle, "the rich get richer and the poor get poorer": a vowel that has a higher degree of some property is more susceptible to processes that increase that property, and a vowel with a low degree of a property is more susceptible to processes that weaken or remove that property.

This means that a child who substitutes [ə] for /e/ will ordinarily also substitute nonpalatal vowels for /ɛ/ and for /æ/. Because lax vowels are less palatal than their tense counterparts and lower vowels are less palatal than their higher counterparts, /ɛ/ and /æ/ are implicationally favored for depalatalization. Other things being equal, we would expect a child who raises /ɛ/ to [ɪ] (increasing its palatality) also to raise /e/ to [i]. Of course, other things are not always equal—in English, for example, the vowel we might analyze as /e/ is a diphthong, [ei̯] or [ɛi̯], and is likely to be perceived as such. The dissimilative forces which underlie diphthongization may counteract the application of raising for this vowel.

In the following sections, I sketch some fortitive vowel processes and illustrate their implicational conditions with examples from the world's languages. Where possible, I give examples of their application in children's substitutions. Note that in the children's substitutions, the implications are maintained.

Context-Free Fortitions: Lowering and Raising

Lowering increases sonority, and it is implicationally favored for vowels that are relatively high in sonority and weak in color. It applies most strongly to nonpalatal, nonlabial vowels such as /ɨ/ and /ə/, and accounts for their absence in many of the world's languages. Several children described in the literature lower [ə] to [ɑ] either obligatorily (for example, the English learners in Leopold, 1939–1949; Velten, 1943) or optionally (for example, the learner of English and Czech in Vogel, 1975).

Lowering also preferentially affects lax vowels, so that, for example, [ɪ] and [ʊ] are more susceptible to lowering than [i], [u]. Some children, such as Sylvia Major, also lower [ɪ] and [ʊ] to [ɛ] and [ɔ] (Major, 1977). Otomo and Stoel-Gammon (1992) report lowering of /ɪ/ to [ɛ] as a particularly persistent substitution. Bleile (1989) provides an example of this: Jake, at age 2 years to 2 years, 2 months, optionally lowered /ɪ/ to [ɛ].

Across languages, lowering follows similar patterns. It is implicationally favored for vowels that are neither palatal nor labial. For example, the difference between short and long /ɑ/ is realized in many languages with an added difference of quality: Short /ɑ/ is [ə] and long /ɑ:/ is [ɑ:] in Sanskrit and in Hawaiian. Both /ə/ and /ə:/ are optionally lowered to [ɑ] and [ɑ:] in Kolami (Emeneau, 1955, 7). In languages which lack an /ə/, this is typically borrowed as [ɑ], as in Japanese borrowings from English (Ohso, 1972). Lowering also favors lax vowels in synchronic alternations, in language histories, and in variation. Eastern Ojibwa short (lax) /ɪ/, /ʊ/ (phonetically [ɪ], [ʊ]) are lowered to [ɛ] and [ə] (the [ə] from [ʊ] is unrounded) in final position (Bloomfield, 1956, 4–7). In the Sacapultec dialect of Quiché, lax vowels are lowered optionally, so [ɪ] ~ [ɛ], [ʊ] ~ [ɔ], [ɛ] ~ [ɑ] and [ɔ] ~ [ɑ] (Campbell, 1977, 16–17). Modern Icelandic lengthened [ɪː] and [ʏː] are variably lowered to [ɛː] and [ɔː] (Einarsson, 1945, 11), and in southern and western 15th-century Swedish, lax /ɪ/ and /ʊ/ lowered to /e/ and /o/ (Haugen, 1976, 258).

Long or lengthened vowels are especially susceptible to lowering: in West Greenlandic Eskimo (Pyle, 1970, 133), and in Pashto (Shafeev, 1964, 34), long vowels are lowered, so that [ɪ] and [ʊ] alternate with [ɛː] and [ɔː]. Vowels are also especially susceptible to lowering when adjacent to a glide of like color (labial vowels lower near labial glides, palatal vowels lower near palatal glides); examples abound in diphthongizations (see "Context-Sensitive Fortitions: Dissimilation"). Although palatal and labial vowels may lower in parallel, lowering need not affect both. In Dagur, for example, Altaic *u became /o/, but *i did not lower (Poppe, 1955, 31).

Raising decreases sonority, but it increases a vowel's color, and fortitive raising (such as raising in stressed or accented positions, under emphasis, and so on) only affects palatal or labial vowels—[ɑ] is not raised to [ə], nor [ə] to [ɨ], in stressed or lengthened positions. Children often raise palatals and labials: Joan raised English [o] to [u], while lowering [ə] to [ɑ] (Velten, 1943, 288), and Linda raised Estonian [e] and [o] to [i] and [u] (Vihman, 1971, 63).

Across languages, only palatal and labial vowels are raised, and tense vowels are favored for raising. In the English Great Vowel Shift, tense palatals and labials were raised, but raising may affect only palatal vowels, as when Old Gutnish æ > e, æː > eː, eː > iː, ø > y, œː > yː (Noreen, 1913, 140–141, 149–150). Note that labiopalatals were included. Raising may affect only labial vowels; this happened in the history of French (Pope, 1934, 90, 210), and in São Miguel Portuguese (Rogers, 1948, 13). In both, in checked syllables, [ɒ] > [o], [o] > [u].

When raising applies dissimilatively, it affects vowels that are adjacent to achromatic or lax vocoids (see "Context-Sensitive Fortitions: Dissimilation").

Context-Free Fortitions: Coloring

Context-free palatalization and labialization affect achromatic vowels, and they are especially applicable to higher vowels. If a low vowel such as [ɑ] is labialized or palatalized, a higher achromatic vowel will undergo the process as well, but the reverse implication does not hold. As a result, many languages have an /ɑ/ vowel but lack nonlow, nonpalatal, nonlabial vowels, such as /ɨ/ and /ə/. Palatalization and labialization appear most clearly in children's speech where a child substitutes [æ] or [ɒ] for /ɑ/, but colorings also occur in very early speech, when children may use a low vowel such as [ɑ] for adult low vowels, and a single high vowel, [i] or [u], for all others (for example, Leopold 1939; Velten 1943). In a further variation of this kind of pattern, we find Linda replacing Estonian /ə/ with [i] or [u]—palatalizing or labializing it, and also raising the result just as she raised /e/ and /o/ (Vihman, 1971).

Among the world's language histories, we find a number of examples of context-free palatalization; these include Yellow Lahu, where Black Lahu /ɨ/ and /ə/ have merged with /i/ and /e/, but /ɑ/ remains nonpalatal (Matisoff, 1973, 12), and Southern Welsh, where /ɨ/ has become /i/, but /ə/ has not become /e/ (Bowen and Jones, 1960, 12). We also find that /ɨ/ became /i/ in Northern Irish (Sommerfelt, 1968, 495), Common Mongolian (Poppe, 1955, 33), and the Özbek dialects of Turkic (Menges, 1968, 79). Palatalization may affect all vowel heights, even low vowels, as when [ɑ:] became [æ:] in Classical Greek (Allen, 1968, 70). Palatalization applied generally to short vowels in Old English, when West Germanic /ɑ/ became /æ/ (Campbell, 1959, 52), and labialization was general for long vowels, as /ɑ:/ became [ɒ:] in Middle English (Jones, 1989, 130–131). We also see labialization where Gutob-Remo /*ɨ/ became /u/ in the Mundlipada dialect of Remo (Zide, 1965, 44), and where the "enunciative" vowel of Dravidian, elsewhere [ɨ], became [u] in Kannada and Telugu (Bright, 1975, 41).

Context-Free Fortitions: Bleaching

Depalatalization and delabialization can be grouped under the term *bleaching*, because both result in the loss of vowel color (as well as an increase in sonority). Sylvia, for example, optionally depalatalized or delabialized English low and mid lax vowels: [bæf] ~ [bɑf] *bath*, [mɔ] ~ [mə] *more*, [mɑrsɛlo] ~ [mɑrsɑlo] *Marcello* [mɑrsɛlo] (Major, 1977). Y, a learner of French, depalatalized /y/ to [u] (Pupier, 1977, 81). Linda seems usually to have depalatalized Estonian /y/ to [u], but occasionally delabialized /y/ and /y:/ to [i] and [i:], and she delabialized and raised /ø:/ to [i:] (Vihman, 1971).

The weaker the vowel color, the more susceptible it is to depalatalization or delabialization, so lower vowels, lax vowels, and vowels with mixed color (labiopalatals) are more susceptible. Thus, in 12th-century English æ > ɑ , but e did not depalatalize (Campbell, 1959, 52–58), and when Indo-European *e and *o merged as /ɑ/—phonetically [ə] (Allen, 1953, 58)—in Sanskrit, *i and *u remained palatal and labial (Burrow, 1965, 103). In Chinautla (Pokomam), lax [ɔ], [ɛ] become [ə], but tense [o:], [e:] remain (Campbell, 1977, 21–22), and in Sacapultec (Quiché) [ɛ], [ɔ] (from lax [ɪ], [ʊ]) optionally become [ə] (Campbell, 1977, 22). Labiopalatal vowels, which have two colors, are particularly susceptible to depalatalization or delabialization. In Lithuanian Yiddish (Sapir, 1915, 259–260), and in the German dialects of Darmstadt, Alsace, Upper Austria, and Luxemburg (Keller, 1961, 125–126, 167–168, 203, 256–257), Middle High German labiopalatal /y/ and /ø/ were delabialized to /i/ and /e/. In Monguor (Poppe, 1955, 49–50) and the "Iranized" Turkish dialects of Özbek (Menges,

1968, 80), labiopalatal /y/ and /ø/ are depalatalized to /u/ and /o/. Height is still relevant in delabialization and depalatalization of labiopalatals: Old English short and long /ø(:)/, became /e(:)/ very early, while /y(:)/ remained /y(:)/ (Campbell, 1958, 76–77).

In diphthongization, depalatalization or delabialization also apply dissimilatively, causing loss of a color when there is a vowel or glide of like color in the environment (see "Context-Sensitive Fortitions: Dissimilation"). Where both depalatalization and delabialization apply fully, we find languages with distinctions only in vowel height, such as Gude, with /ɨ, a/ (Hoskison, 1974) or Kabardian, with /ə, a/ (Kuipers, 1960).

Context-Free Fortitions: Tensing and Laxing

Tenseness may be defined as a high degree of color for a given degree of vowel height, and laxness as weakness of color; thus [i] is more palatal than [ɪ], [u] is more labial than [ʊ], and so on. Nonpalatal, nonlabial vowels, having no color, are by definition lax. Higher vowels are more susceptible to tensing, lower vowels to laxing. Hildegard substituted tense [i] for English [ɪ] (Leopold, 1939).

The application of tensing and laxing is clearly evident from cross-language comparison of phoneme inventories, where we find /e/ - /ɛ/ and /o/ - /ɔ/ contrasts far more widespread than contrasts of /i/ - /ɪ/ or /u/ - /ʊ/. Among the world's languages, potential tense-lax contrasts of high vowels are usually merged in favor of tense /i/ and /u/; potential contrasts of mid vowels *may* be merged as /ɛ/ or as /e/, and as /ɔ/ or /o/ (although the tense-vowel letter is usually chosen), but many languages maintain midtense versus midlax contrasts. Long vowels appear to favor tenseness; in many languages, the colored long vowels are tense and the colored short vowels are lax (note Spanish [ɛ, ɔ] in closed and [e, o] in open syllables. Of course, in many languages, long and short vowels have the same quality. Tensing (especially applicable before glides that lack color or have opposite color) and laxing (especially before like-colored glides) are also evident in diphthongization, where the first step of a diphthongization may consist of tensing or laxing part of the vowel's duration, (with further dissimilation to follow): for example, [uṷ] > [ʊṷ] (> [iṷ]), or [eẹ] > [eɛ] (> [eə̣]).

Context-Sensitive Fortitions: Dissimilation

In children's speech, as in adult languages, diphthongs arise from single vowels, from the vocalization of consonants, and from consonant loss that makes two vowels adjacent. A long or lengthened vowel is like a vowel followed by a nonsyllabic copy of itself: [e:] equals [eẹ]. Diphthongs (two vowel qualities within a single syllable) often arise when one part of a vowel undergoes a change and the rest does not. This may occur by raising ([eẹ] > [eị]), or lowering ([eẹ] > [æẹ]), or bleaching ([eẹ] > [ʌẹ]), or laxing ([eẹ] > [ɛẹ]), and it is a dissimilation. Diphthongs are especially susceptible to further dissimilation; they allow the maximization of both sonority and color (or the maximization of conflicting colors).

Bleile (1989) describes diphthongization of /æ/ to [aị] in the speech of 2-year-old Kylie, an American English learner: *hand* [haịn], and *flag* [faịk]. Kylie also dissimilates /ɛị/ to [aị]: *play* [paị], *paper* [paịpə]. Sylvia Major diphthongized both palatal and labial vowels in English: [peịŋki] *Pinky*, [spoụn] *spoon*, [dɑụli] ~ [dæụli] *dolly*, [seị] *see* (but not in Portuguese: only [se], not *[seị], for *(vo)sé* "you"). She also dissimilated /aị, aụ/ to [ɒị, æụ], or [ɔị, ɛụ], as in [ɣɔịt nɛụ] *right now*. Moreover, Sylvia's lax and low vowels /ɪ, ɛ, ʊ, ɔ, æ/ variably acquired a schwa offglide, and the vowels were sometimes tensed or raised, for example, [dɔẹg, doẹg] *dog*, [hɛẹd, heẹd] *head* (Major, 1977).

Fortitive processes are subject to the same implicational conditions in dissimilative applications as in context-free applications; for example, if the syllabic of [uụ] is delabialized to [iụ], then that of [oụ] must also be delabialized to [əụ], because delabialization is especially applicable to lower vowels. Diphthongization and dissimilation within diphthongs occur most often in long or stressed syllables, especially in slow or emphatic speech. For example, for my daughter Elizabeth, a word such as *no!* usually [noụ] or [nəụ] may become [naụ] (by lowering) or [nɛụ] (by palatalization) or even [naụ] (by both) under extreme emphasis.

In many accents of English, the adult vowels vary between monophthongal and diphthongal manifestations, depending on accent and other lengthening conditions: Even in quite conservative dialects, based on Received Pronunciation and General American (Wells, 1983), [i:] ([iị]) varies with [ɪị] or [iị] and [u:] ([uụ]) varies with [ʊụ] or [iụ] or even [ɪụ], so it is hardly surprising if we find diphthongizations in children's speech. Monophthongal vowels may diphthongize in children's speech, as in adult speech, by dissimilation within the monophthong (/e:/ becomes [eị], /ɛ:/ becomes [ɛə]), or by partial assimilation of monophthongs to adjacent consonants (/æ:ʃ/ becomes [æiʃ]—see previous text).

There are additional sources of diphthongs in children's speech, which may lead to dissimilative changes that might seem unexpected. Approximants may become vowels, which may form diphthongs. English approximant /r/ seems to have rhotic, palatal, and labial qualities. Syllabic [ɹ] may lose its rhotic quality and become [y] or [œ] (as in my daughter's pronunciation of *Ernie and Bert* as [œni ən bœp] (2 years, 1 month)). If /r/ also loses palatality or labiality it may become [ʊ] or [ɔ] (*Ernie* as [ʊni] or [ɔni]) or [i] (*bird* as [bi]). Two-year-old Kylie pronounced /ar/ as [aị] in *cards* [taịz], *market* [maịkɪt] (Bleile, 1989). Menn's subject Jacob also substituted [ị] for some postvocalic /r/'s: *horse ~horsie* [hɔịs]~

[haiçi]∼ [həiçi] and *more* [mwɔi] (Menn, 1978). And if /r/ loses rhoticity, palatality, and labiality, it becomes [ə], as it does in unstressed syllables for many children (and adults). When syllabic [l] loses its laterality it often becomes [u] or [o], because it is usually velarized when syllabic.

Consonantal [ɹ] and [l] may become the glides ([ɣ, i, u] or [ɥ, j, w]) that correspond to these vowels. If an [ɹ] or [l] becomes a glide, the adjacent vowel may dissimilate: For example, if [ł] becomes [u] in words such as *tell* and *belly*, the preceding [ε] may lower, yielding [tau] and [baui] or [bawi]. In fact, dissimilative lowering may occur before [ł], even if it does not lose its laterality. And [ɹ], whether or not it is de-rhotacized and bleached to [ə], may also condition a variety of diphthongizations and dissimilations: Vowels often develop schwa offglides before [ɹ], as is standard in Received Pronunciation (where *steering, fairy* are [stiəɹɪŋ, fεəɹi]). Alternatively, they may become lax, as in General American ([stɪɹɪŋ, fεɹi]), or tense, as in some East Coast U.S. dialects with ([stiɹɪŋ, feɹi]).

Diphthongs may also arise in children's speech when intervocalic consonants are lost, for example, Hildegard's [bai] for *buggy* (Leopold, 1939), Jacob's [bæi] for *battery* (Menn, 1978, 278). Dissimilation within the diphthong may follow. My daughter's pronunciation of words such as *butter* (adult [bərɹ]) varied considerably (2 years, 1 month), from emphatic [bədi] to less careful [bəri] or [bəi] to [bai]. This [ai] pronunciation, the result of dissimilation of [ə] from the following [i], also occurred in words such as *bunny* and *funny*, where the /n/ was deleted: [bai, fai].

Diphthongs may in turn be resolved into disyllabic sequences. Bleile (1989) describes two children who insert [ə] after a final /au/; one of them also inserts [ə] after final /ɔi/ as well.

Context-Sensitive Lenitions: Monophthongization

Monophthongization is a context-sensitive substitution in the sense that it occurs by the complete mutual assimilation of the parts of a diphthong; when /ai/ becomes [æ], the [a] assimilates to the palatality of the following [i], and the [i] assimilates to the openness of the preceding [a]. Many children, such as Sylvia, start out with all monophthongs (Major, 1977). Others, such as Linda, may monophthongize more similar sequences such as /ei/ and /ɔi/ but allow less similar sequences such as /ai/ to remain diphthongal (Vihman, 1971). Hildegard also monophthongized /εi/ and /ou/, but pronounced /ai/ and /au/ as diphthongs (Leopold, 1939). Monophthongization of palatal and labial diphthongs is not always symmetrical. Amahl monophthongized /εi/ in *rain* to [e], /ɔi/ in *noisy* to [ɔ:], and /aiə/ in *fire* to [æ:]; /ou/ in *soap* was at first variably monophthongized to [u:], but it later remained diphthongal [əu] (Smith, 1973).

Monophthongization is often associated with shortening; a syllabic-plus-offglide is equivalent to a long vowel in most languages, while a simple syllabic can be short. So monophthongizations such as /ei̯/ > [e] are sometimes seen simply as glide loss, and monophthongizations such as /ou̯/ > [u], as loss of the syllabic and reassignment of syllabicity to the [u̯]. We could also say that if /ei̯/ monophthongizes to [e], the [i̯] assimilates to the height of the [e], and if /ou/ monophthongizes to [u], the [o] assimilates to the height of the [u̯]; in both cases, shortening may or may not occur.

The similarity principle (segments that are similar are implicationally favored for further assimilation) predicts that [ei̯] is more susceptible to mutual assimilation than [oi̯] or [ai̯]. The similarity principle appears to govern monophthongization, so there is reason to regard monophthongization as complete assimilation. A child who monophthongizes [ei̯] to [e] or [ou̯] to [u] may be able to say the less-similar sequences, [ai̯] or [au̯], as Amahl could (Smith, 1973).

Other Lenitive Processes: Reduction and Harmony

In children's speech, as in adult languages, vowel reduction is related to speech timing. In adult languages, we expect that where syllables have relatively equal timing, we will find full vowels. Unless syllables are considerably shortened, we will not find the loss of sonority and color, and the limitation to a small set of possible vowel qualities, which mark the unstressed syllables of languages such as English or Khmer. Vihman notes that "a correlation between rate of articulation and children's age is commonly reported" (1996, 213). Thus, it does not seem coincidental that Allen and Hawkins (1978) found that the 3-year-old English learners they studied did not reduce syllables as generally as adult speakers do, although there was considerable variation across children. Allen and Hawkins (1978, 174) comment that children's earliest words "typically have only heavy syllables" with "peripheral (noncentral) vowels and rather fully articulated consonants." It seems that reduction may occur if unstressed, shortened syllables appear in a child's speech, but that in many cases, unstressed syllables are deleted entirely. If they survive, they are not articulated quickly enough to reduce. Allen and Hawkins (1980, 231) also note that because unstressed syllables are often entirely absent in the speech of 1 and 2 year olds, their speech may appear to be syllable-timed.

This appearance (or percept) of syllable timing might lead us to expect that vowel harmony, an assimilative phenomenon associated with syllable- or mora-timed languages, would be fairly pervasive in children's speech. But vowel harmony is less common in children than we might expect. There are cases where an epenthetic or paragogic vowel shares the features of a preceding vowel: Ross (1937) gives examples from one English-speaking child, and Chervela (1981) cites a number of examples in Telugu learners. Reduplication may result in matching vowels in consecutive syllables (Ingram, 1971; Vihman, 1996), as an unstressed syllable may reduplicate an adjacent stressed or unstressed syllable (Drachman and Malikouti-Drachman, 1973), but children who spread the values of palatality or labiality across whole multisyllabic words, as in the vowel harmony systems of languages such as Turkish or Finnish, are to my knowledge unreported.

Variation

Children may eliminate any particular difficulty by means of a range of processes: For example, the particular combination [nonhigh, nonlow, nontense, palatal] presents a certain difficulty, so [ɛ] may be raised, or lowered, or tensed, or depalatalized. Because vowels are simultaneous combinations of conflicting features, and increasing one feature, like palatality, results in the weakening of another, like sonority (and vice versa), it might seem that virtually any change can be motivated. Certainly we cannot predict the order of acquisition of vowels in general. (If we could, we might also expect the vowel inventories of the languages of the world to be in entirely subset relationships. In comparing vowel inventories, we do find some seductively subsetlike partial patterns, but these do not turn out to be universal.)

Yet there are some predictions that can be made, not necessarily about the order of acquisition of particular vowel qualities or even particular feature oppositions, but rather about the substitution patterns that may occur within the speech of an individual child. For example, if [ɛ] is tensed, we may expect that in similar circumstances [ɪ] will be tensed as well (because higher vowels are more susceptible to tensing); if [ɛ] is depalatalized, we can have no such expectation about [ɪ] (lower vowels are more susceptible to depalatalization). We expect substitutions to conform to implicational conditions on processes because these implicational conditions reflect the phonetic motivations—articulatory or perceptual—of the processes. If a child unrounds [u] to [ɨ] (losing labiality, increasing sonority), we can expect unrounding of [ɒ] to [ɑ], because the phonetic basis of the latter substitution is the same as that of the former, but stronger. There is less labiality to lose, and more sonority to increase.

Variation within the speech of individual children has previously been noted. Children lack articulatory control and experiment with different substitutions, particularly in the early stages of word production. By the time the child settles on consistent substitutions in consonants, the vowels in his or her speech may be reasonably accurate. Nevertheless, some variation remains. As in adults, process application may vary with effort and with attention paid to speech; Elbers and Wijnen (1992), note the effects of effort. Process application may also vary with affect. For example, my daughter Elizabeth's pronunciations of her own name at age 3 ranged from hyperarticulate, emphatic [iˈjazəbɪs], with full vowels and lowering of the stressed (lax) vowel, to hypoarticulate, too-sleepy-to-talk ['miββiɸ], with vowel reduction, unstressed vowel deletion, and consonant place harmony. It is important to note that variation confirms the phonetic character of substitutions, because it reveals how different demands on the child's abilities may elicit different substitutions as responses.

The ability (or desire) to produce a sound or sound sequence in one set of circumstances does not necessarily extend to all circumstances. Words may be more accurately produced in imitation than in spontaneous utterances. This is sometimes used to argue for inaccuracy or incompleteness of a child's lexical representations, but imitation may involve increased effort and attention to pronunciation, and spontaneous productions require the organization of sequences of articulations to combine with the effort of lexical recall.

Imitated forms are also used to argue against the characterization of substitutions as expressions of "inability." Obviously, if a child pronounces a particular sound or combination under some conditions, he or she has the phonetic ability to pronounce it, but he may not be able to pronounce it under all conditions. If substitutions occur, they may still be phonetically motivated. Consider that all English-speaking adults can say [prɛzɪdɛ̃nt əv ði junaɪ̯tɛd stɛɪ̯ts], but there is still phonetic motivation for the substitutions that result in (American) [prɛzdɲaɪ̯dstɛɪ̯ts] in connected speech. We may even claim that American adults are *unable* to use the hyperarticulate form in all circumstances, as they are unable to avoid pronunciations such as [kɪɾi] in connected speech, even though they are capable of saying [kɪti] in hyperarticulate speech.

Conclusion

The general cross-linguistic and cross-child patterns that we find cannot be attributed to a simple principle such as maximal dispersion, which predicts that any given number of vowel phonemes will be distributed within vowel space so as to maximize the sum of their differences. This principle predicts that the expected three-vowel system will be /i, ɑ, u/ and the most common five-vowel system /i, e, ɑ, o, u/—but the predictions of the principle do not correspond to the actual vowel systems of the world's languages very much beyond this. Further, this principle alone gives no way to account for vowel systems (such as /ɨ, ə, ɑ/ or /e, o, a/), which are not maximally dispersed. Vowel systems, like consonant systems, are based on feature contrasts, and they are constrained by the application of processes which are implicationally conditioned to apply where their phonetic motivation is strongest.

Bloomfield (1933), in discussing sound change, described a wide variety of changes in the histories of languages, and he pointed to an array of phonetic motivations which seem to underlie these changes. Then, at the end of the discussion, he rejected the idea that these changes are phonetically motivated, on the grounds that if sound change were phonetically motivated, all languages would develop toward a single optimal phonology, and all would end up alike. Bloomfield, however, did not consider that speakers' learning is the key to the paradox. Children, who at first submit to their phonetic inclinations, learn, in developing their abilities, to control articulation and thereby inhibit some phonetically motivated substitutions in order to perceive and pronounce the sounds and sequences of a particular language.

Most children's vowel substitutions seem to escape notice, with the result that the data we have on normal vowel development does not show nearly the variety that vowel substitutions in the world's languages would lead us to expect to find in children. In fact, it seems likely that most instances of apparently abnormal vowel development—unusual substitutions—are likely not to be abnormal at all, except perhaps in being too persistent. In the case of vowels, it is speech pathologists rather than developmental linguists who are in the best position to discover and publish the facts regarding what children do about vowels they can't pronounce. My aim has been to show that the vowel systems of the world suggest that normal children might take many different paths to the mastery of the vowels of their languages.

Notes

1. A phonological substitution here is meant to include any change of a single phonetic or phonological feature: Devoicing of [d] to [t], or assimilation of [np] to [mp] are all substitutions. Some substitutes (outputs) may be the result of multiple substitutions. If /l/ becomes [d], it is delateralized as well as stopped. If /ɑi̯/ is pronounced as [æ], the /ɑ/ assimilates the palatality and tenseness of [i̯], and the [i̯] assimilates the lowness of /ɑ/.

2. For a consonant example, Fey and Gandour (1982, 80) described a process of postnasalization of word-final voiced stops in the speech of a 21-month-old English-speaking boy. They claimed that this must be an idiosyncratic, discovered rule rather than a natural one, because they knew of no phonological system that derives a phonetic sequence of stop plus nasal from an underlying voiced stop. But postnasalization of voiced stops, while somewhat uncommon, does occur in such languages as Mundari (Osada, 1992) and Temiar (Benjamin, 1976) as a regular allophonic process.

References

Aitcheson, J., and Chiat, S. (1981). Natural phonology or natural memory? The interaction between phonological processes and recall mechanisms. Language and Speech, 24, 311–326.

Allen, W. S. (1953). Phonetics in ancient India. London: Oxford University Press.

Allen, W. S. (1968). Vox Graeca. Cambridge, England: Cambridge University Press.

Allen, W. S. (1970). Vox Latina. Cambridge, England: Cambridge University Press.

Allen, G. D., and Hawkins, S. (1978). The development of phonological rhythm. In A. Bell and J. B. Hooper (Eds.), Syllables and segments (pp. 173–185). Amsterdam: North-Holland.

Allen, G. D., and Hawkins, S. (1980). Phonological rhythm: Definition and development. In G. H. Yeni-Komshian, J. F. Kavanagh, and C. A. Ferguson (Eds.), Child phonology, Vol. 1: Production. New York: Academic.

Alves, M. (2000). A Pacoh analytic grammar. Ph. D. dissertation, University of Hawaii, Honolulu.

Aslin, R. N., Pisoni, D. B., Hennessy B. L., and Perey, A. J. (1981). Discrimination of voice onset time by human infants: New findings and implications for the effect of early experience. Child Development, 52, 1135–1145.

Bassi, C. (1983). Development at 3 years. In J. V. Irwin and S. P. Wong (Eds.), Phonological development in children: 18 to 72 months (pp. 87–105). Carbondale: Southern Illinois University Press.

Baudouin de Courtenay, J. [1895]. An attempt at a theory of phonetic alternations. In E. Stankiewicz (Ed. and Trans., 1972), A Baudouin de Courtenay anthology (pp. 144–212). Bloomington: Indiana University Press.

Benjamin, G. (1976). An outline of Temiar grammar. In P. N. Jenner, L. C. Thompson, and S. Starosta (Eds.), Austroasiatic studies I, (pp.129–187). Honolulu: University Press of Hawaii.

Bernhardt, B. H., and Stemberger, J. P. (1998). Handbook of phonological development. New York: Academic.

Best, C. T., McRoberts, G. W., and Sithole, N. M. (1988). The phonological basis of perceptual loss for non-native contrasts: Maintenance of discrimination among Zulu clicks by English-speaking adults and infants. Journal of Experimental Psychology: Human Perception and Performance, 14, 345–360.

Bleile, K. M. (1989). A note on vowel patterns in two normally developing children. Clinical Linguistics and Phonetics, 3, 201–212.

Bloomfield, L. (1933). Language. New York: Holt.

Bloomfield, L. (1956). Eastern Ojibwa. Ann Arbor: University of Michigan Press.

Bond, Z. S., Petrosino, L., and Dean, C. R. (1982). The emergence of vowels: 17 to 26 months. Journal of Phonetics, 10, 417–422.

Bowen, J. T., and Rhys Jones, T. J. (1960). Teach yourself Welsh. London: English Universities Press.

Bright, W. (1975). The Dravidian enunciative vowel. In H. F. Schiffman and C. M. Eastman (Eds.), Dravidian phonological systems, (pp. 11–46). Seattle: University of Washington Press.

Buhr, R. (1980). The emergence of vowels in an infant. Journal of Speech and Hearing Research, 23, 73–94.

Burrow, T. (1965). The Sanskrit language. London: Faber and Faber.

Campbell, A. (1959). Old English grammar. Oxford: Oxford University Press.

Campbell, L. (1977). Quichéan linguistic prehistory. University of California Publications in Linguistics, 81. Berkeley: University of California Press.

Chervela, N. (1981). Medial consonant cluster acquisition by Telugu children. Journal of Child Language, 8, 63–73.

Davis, B., and MacNeilage, P. (1990). Acquisition of correct vowel production: A quantitative case study. Journal of Speech and Hearing Research, 33, 16–27.

de Boysson-Bardies, B., Sagart, L., and Durand, C. (1984). Discernable differences in the babbling of infants according to target language. Journal of Child Language, 11, 1–15.

Diffloth, G. (1980). The Wa languages. Linguistics of the Tibeto-Burman Area 5, 1–182.

Dinnsen, D. A. (1984). Methods and empirical issues in analyzing functional misarticulations. In M. Elbert, D. A. Dinnsen, and G. Weismer (Eds.), Phonological theory and the misarticulating child, AHSA Monograph No. 22 (pp. 5–17). Rockville, Md.: American Speech-Language-Hearing Association.

Donegan, P. (1978). On the natural phonology of vowels. Ohio State University dissertation. OSU Working Papers in Linguistics No. 23. (1985). New York: Garland.

Donegan, P. (1995). The innateness of phonemic perception. In V. Samiian (Ed.), WECOL 7 (Proceedings of the 24th Western Conference on Linguistics), (pp. 59–69). Fresno, Calif.: Western Conference on Linguistics.

Donegan, P., and Stampe, D. (1979). The study of natural phonology. In D. A. Dinnsen (Ed.), Current approaches to phonological theory (pp. 126–173). Bloomington: Indiana University Press.

Drachman, G., and Malikouti-Drachman, A. (1973). Studies in the acquisition of Greek as a native language: I. Some preliminary findings on phonology. Ohio State University Working Papers in Linguistics, 15, 99–114.

Eilers, R. E., Gavin, W. J., and Oller, D. K. (1982). Cross-linguistic perception in infancy: Early effects of linguistic experience. Journal of Child Language, 9, 289–302.

Eilers, R. E., Gavin, W. J., Oller, D. K., et al. (1979). Speech perception in the language-innocent and the language-wise: The perception of VOT. Journal of Child Language, 6, 1–18.

Eimas, P. D. (1974). Auditory and linguistic units of processing of cues for place of articulation by infants. Perception and Psychophysics, 16, 513–521.

Eimas, P. D. (1975). Auditory and phonetic coding of the cues for speech: Discrimination of the [r-] distinction by young infants. Perception and Psychophysics, 18, 341–347.

Eimas, P. D., Siqueland, E.R., Jusczyk, P., and Vigorito, J. (1971). Speech perception in infants. Science, 171, 303–306.

Einarsson, S. (1945). Icelandic: Grammar, texts, glossary. Baltimore: Johns Hopkins University Press.

Elbers, L., and Wijnen, F. (1992). Effort, production skill, and language learning. In C. A. Ferguson, L. Menn, and C. Stoel-Gammon (Eds.), Phonological Development (pp. 337–368). Timonium, Md.: York Press.

Emeneau, M. B. (1955). Kolami, a Dravidian language. University of California Publications in Linguistics, 12. Berkeley: University of California Press.

Ferguson, C. A., and Farwell, C. B. (1975). Words and sounds in early language acquisition: English initial consonants in the first fifty words. Language, 51, 419–439.

Fey, M. E., and Gandour, J. (1982). Rule discovery in phonological acquisition. Journal of Child Language, 9, 71–81.

Fry, D. B. (1966). The development of the phonological system in the normal and deaf child. In F. Smith and G. A. Miller (Eds.), The Genesis of Language (pp. 187–206). Cambridge, Mass.: MIT Press.

Gierut, J. A., Cho, M-H., and Dinnsen, D. A. (1993). Geometric accounts of consonant-vowel interactions in developing systems. Clinical Linguistics and Phonetics, 7, 219–236.

Hare, G. (1983). Development at 2 years. In J. V. Irwin and S. P. Wong (Eds.), Phonological development in children: 18 to 72 months (pp. 55–85). Carbondale: Southern Illinois University Press.

Haugen, E. (1976). The Scandinavian languages. Cambridge, Mass.: Harvard University Press.

Hoskison, J. (1974). Prosodies and verb stems in Gude. Linguistics, 141, 17–26.

Huffman, F. E. (1990). Burmese Mon, Thai Mon, and Nyah Kur: A synchronic comparison. Mon-Khmer Studies, 16–17, 31–84.

Hutcheson, J. W. (1974). A natural history of complete consonantal assimilations. Ph.D. dissertation, Ohio State University.

Ingram, D. (1971). Phonological rules in young children. Stanford Papers and Reports on Child Language Development, 3, 31–50.

Irwin, J. V., and Wong, S. P. (1983). Phonological development in children: 18 to 72 months. Carbondale: Southern Illinois University Press.

Jakobson, R. (1941). Kindersprache, aphasie, und allgemeine lautgesetze. In A. R. Keiler (Trans., 1968), Child language, aphasia, and phonological universals. The Hague: Mouton.

Jakobson, R., and Halle, M. (1956). Fundamentals of language. The Hague: Mouton.

Jones, C. (1989). A history of English phonology. London: Longman.

Jusczyk, P. W. (1992). Developing phonological categories from the speech signal. In C. A. Ferguson, L. Menn, and C. Stoel-Gammon (Eds.), Phonological Development (pp. 17–64). Timonium, Md.: York Press.

Jusczyk, P. W, and Thompson, E. (1978). Perception of a phonetic contrast in multisyllabic utterances by two-month-old infants. Perception and Psychophysics, 23, 105–109.

Keller, R. E. (1961). German dialects: Phonology and morphology, with selected texts. Manchester, England: Manchester University Press.

Kent, R. D. (1992). The biology of phonological development. In C. A. Ferguson, L. Menn, and C. Stoel-Gammon (Eds.), Phonological Development (pp. 65–90). Timonium, Md.: York Press.

Kornfeld, J. R. (1971). Theoretical issues in child phonology. Papers from the Seventh Regional Meeting of the Chicago Linguistic Society, 454–468. Chicago: Chicago Linguistic Society.

Kuhl, P. K. (1980). Perceptual constancy for speech-sound categories in early infancy. In G. H. Yeni-Komshian, J. F. Kavanagh, and C. A. Ferguson (Eds.), Child phonology, Vol. 2: Perception. New York: Academic.

Kuhl, P. K. (1983). Perception of auditory equivalence classes for speech in early infancy. Infant Behavior and Development, 6, 263–285.

Kuhl, P. K. (1991). Human adults and neonates show a "perceptual magnet effect" for the prototypes of speech categories; monkeys do not. Perception and Psychophysics, 50, 93–107.

Kuhl, P. K., and Miller, J. (1982). Discrimination of auditory target dimensions in the presence or absence of variation in a second dimension by infants. Perception and Psychophysics, 31, 279–292.

Kuipers, A. H. (1960). Phoneme and morpheme in Kabardian. The Hague: Mouton.

Larkins, P. (1983). Development at 4 years. In J. V. Irwin and S. P. Wong (Eds.), Phonological development in children: 18 to 72 months (pp. 107–132). Carbondale: Southern Illinois University Press.

Lassettre, P. (1995). Process effects in non-processual phonology. University of Hawaii Working Papers in Linguistics, 27, 37–54.

Leopold, W. (1939, 1947, 1949, 1949). Speech development of a bilingual child, 4 vols. Evanston, Ill.: Northwestern University Humanities Series, vols. 6, 11, 18, 19.

Lieberman, P. (1980). On the development of vowel production in young children. In G. H. Yeni-Komshian, J. F. Kavanagh, and C. A. Ferguson (Eds.), Child phonology, Vol. 1: Production (pp. 113–142). New York: Academic.

Lindblom, B. (1992). Phonological units as adaptive emergents of lexical development. In C. A. Ferguson, L. Menn, and C. Stoel-Gammon (Eds.), Phonological development (pp. 131–163). Timonium, Md.: York Press.

Locke, J. L., and Pearson, D. M. (1992). Vocal learning and the emergence of phonological capacity. In C. A. Ferguson, L. Menn, and C. Stoel-Gammon (Eds.), Phonological development (pp. 91–129). Timonium, Md.: York Press.

Lohuis-Weber, H., and Zonnefeld, W. (1996). Phonological acquisition and Dutch word prosody. Language Acquisition, 5, 245–283.

Macken, M. A. (1979). Developmental reorganization of phonology: A hierarchy of basic units of acquisition. Lingua, 49, 11–49.

Macken, M. A. (1980). The child's lexical representation: The "puzzle-puddle-pickle" evidence. Journal of Linguistics, 16, 1–17.

Macken, M. A., and Barton, D. (1980). The acquisition of the voicing contrast in English: A study of voice onset time in word-initial stop consonants. Journal of Child Language, 7, 41–74.

Major, R. C. (1977). Phonological differentiation of a bilingual child. Ohio State University Working Papers in Linguistics, 22, 88–122.

Matisoff, J. A. (1973). The grammar of Lahu. University of California Publications in Linguistics, 75. Berkeley: University of California Press.

Meltzoff, A. N., and Moore, M. K. (1977). Imitation of facial and manual gestures by human neonates. Science, 198, 75–78.

Menges, K. H. (1968). The Turkic languages and peoples. Wiesbaden: Harassowitz.

Menn, L. (1976). Pattern, control and contrast in beginning speech. University of Illinois, Ph.D. dissertation (1978). Bloomington: Indiana University Linguistics Club.

Menyuk, P., Menn, L., and Silber, R. (1986). Early strategies for the perception and production of words and sounds. In P. Fletcher and M. Garman (Eds.), Language Acquisition (pp. 198–223). Cambridge, England: Cambridge University Press.

Myers, S. (1997). Expressing phonetic naturalness in phonology. In I. Roca (Ed.), Derivations and constraints in phonology (pp. 125–152). Oxford: Clarendon Press.

Noreen, A. (1913). Geschichte der nordischen Sprachen. Strassburg: Trübner.

Ohso, M. (1972). A phonological study of some English loan words in Japanese. Ohio State University Working Papers in Linguistics, 14, 1–26.

Oller, D. K., and Eilers, R. E. (1988). The role of audition in infant babbling. Child Development, 59, 441–449.

Osada, T. (1992). A reference grammar of Mundari. Tokyo: Institute for the Study of Languages and Cultures of Asia and Africa, Tokyo University of Foreign Studies.

Otomo, K., and Stoel-Gammon, C. (1992). The acquisition of unrounded vowels in English. Journal of Speech and Hearing Research, 35, 604–616.

Paschall, L. (1983). Development at 18 months. In J. V. Irwin and S. P. Wong (Eds.), Phonological development in children: 18 to 72 months (pp. 73–81). Carbondale: Southern Illinois University Press.

Polka, L., and Werker, J. F. (1994). Developmental changes in perception of non-native vowel contrasts. Journal of Experimental Psychology: Human Perception and Performance, 20, 421–436.

Pollock, K., and Keiser, N. (1990). An examination of vowel errors in phonologically disordered children. Clinical Linguistics and Phonetics, 4, 161–178.

Pope, M. K. (1934). From Latin to modern French. Manchester, England: Manchester University Press.

Poppe, N. (1955). Introduction to Mongolian comparative studies. Mémoires de la société Finno-Ougrienne, 110.

Prince, A., and Smolensky, P. (1993). Optimality theory: Constraint interaction in generative grammar. Technical Report No. 2, Rutgers University Center for Cognitive Science. Piscataway, N.J.: Rutgers University.

Pupier, P. (1977). Quelques observations sur l'acquisition de la phonologie par des enfants montréalais de 2 ans. Rechereches Linguistiques à Montréal, 9. Montréal: L'association Linguistique de Montréal.

Pyle, C. (1970). West Greenlandic Eskimo and the representation of vowel length. Papers in Linguistics, 3, 115–146.

Rogers, F. M. (1948). Insular Portuguese pronunciation: Porto Santo and eastern Azores. Hispanic Review, 17, 47–70.

Ross, A. S. C. (1937). An example of vowel-harmony in a young child. Modern Language Notes, 52, 508.

Sapir, E. (1915). Notes on Judaeo-German phonology. The Jewish Quarterly Review, n.s., 6, 231–266. In D. G. Mandelbaum (Ed.) (1949), Selected writings of Edward Sapir (pp. 252–272). Berkeley: University of California Press.

Sapir, E. (1933). La réalité psychologique des phonèmes, Journal de Psychologie Normale et Pathologique, 30, 247–265. In D. G. Mandelbaum (Ed.) (1949), reprinted as The psychological reality of phonemes, selected writings of Edward Sapir (pp. 46–60). Berkeley: University of California Press.

Shafeev, D. A. (1964). A short grammatical outline of Pashto. Translated and edited by H. H. Paper. Bloomington: Indiana University Press.

Smith, B. L., Macaluso C., and Brown-Sweeney, S. (1991). Phonological effects shown by normal adult speakers learning new words: Implications for phonological development. Applied Psycholinguistics, 12, 281–298.

Smith, N. V. (1973). The acquisition of phonology. Cambridge, England: Cambridge University Press.

So, L. K. H., and Dodd, B. J. (1995). The acquisition of phonology by Cantonese-speaking children. Journal of Child Language, 22, 473–495.

Sommerfelt, A. (1968). Phonetics and sociology. In B. Malmberg (Ed.), Manual of phonetics. Amsterdam: North Holland.

Stampe, D. (1969). The acquisition of phonetic representation. In R. I. Binnick, A. Davison, G. M. Green, and J. L. Morgan (Eds.), Papers from the 5th Regional Meeting of the Chicago Linguistics Society (pp. 443–454). Chicago: Chicago Linguistics Society.

Stampe, D. (1973). A dissertation on natural phonology. University of Chicago Ph. D. dissertation. With annotations (1979). New York: Garland.

Stampe, D. (1987). On phonological representations. In W. Dressler, H. C. Luschutzky, O. E. Pfeiffer, and J. R. Rennison (Eds.) (1984), Phonologica (pp. 287–300). Cambridge, England: Cambridge University Press.

Stevens, K., and Keyser, S. J. (1989). Primary features and their enhancement in consonants. Language, 65, 81–106.

Stoel-Gammon, C., and Dunn, C. (1985). Normal and disordered phonology in children. Baltimore: University Park Press.

Templin, M. (1957). Certain language skills in children. Institute of Child Welfare Monograph Series 26. Minneapolis: University of Minnesota Press.

Trehub, S. E. (1976). The discrimination of foreign speech contrasts by infants and adults. Child Development, 47, 466–472.

Velten, H. V. (1943). The growth of phonemic and lexical patterns in infant language. Language, 19, 281–292.

Vihman, M. M. (1971). On the acquisition of Estonian. Stanford Papers and Reports on Child Language Development, 3, 51–94.

Vihman, M. M. (1992). Early syllables and the construction of phonology. In C. A. Ferguson, L. Menn, and C. Stoel-Gammon (Eds.), Phonological development (pp. 393–422). Timonium, Md.: York Press.

Vihman, M. M. (1996). Phonological development: The origins of language in the child. Cambridge, Mass.: Blackwell.

Vogel, I. (1975). One system or two: An analysis of a two-year-old Romanian-English bilingual's phonology. Stanford Papers and Reports on Child Language Development, 9, 43–62.

Wells, J. C. (1983). Accents of English (3 vols). Cambridge, England: Cambridge University Press.

Werker, J. F., Gilbert, J. H. V., Humphrey, K., and Tees, R. C. (1981). Developmental aspects of cross-language speech perception. Child Development, 52, 349–353.

Werker, J. F., and Lalonde, C. E. (1988). Cross-language speech perception: initial capabilities and developmental change. Developmental Psychology, 24, 672–683.

Werker, J. F., and Pegg, J. E. (1992). Infant speech perception and phonological acquisition. In C. A. Ferguson, L. Menn, and C. Stoel-Gammon (Eds.), Phonological development (pp. 285–311). Timonium, Md.: York Press.

Werker, J. F., and Tees, R. C. (1984). Cross-language speech perception: Evidence for perceptual reorganization during the first year of life. Infant Behaviour and Development, 7, 49–63.

Wolfe, V. I., and Blocker, S. D. (1990). Consonant-vowel interactions in an unusual phonological system. Journal of Speech and Hearing Disorders, 55, 561–566.

Zide, N. H. (1965). Gutob-Remo vocalism and glottalized vowels in Proto-Munda. In G. B. Milner and E. Henderson (Eds.), Indo-Pacific linguistic studies (part 1, pp. 43–53). Amsterdam: North Holland.

2

The Contribution of Phonetics to the Study of Vowel Development and Disorders

Sara J. Howard
Barry Heselwood

Now we must pull ourselves together, for we have come to the vowels, and they are very troublesome. (Rippmann, 1911, 32)

As Ball (1993, 66) observes, "vowels are not as easy to classify as consonants." Nor are they easy to describe generally in terms of their articulatory and acoustic correlates, and, furthermore, they pose particular problems for perceptual analysis and transcription. Rippmann, it seems, had a point! This chapter will consider some phonetic approaches to vowel description from both instrumental and perceptual perspectives and will examine evidence from speech development and impaired speech. This helps to illuminate some of the particular challenges and problems posed by vowel description and classification.

Vowels: A Working Definition

First, we need to provide a working definition for the scope of the term *vowel* as used in this chapter. As we shall see, even providing a simple but unambiguous definition is not straightforward. The problem relates in large part to the difference between phonetic and phonological usages of the term. As many authors have noted, from a phonetic perspective vowels can be described as resonant segments that are produced with an unobstructed laminar airflow escaping centrally through the vocal tract (Ball and Rahilly, 1999; Ladefoged,

1993; Laver, 1994). In contrast, consonants involve some degree of constriction in the vocal tract which either blocks the airflow momentarily, causes it to become turbulent, or diverts it from a central oral path. Phonologically, on the other hand, vowels are viewed from distributional and functional perspectives, and can be described as those segments which may occupy the center or nucleus of a syllable, as opposed to consonants, which occur in marginal positions in a syllable (onsets and codas).

Ball and Rahilly (1999, 43) point out that, "these two approaches to defining consonants and vowels overlap in the majority of cases." But, as they observe, some sounds appearing to match a phonetic description of the category of vowels (such as /j/ and /w/), have distribution patterns placing them in the consonant category, according to a phonological perspective. Catford (1977) provides a long discussion on the ambiguous relationship of approximants and vowels, noting inter alia that /j/ and /w/ are differentiated phonetically from the high vowels /i/ and /u/ on durational grounds, and are very similar in terms of articulatory stricture. Similarly, some sounds we would happily term consonants on the grounds of their phonetic characteristics may occur as syllable nuclei ([l̩] and [n̩] , often termed *syllabic consonants*). Because of this potential ambiguity, Pike (1947) suggested a two-way categorization, reserving the terms *vowel* and *consonant* to reflect a segment's phonological behavior, and using the terms *contoid* and *vocoid* to imply phonetic characteristics of segments. In this way, one might distinguish four sets of sounds: contoid consonants (such as [p], [s]), vocoid vowels (such as [i], [a]), contoid vowels (such as [l̩], [n̩]) and vocoid consonants (such as [j], [w]). In this chapter, we will restrict our use of the term *vowel* to those segments complying with both the phonetic and phonological definitions of vowel given above; in other words, to segments described by Pike (1947) as vocoid vowels.

Studying the Phonetics of Vowels

In the discussions later in this chapter, references will be made to properties of vowels in the articulatory, acoustic, and auditory domains. Before embarking on those discussions, it will be useful to briefly review some of the principal means at our disposal for investigating these properties.

The Articulatory Domain

Clark and Yallop (1995, 22) observe that, "the major challenge in describing the articulation of vocalic sounds is to define the position of the tongue," and the majority of the following instrumental techniques, when applied to the task of vowel description, aim to provide different types of information on the location and movement of the tongue during vowel description.

Electropalatography (EPG) is a technique that provides information on patterns of contact between the tongue and the palate in the region from the rear of the front teeth (the Kay Palatometer: Fletcher, McCutcheon and Wolf, 1975; and the Rion Palatograph: Fujimura, Tatsumi, and Kayaga, 1973) or the alveolar ridge (the Reading EPG: for a review of different versions, see Hardcastle and Gibbon, 1997) to the margins of the hard and soft palate. In our phonetic definition of vowels described previously, we said that they require an unobstructed airflow, which means that we would not expect lingualpalatal contact in the central part of the palate. However, particularly for close vowels (such as /i/, /ɪ/) and for the latter stages of closing dipththongs (such as /ɔɪ/, /aɪ/), there are clear patterns of contact between the sides of the tongue and the lateral margins of the palate. Hardcastle and Gibbon (1997) state that there will be little discernible contact for open vowels or for back vowels, although Byrd (1995) suggests that the raising of the back of the tongue for a vowel such as /u/ results in a lateral lingualpalatal contact pattern in the posterior region of the palate. Figure 2-1 shows lingualpalatal contact patterns for the high vowels /i/ and /u/ and the closing diphthong /aɪ/ in Southern Standard British English.

Although EPG appears to be a technique with relatively little to offer in the study of normal vowel production, it has provided interesting insights into the production of vowels in speakers with impaired speech. Yamashita, Michi, Imai, and colleagues (1992) describe the speech of a 6-year-old child with a history of cleft palate, who maintained strictures of central lingualpalatal contact over extensive areas of the palate during productions perceptually identified as the vowel /i/. Howard (2001) also used EPG to identify a similar phenomenon extending over a larger set of vowel articulations in an adolescent with cleft palate speech.

Electromagnetic articulography (EMA) uses electromagnetic transmitter and receiver coils attached to active and passive articulators in the vocal tract to track range and velocity of movement of the active articulators and changing vocal tract configurations over time (Perkell, Cohen, Svirsky, et al., 1992; Schönle, Grabe, Wenig, et al., 1987; Stone, 1997). Using a system of fixed reference points, up to five coils can be attached to the upper and lower lips, the tip or blade and dorsum of the tongue, the mandible, and even the soft palate to provide a representation of the time course of articulatory movements in the midsagittal plane.

This is a relatively new technique, but it has already been used to examine aspects of normal and impaired speech production, and has been combined with EPG to give information about lingual activity across different dimensions. Clearly, by providing a detailed examination of articulator coordination, it has enormous potential in the study of normal and atypical vowel production. The simultaneous monitoring of different articulators means that the complex

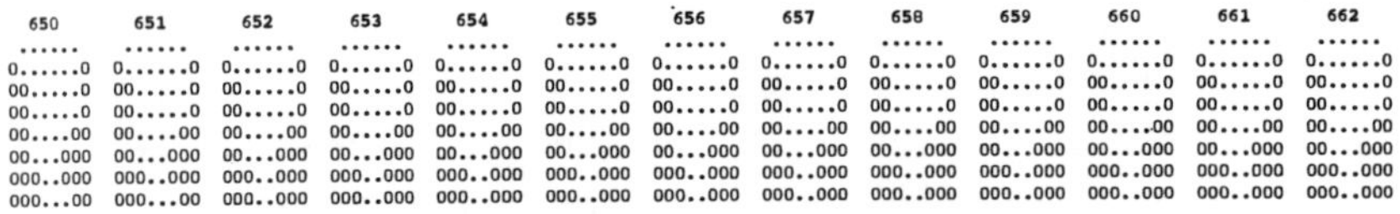

```
 650       651       652       653       654       655       656       657       658       659       660       661       662
.......   .......   .......   .......   .......   .......   .......   .......   .......   .......   .......   .......   .......
0......0  0......0  0......0  0......0  0......0  0......0  0......0  0......0  0......0  0......0  0......0  0......0  0......0
00.....0  00.....0  00.....0  00.....0  00.....0  00.....0  00.....0  00.....0  00.....0  00.....0  00.....0  00.....0  00.....0
00.....0  00.....0  00.....0  00.....0  00.....0  00.....0  00.....0  00.....0  00.....0  00.....0  00.....0  00.....0  00.....0
00....00  00....00  00....00  00....00  00....00  00....00  00....00  00....00  00....00  00....00  00....00  00....00  00....00
00...000  00...000  00...000  00...000  00...000  00...000  00...000  00...000  00...000  00...000  00...000  00...000  00...000
000..000  000..000  000..000  000..000  000..000  000..000  000..000  000..000  000..000  000..000  000..000  000..000  000..000
000..00   000...00  000..000  000..000  000..000  000..000  000..000  000..000  000..000  000..000  000..000  000..000  000..000
```

Figure 2-1a

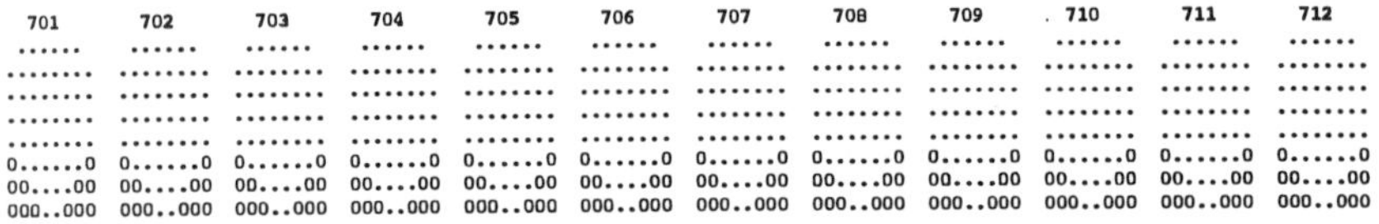

```
 701       702       703       704       705       706       707       708       709      . 710      711       712
.......   .......   .......   .......   .......   .......   .......   .......   .......   .......   .......   .......
........  ........  ........  ........  ........  ........  ........  ........  ........  ........  ........  ........
........  ........  ........  ........  ........  ........  ........  ........  ........  ........  ........  ........
........  ........  ........  ........  ........  ........  ........  ........  ........  ........  ........  ........
........  ........  ........  ........  ........  ........  ........  ........  ........  ........  ........  ........
0......0  0......0  0......0  0......0  0......0  0......0  0......0  0......0  0......0  0......0  0......0  0......0
00....00  00....00  00....00  00....00  00....00  00....00  00....00  00....00  00....00  00....00  00....00  00....00
000..000  000..000  000..000  000..000  000..000  000..000  000..000  000..000  000..000  000..000  000..000  000..000
```

Figure 2-1b

```
 180       181       182       183       184       185       186       187       188       189       190       191       192
.......   .......   .......   .......   .......   .......   .......   .......   .......   .......   .......   .......   .......
........  ........  ........  ........  ........  ........  ........  ........  ........  ........  ........  ........  ........
........  ........  ........  ........  ........  ........  ........  ........  ........  ........  ........  ........  ........
........  ........  ........  ........  ........  ........  ........  ........  ........  ........  ........  ........  ........
........  ........  ........  ........  ........  ........  ........  ........  ........  ........  ........  ........  ........
........  ........  ........  ........  ........  ........  ........  ........  ........  ........  ........  ........  ........
........0  ........  ........  ........  ........  ........  ........  ........  ........  ........  ........  0.......  0......0

 193       194       195       196       197       198       199       200       201       202       203       204       205
.......   .......   .......   .......   .......   .......   .......   .......   .......   .......   .......   .......   .......
........  ........  ........  ........  ........  ........  ........  ........  ........  ........  ........  ........  0.......
........  ........  ........  ........  ........  ........  ........  ........  ........  0.......  0.......  0......0  0......0
........  ........  ........  ........  ........  ........  ........  0......0  0......0  00.....0  00.....0  00....00  00....00
........  ........  ........  ........  ........  0......0  0......0  00....00  00....00  00....00  00....00  00....00  00....00
........  ........  ........  0.......  0......0  0......0  00....00  00....00  00....00  00....00  00....00  00....00  00....00
0......0  0......0  0......0  0......0  0.......0  00.....0  00....00  00....00  00....00  00....00  00....00  00....00  00....00
```

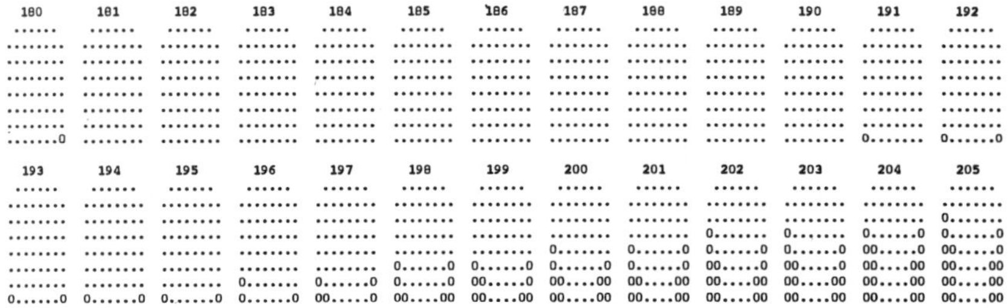

Figure 2-1c

Figure 2-1a-c   Lingualpalatal contact patterns for the English [iː], [uː], and [aɪ] vowels in a) BEE, b) BOO, and c) BUY.

interrelationships between lip, tongue, and jaw movements in vowel articulation can be examined. However, because of its present high cost, and the problems it presents for use with young children, this may mean that, for the time being, not much insight into developmental vowel disorders will be gained through EMA.

X-ray and ultrasound imaging are two techniques that, for reasons of safety and of cost, are less readily available for the phonetic study of speech production. Both, however, have been used to investigate the articulatory properties of vowels. X-rays can provide both static and dynamic images of the movements of the vocal organs during speech production, and can sample data from various different spatial perspectives. For investigating vowel production, a dynamic, midsagittal view provides the best information on tongue position and movement and on its relationship with other articulators, including the lips, jaw, and velum. Ball and Gröne (1997) and Stone (1997) give clear accounts of the technique, outlining methodological problems and pitfalls, including the difficulty of disentangling overlapping images of different parts of the vocal tract (tongue, teeth, lips, bone, and so on) and identifying precisely which part of an articulator is revealing itself in the image. For example, is the image of the edge of the tongue in a given data sample showing the centre of the tongue or one of its lateral margins?

Such questions may, however, be more problematic for the study of consonant articulations than vowels. Certainly, x-ray data has provided us with a considerable body of useful information about vowel production. It has been used to identify both the highest point of the tongue and also the point of closest lingual constriction in the vocal tract (not always the same thing), and to relate tongue strictures to spatial adjustments of the mandible and velum (Kent and Moll, 1972; Perkell, 1996; Wood, 1979). Ultrasound imaging has great potential in the description of vowel production because it is a technique that maps the cross-sectional shape of the vocal tract more completely than other techniques. Ultrasound uses the sound wave reflections that occur at boundaries between tissues or surfaces with different densities (Stone, 1997), and maps data over complex spatial configurations and dimensions. It has been used to explore lingual and mandibular activity in vowel production and in consonant-vowel coarticulation (Stone, Shawker, Talbot, and Rich, 1988; Stone and Vatikiotis-Bateson, 1995).

Electromyography (EMG) detects muscle activation by measuring electrical potential (Gentil and Moore, 1997; Stone, 1997). Small electrodes are attached to the surface of the articulators and detect electrical activity as muscle fibers contract. Increased electrical potential can show that a muscle is being innervated even if there is no observable movement of the related organ. This makes it possible to infer the speakers's intention to employ a particular articulator. Because it is possible to place electrodes on a number of discrete sites and collect simultaneous information from muscles of the lips, tongue, and jaw, this technique, like EMA discussed previously, has the potential to provide information about the coordination of different articulators in vowel production.

Gentil and Moore (1997) and Stone (1997), however, outline some of the technical problems associated with EMG making data collection and interpretation potentially difficult. These include the challenge of accurate electrode positioning to avoid obstructions such as bone or folds of skin, and the difficulty of pinpointing precisely the particular muscle or bundle of muscles to be investigated. Stone (1997, 32) cautions that when using EMG to explore aspects of lingual activity, obviously a focus of particular interest in the study of vowel production, because of the complex configuration of the lingual musculature, "it is almost impossible to be sure that the signal comes from the muscle of interest." The need for administration under medical supervision severely inhibits widespread availability and use of EMG. However, studies examining vowel production in normal and impaired speech production have used EMG. Alfonso and Baer (1982); Baer, Alfonso, and Honda (1988); Gentil and Moore (1997); Honda, (1996); McGarr and Harris (1983); and Shankweiler, Harris, and Taylor (1968) argue that the technique has a valuable role to play in analyzing impaired speech production.

Electrolaryngography (ELG) derives a waveform indicating degrees of vocal fold approximation during the glottal cycle. The efficiency of laryngeal function in voicing affects the quality of resonance in the supralaryngeal chambers (Abberton, Howard, and Fourcin, 1989), which may also affect the perceptual analysis of vowel quality (Lotto, Holt, and Kluender, 1997), particularly at high levels of fundamental frequency (Sundberg and Gauffin, 1979).

The Acoustic Domain

Spectrography is the prime technique for making acoustic measurements of speech production. The speech spectrograph is capable of providing detailed quantitative information regarding speech waveform, including intensity, frequency, duration, and spectral analysis (Kent and Read, 1992). It is not surprising, therefore, that the technique has proved extremely popular for the investigation of normal vowel production, vowel development, and vowel disorders. As Baken (1987, 353) notes in discussing vowels, "the sound spectrograph, by making them readily observable, unleashed a flood of research into their characteristics and significance."

Formant structure and duration, two aspects of vowel production, have proved particularly popular in spectrographic analysis. The acoustic structure of vowel productions can normally be adequately specified by measuring the center frequency of the first three or four formant resonances (Fant, 1956), with the first two often being sufficient (Kent and Read, 1992), particularly in languages such as English that do not contain vowel distinctions that depend solely on contrasts in lip position (Ladefoged, 2001). It is important to know that formant measurements and comparisons between them are seen as relative, not absolute values, because they relate to the dimensions of the vocal tract varying between individual speakers.

Vowel duration values, meanwhile, are usually obtained by measuring from the onset of the second formant (F2) to its offset, although Blomgren and Robb (1998) point out the difficulties in determining vowel duration. Farmer (1997) provides a comprehensive review of the use of spectrography in clinical phonetic analysis, revealing how it has been used to study vowel production across a wide range of speech impairments. In this chapter, we will also make extensive reference to spectrographic studies of vowel development and vowel disorders, as well as the production of vowels by normal speakers (Figure 2-2).

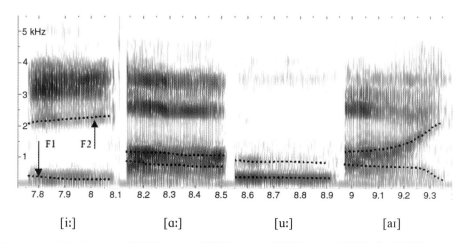

Figure 2-2 Spectrograms of the English FLEECE, BATH, GOOSE and PRICE vowels produced between glottal stops in a near-RP accent, showing formant structure.

The Auditory Domain

Measuring formants and tracking articulator movements are undeniably valuable sources of information that can shed light on why particular vowel productions sound the way they do, and, in the context of disordered speech, do not sound the way we think they should. However, perceptual analysis is indispensable if we wish to regard vowel sounds, or any speech sounds, as speech *sounds*, that is, as phenomena that impinge on listeners' consciousness and carry linguistic information. The question as to whether a particular vowel production *sounds* like a realization of English /i/ or /u/ can only be answered by listening to it, not by measuring its formants or obtaining information about the speaker's tongue and lip movements. For this reason, we need to know how the auditory experience of sound compares to its acoustic structure.

Formants are clearly important determinants of our perceptual experience of vowels as shown by neurograms of the peripheral auditory system's phase-locked responses to amplitude peaks corresponding to formant frequencies (Delgutte, 1997; Hayward, 2000). However, it is not clear how this determination takes place and what other factors may be involved. Psychoacoustic research literature states that the auditory system treats the lower end of the frequency spectrum differently from the upper end, devoting approximately two thirds of its resolving power to frequencies below approximately 3kHz, with the remaining one third having to contend with all the higher frequencies. For speech, that means up to approximately 10kHz (Figure 2-3).

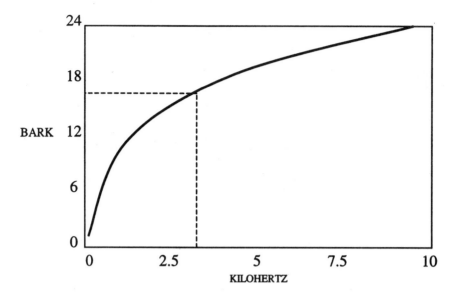

Figure 2-3   Approximate relationship of the auditory Bark scale and the acoustic Hertz scale. The dotted lines show the lower third of the speech acoustic range mapping onto two thirds of the auditory system's resolution power as represented by the Bark scale. Diagram based on Johnson (1997), p. 55.

Perceptual-auditory units have been developed to reflect these responses. The most commonly used are the Barks, related to Hertz by the Z-scale (Zwicker and Terhardt, 1980), and are derived from experimental data suggesting that the basilar membrane behaves like a series of discrete but overlapping frequency-band detectors, with the band increasing in size with increased frequency. The ERB-rate scale (equivalent rectangular bandwidth) is, in effect, very similar, but is claimed to be more accurate for lower frequencies (Hayward, 2000; Moore and Glasberg, 1983).

The 0–3kHz part of the spectrum contains the ranges in which F1 and F2 vary across vowel qualities (c. 200–1,000Hz and c. 700–2,500Hz, respectively, in adult males) and indicates that these formants will be resolved more clearly than the higher formants which are known to play less of a role in vowel perception. However, things are not as straightforward as we might wish them to be in this respect. Frequency resolution decreases continuously, although not at a uniform rate, as frequency increases. One result is that the first three or four harmonics of a vowel are probably resolved separately (those that contribute their energy to F1). The question then arises whether F1 is a real percept, and, if so, how are the harmonics integrated after resolution?

To further complicate matters, although F2, F3, and F4 are resolved separately in peripheral processing, in central auditory processing they become integrated when F2 is high (Bladon, 1983; Hayward, 2000). What might actually be perceived in this case is referred to as F2′ (F2 prime) and is explained as the weighted integration of F2, F3, and F4 (Chistovich, Sheikin, and Lublinskaja, 1979). By applying Z and ERB-rate scales to spectrographic data, it is possible to derive cochleagrams which purport to represent the spectral components of vowels in a more perceptually realistic way (Johnson, 1997).

It is necessary to keep these factors in mind when relating spectral and spectrographic data to vowel qualities.

Perceptual Analysis

Perceptual analysis is, no doubt, the most commonly used source of information about speech sounds, particularly in clinical settings. While listening may seem an easy, well-practised, and low-budget procedure, there are a number of pitfalls awaiting the unwary analyst. If developmental or disordered vowel data collected by perceptual analysis are to be valid and reliable, some of these difficulties need to be addressed. We need to make informed decisions about the advantages and disadvantages of different approaches, even in deciding how to sample and how to record speech data. We need to be aware that in recorded speech the fidelity of the acoustic signal is not always high. Poor equipment, problems with positioning of microphones, and excessive background noise, can affect recordings made in speech and language therapy (SLT) clinics or schools. Should transcription, then, be carried out live *in situ*, or should audio and video recordings be used?

For speech data generally, and for the disambiguation of aspects of vowel production, such as lip posture and jaw position, we should listen to Kelly and Local (1989, 35). They caution that, "in doing phonetic transcription it is important to pay attention to at least part of what a speaker can be *seen* to be doing" (our italics), thus having some recourse to visual data in our collection of the speech sample. We also should realize that one condition which provides visual information, real-time speech production, simply happens too quickly for us to make reliable perceptual judgements about it. Amorosa, von Benda, Wagner, and Keck (1985) argue that live transcription, unsupplemented by subsequent reference to audio or video recordings, cannot provide a reliable basis for even the most superficial phonological analyses of developmental speech disorders. They observe that the time pressure of live transcription resulted in a significant normalization of the data towards the expected forms.

This, in turn, brings us to another problem with transcription, how the listener's expectations regarding speech output affect their transcription accuracy. Laver (1994, 556) remarks that the most challenging type of speech output for a listener to transcribe is material from his or her own native language. Because the native phonologic system is so effective, "listeners tend to force the new material through the perceptual grid of the phonological categories of their own language." This will apply, of course, to all speech data, including speech that differs from normal native language categories by virtue of being immature, impaired, or merely from a different social or regional accent from the listener.

This not only encourages the phenomenon of phonemic false evaluation (Buckingham and Yule, 1987), whereby speech material not readily conforming to native segmental categories might be incorrectly categorized and inaccurately transcribed; it also means that if the listener knows the target word or utterance, they are likely to normalize or transcribe towards that form (Oller and Eilers, 1975). Ingrisano, Klee, and Binger (1996, 46) note, rather alarmingly, that, "transcribers in contextual conditions don't seem to recognise utterances as unintelligible, rather, they loosely transcribe 'what it is they think they heard'." Oller and Eilers (1975) suggest that knowing the target utterance can lead listeners to add or to omit elements of their transcription with no supporting evidence in the acoustic data. This effect can be seen in the perceptual analysis of vowel data. Pye, Wilcox, and Siren (1988) note that when the vowels [ɪ] and [ə] occur in unstressed syllables, they are frequently added or omitted in the transcription of children's speech.

The literature on the perceptual analysis of vowels is not extensive, reflecting, in part, an apparent imbalance between transcription practices for consonants and vowels. A number of authors have observed that frequently consonants are subject to narrow transcription, but vowels, even in the same data, are transcribed broadly (Ball, 1988; Ball, 1991; Crystal, 1982; Grunwell, 1987). Butcher (1989) suggests that vowels have not customarily been transcribed in detail because of the technical difficulties of transcription, in contrast to consonants. Vieregge and Maassen (1999) support this position, noting that in atypical developmental data, vowels are harder to transcribe than consonants.

The avoidance of narrow vowel transcription may be, in part, responsible for the widespread belief that vowel impairments are rare. Ball (1991) argues that the routine narrow transcription of vowels might prove extremely important in analyzing disordered sound systems in order to capture clinically significant consonant-vowel interactions and coarticulations. Local (1983), in a single case study of vowel development in a child from the North East of Britain, demonstrates convincingly how the use of narrow transcription can illustrate subtle but significant variation in vowel productions. He suggests this is "something to be accounted for and not something troublesome to be got rid of at any cost."

Regarding the level of perceptual difficulty of different types of vowels, Pye, Wilcox, and Siren (1988) suggest that diphthongs are relatively easier to transcribe than monophthongs. This observation might relate, in part, to the comment by Norris, Harden, and Bell (1980) that, in general, segments with longer durations are easier than their shorter counterparts. Maassen, Offeringa, Vieregge, and Thoonen (1996) mention that, in their studies of the transcription of developmentally disordered speech production in Dutch, low vowels were easier to transcribe than central vowels. This observation has intriguing parallels with the normal developmental order of emergence of vowels in speech development (Kent and Miolo, 1995; Stoel-Gammon, 1985), and also with the frequent occurrence of peripheral versus central vowels in the languages of the world (Ladefoged and Maddieson, 1996; Schwartz, Boë, Valée and Abry, 1997). An interesting study by Lotto, Holt, and Kluender (1997) suggests that voice quality can affect the perceptual analysis of vowels. Listeners in their study identified significantly more synthesized vowels with breathy voice quality as high vowels, in comparison with vowels having modal voice quality.

Despite the problems outlined above, we should recognize that perceptual analysis is important for two reasons. First, it completes the bridge between the speaker and the hearer in the sense that, without perceptual judgements, we are dealing with phenomena devoid of communicative value. We don't speak palatograms or hear spectrograms, neither is a vowel simply the sum of the measurements we can make in the various domains. Second, it engages us more fully with the data so we are less likely to miss significant details and more likely to detect possible patterns. We can then go on to investigate instrumentally, if we think it might prove fruitful. To turn one's back on perceptual analysis because of its methodological imperfections is tantamount not only to deciding not to listen to the data but to rely entirely on instruments. We need to remember that the role of instruments is to fill in the details in certain parts of the whole picture, not just to define the whole picture.

Description, Classification, and Transcription of Vowels in Normal and Disordered Speech

When we wish to denote a vowel in transcription, there are four basic questions to consider.

- What taxonomic framework should we use for classifying vowels?
- What does a vowel symbol denote in terms of articulatory, acoustic, and auditory properties?
- Should we use vowel symbols with language-independent values, or the values they have in the accent of the speaker's speech community?
- Are the available transcriptional conventions adequate for normal and clinical vowel data?

Description and Classification

As Ladefoged observed, "What are phoneticians really doing when they describe a vowel sound by allocating it to a certain box in their scheme of categories, or a certain point on their vowel diagrams?" (Ladefoged, 1967, 53). To begin with, it might be useful to distinguish between description and classification, a distinction that isn't always made yet has some important implications. We can describe sounds in as little or as much detail as we like, and we can use any property as a descriptor, for example, [a] can be described just as sonorant, or as having an F2 value of approximately 1,720Hz in adult males (Peterson and Barney, 1952). We can attempt to give a near-exhaustive description of the whole vocal tract during its production, including such observations as pharyngeal width, position of tongue tip, and convexity of the tongue surface. Description can also include dynamic accounts of vocal tract activity during speech production.

Classification, on the other hand, takes an essentially static view. It requires a parsimonious set of categories to which vowels and consonants are assigned, and those categories have to be set up according to certain principles. For speech sounds, categories are based on judging what are the significant aspects of their production. For example, pharyngeal width is not regarded as significant in the production of [t], but position of the tongue tip is, so it is incorporated into the classification.

It should be clear that, as far as description is concerned, there is no reason to treat consonants and vowels any differently: the same vocal organs are involved in both and their actions can be described in the same terms. However, they have traditionally been assigned to categories in different classifications because of particularities in their production. Consonants involve identifiable strictures, and both the location and the degree of that stricture have been set up as classificational criteria with a nomenclature derived largely from the superior speech organs: alveolar, palatal, velar, and so on.

By contrast, vowels have been classified according to the location of the highest point of the tongue in a two-dimensional space defined by the axes close-open (or high-low) and front-back.

A third classificatory dimension is provided by the rounded-spread axis of lip posture. The reason for this difference is probably twofold: The highest point of the tongue for many vowels is too far away from any of the superior organs for its approximation to them to be readily conceptualised as a stricture, and the quality of the vowel cannot be attributable simply to that approximation; rather, it is attributable to the distribution of volume throughout the whole supralaryngeal vocal tract. In fact, this last point applies to sonorant consonants, too, and also in a modified sense to obstruents insofar as the vocal tract dimensions in front of the stricture contribute to the quality of frication in stop-bursts and fricatives (Stevens, 1998).

Ladefoged (1967) outlined attempts at vowel classification in European, and especially British, phonetics dating back to the early 17th century, showing how early descriptions were limited in the number of descriptive parameters used. In the late 19th century, Bell (cited in Ladefoged, 1967) devised a method of description including categories for tongue position along both the vertical and horizontal parameters and making reference to the position of the lips.

The most well-known framework for vowel classification, however, is probably the Cardinal Vowel system. Although the system has attracted much criticism over the years, (for example, Butcher (1982, 50) described it as, "theoretically inadequate and scientifically redundant,") it is still widely used today. Ladefoged (1993) observes that it has aided in a more precise description of accents and languages of the world than any other method currently available. The Cardinal Vowel system was developed in the early 20th century by Daniel Jones to replace the system of three-term articulatory labels, such as close, back, rounded, which had proved too imprecise for adequate classification (Abercrombie, 1967). Jones observed that the consonants of a foreign language "are as a rule best acquired by directing attention to tactile and muscular sensations, whereas in learning *vowels* it is necessary to direct attention more particularly to the acoustic qualities of the sounds" (Jones, 1972, 26). He began by defining two articulatory positions at opposite ends of the vocal tract's vowel space and noting the vowel qualities associated with them (Table 2-1).

From these he derived six further vowel qualities, giving a front series of four and a back series of four which he termed the Primary Cardinal Vowels (Table 2-2), and, plotting them onto a vowel quadrilateral (Figure 2-4).

Table 2-1   Anchor Vowels

Articulatory position	*Vowel*
tongue: close front, *lips*: spread	[i], CV 1
tongue: open back, *lips*: not rounded	[ɑ], CV 5

Table 2-2   The Primary Cardinal Vowels

Front series	*Back series*
i e ɛ a	u o ɔ ɒ

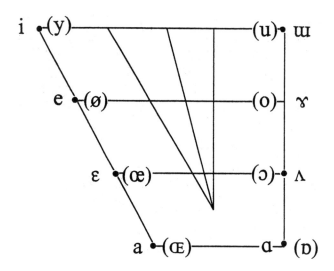

Figure 2-4   Traditional vowel quadrilateral, showing Primary and Secondary Cardinal Vowels (primary to left, secondary to right, rounded vowels in brackets)

Both the front and back routes from [i] to [ɑ] involved what Jones described as equal degrees of acoustic separation, that is the steps from one vowel to the next should be judged auditorily equal. Further Cardinal Vowels were derived by changing the lip shape from spread to rounded and vice versa, or from neutral to rounded, and by specifying vowels in the central areas of the vowel space. All these together are called the secondary Cardinal Vowels.

Ladefoged (1967) noted an ambivalence in Jones' account. On the one hand, he stresses the acoustic relations as the defining ones and is adamant that "The values of Cardinal Vowels cannot be learnt from written descriptions; they should be learnt by oral instruction from a teacher who knows them" (Jones, 1972, 34). On the other hand, he is drawn into specifying for each vowel in the series what he terms an *approximate* tongue and lip position, but given with more exactness than approximate suggests. He also compares the degree of tongue movement required in the front and back series to attain acoustic equidistance, and goes so far as to refer to the Cardinal Vowels as, "a set of fixed vowel-sounds having known acoustic qualities *and known tongue and lip positions*" (Jones, 1972, 28, italics added).

Ladefoged and Maddieson (1996) remind us, however, that tongue height is a difficult parameter to use with confidence, because for the back vowels it is not only the height of the tongue, but also the relative height of the soft palate that must be taken into account. Stevens and House (1955; 1961) pointed out that the location of the most significant tongue stricture in many vowels is not at the point of maximum lingual elevation but occurs in the pharyngeal cavity. Wood

(1979) uses x-ray evidence to confirm that these constrictions lie outside the vowel space originally proposed by Jones.

It might also be argued that the lip positions for the Cardinal Vowels are underspecified in Jones' original accounts. He describes Cardinal Vowels 1 to 5 as having spread or neutral lips, and Cardinal Vowels 6, 7, and 8 as having open, indeterminate, and close lip-rounding, respectively. Catford (1988) and Ladefoged and Maddieson (1996) observed that the degree of lip-rounding in the Cardinal Vowel system correlates quite closely with the height of the tongue. However, Catford points out that it is useful to distinguish between different types of lip-rounding: He associates endolabial rounding (lip-pouting, with the rounding formed by the inner surfaces of the lips) with back rounded vowels, and exolabial rounding (lip-pursing, with the rounding formed by the outer surfaces of the lips) with front rounded vowels. These different types of rounding are useful to note in the description of vowels in different accents and languages. Iivonen (1994), for example, describes significant differences in the types of rounding found in Swedish [y:] and [ʉ:].

Given these ambivalences and complications, it is hardly surprising that the practice has remained of interpreting the Cardinal Vowels according to precisely those same three articulatory dimensions that were originally deemed inadequate. In fact, the current International Phonetic Alphabet (IPA) vowel quadrilateral is generally seen as an articulatory space rather than an auditory one, and the arrangement into rounded and unrounded series rather than primary and secondary, (although in practice only affecting the open back vowels) is a shift towards a more explicit articulatory framework.

What is common to the traditional classificatory schemes for consonants and vowels, then, is their articulatory basis even where acoustic-auditory principles have been introduced for vowels. It would therefore seem an advantage, in principle at least, if they could be combined into one framework. Catford (1977) shows how this could be done using a system of polar coordinates in which Cardinal Vowels 1, 8, 7, 6, and 5 form a series of narrow approximants corresponding with consonantal places of articulation (Table-2-3).

Table 2-3   Catford's Vowel System

Vowel	Place of articulation	Homorganic voiced fricative
i	Palatal	j̞
u	Advanced velar	ɣ̟
o	Velar	ɣ
ɔ	Uvular	ʁ
ɑ	Pharyngeal	ʕ

Further vowels are derived by progressively opening the approximation, as in the cardinal system, from close through half-close and half-open to open (Figure 2-5). An important difference between Catford's scheme and the Cardinal Vowel scheme of Jones, however, is that these terms do not have the same interpretation. Jones classes [ɑ] as open, whereas Catford classes it as closed. The difference lies in how the tongue is seen to occupy the vowel space. Jones feels that in the vertical plane the highest point of the tongue is low down compared to [u] and the jaw is open. Catford's proposal invites us to regard the proximity of the tongue root to the rear pharyngeal wall as the salient feature. This is similar to the tongue dorsum's proximity to the velum in the production of [u].

However, Catford advances acoustic reasons concerning the near-universality of the [i u a] point vowel triangle, and physiological reasons concerning the proprioceptive discreteness of tongue-raising and tongue-retracting muscles, to explain why this system is not as advantageous as it might appear. He concludes by saying that, "we must continue to treat vowels differently from consonants for purposes of practical classification. It is equally clear, however, that from a purely theoretical point of view, vowels can be well fitted into the normal taxonomic parameters of location and stricture type if we wish to treat them this

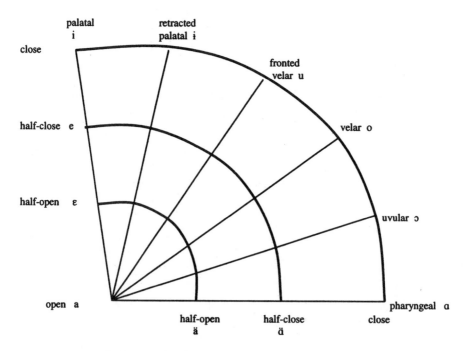

Figure 2-5   Catford's Vowel Schema

way" (Catford, 1977, 186–187). Catford's scheme does not address the relationship of articulatory behaviours to the acoustic or auditory domains. It is difficult to establish such relationships, which to some extent justifies regarding vowels as very different from consonants.

Articulatory, Acoustic, or Auditory?

In 1928, Russell stated that, "phoneticians are thinking in terms of acoustic fact and using physiological fantasy to express the idea" (Ladefoged, 1967, 72). It is important to be clear about the information value of a vowel symbol. Is it denoting the speaker's vocal tract configuration, or its acoustic output in terms of formant resonance patterns, or the phonetically trained listener's auditory impression? Several writers have commented that vowels are auditory qualities to which we attach articulatory labels (Ball, 1993; Catford, 1977; Ladefoged, 1975). We have seen how even Daniel Jones was unable to really free himself from this practice.

Most of the time, the inference from auditory impression to tongue and lip positions in normal speech is likely to be accurate enough for our purposes and can, to a significant but limited extent, be objectively validated by formant frequency measurements. There is a robust inverse relation between the height of F1 and jaw height (Keating, 1983), although this might be less true in the case of back vowels (Stone, 1997), and F2 frequency is indicative of the bulk of the tongue's position along the front-back axis of the vowel space (Stevens, 1998).

It is these relationships that have made it possible to construct formant charts that map onto the traditional vowel quadrilateral (Ladefoged, 1975). There are often practical problems in identifying formants accurately, particularly among close and back vowels (Ladefoged, 1967), that is, the set of vowels that fall into Catford's narrow approximant class (Catford, 1977). Ladefoged (2000) notes that for British and American English, F3 is fairly predictable from the values for F1 and F2 for any given vowel. However in languages such as Swedish, which, unlike English, produce vowel contrasts that have the same tongue position but are distinguished by different lip positions (Iivonen, 1994), F3 assumes a greater importance in looking at the acoustic identity of vowels.

In addition, it has to be noted that the role of F2 as a determinant of auditory quality differs between front and back vowels. If F3 is within 3.5 Bark of F2, that is, if the responses on the basilar membrane to the two formants are within three and a half critical bands (about 4.2 mm in a mature adult) of each other, then what is perceived in this frequency region is a single F2′ (see previous discussion). F3 is only within 3.5 Bark of F2 in front vowels. In back vowels, F3 is further away from F2 and does not contribute to the F2′ percept (Stevens, 1997; 1998).

Insofar as the articulatory-acoustic-auditory relationships are constant, it doesn't much matter if auditory impressions are expressed in articulatory terms, or, indeed, if the articulatory terms are, in Russell's words, a fantasy. But how constant are they, and how safely can we infer from one domain to another? An experiment on the auditory judgement of lip posture in vowels (Lisker, 1989) revealed significant inaccuracies with unrounded [ɯ] (Cardinal 16) judged rounded in 63% of responses, and rounded [y] (Cardinal 9) judged to be rounded in only 44% of responses. This result reinforces fears regarding inter-subjective disagreements and the reliability of vowel transcriptions.

The problem is compounded by the fact that a given set of formant frequencies can be produced by more than one vocal tract shape (Ladefoged, Harshman, Goldstein, and Rice, 1978). Stevens (1989) offers evidence to show that articulatory tolerance is not monotonic with respect to different zones of the vowel space. The point (or quantal) vowels, that is, [i], [ɑ], [u], according to Stevens, remain acoustically stable across a wider range of articulatory variation than nonpoint vowels.

Perkell (1997, 366) attributes the many-to-one relation between vocal tract shape and acoustic output to the phenomenon of *motor equivalence*, meaning that deflections away from a target position for an articulator can be corrected for by compensatory controlled adjustments of other speech organs. A study of normal vowel production in German by Maurer, Gröne, Landis, and colleagues (1993) using EMA confirmed that significantly different vocal tract configurations can produce perceptually identical timbres. They also found that very similar configurations can be responsible for significantly different formant patterns as a function of a varying F0. This agrees with some previous research findings by Carrell, Smith and Pisoni, 1981. Maurer and colleagues found that the degree of articulatory movement is not directly or easily related to the degree of perceived change of vowel quality. These findings led Maurer and colleagues (1993, 141) to state that, "there is no evidence of an imperative relationship between the vocal tract shape and the vowel identity in real vocalizations."

Some caution must be exercised, however, before accepting the validity of Maurer and colleagues's conclusion that the source-filter theory of vowel production (Fant, 1960; Stevens and House, 1961) is contraindicated by their results. They claim to have found a lack of evidence for predictable relationships between vocal tract shape and vowel quality in sustained isolated vowel productions. Two subjects in these productions were instructed to move the articulators around while trying to keep vowel quality constant. In a different task, subjects repeated lexical items in response to the experimenter's productions (rather misleadingly described as spontaneous speech by the authors), and a much more robust relationship was found. From this we might conclude, rather, that there are a number of different configurations that will produce similar output involving adjustments not measured or considered by Maurer and colleagues, such as altering larynx height, lip, and tongue posture in the lateral dimension, and changes of shape and volume in the oropharynx and laryngopharynx (Laver, 1980).

We might also conclude that most of these configurations are not habitually used for producing vowels in spoken German, because in speech much shorter timeslots are available than in deliberately sustained isolated vowels and configurations must accommodate to consonantal context.[1] That is to say, the temporal constraints operating in normally-spoken syllables might favor the use of articulatory-acoustic relationships that are more straightforwardly predictable by the source-filter model.

Interesting in this respect, is Strange's (1989) conclusion that steady states are not crucial for vowel identification and that vowels may be dynamically specified. In fact, vowels rarely attain steady states in speech due to the formant transitions caused by neighboring consonants. We therefore need to consider whether, from an acoustic point of view at least, the term *monophthong* is strictly applicable to most vowel data. It does seem, nonetheless, to retain its validity in the subjective realm of perception, suggesting that transitions might not affect the stability of vowel percepts in central auditory processing. As a complication, however, it has been noted that monophthongs are harder to transcribe than diphthongs (Pye, Wilcox, and Siren, 1988).

Studies of EMG vowel data by Honda and associates, which were produced in a [əp_p] context, have led to the claim that, "Vowels have analogous motor and sensory representations in the anterior and posterior cortical areas" (Honda, 1996, 49), and that the relations between them are robust (Maeda and Honda, 1994). The robustness of this relation, far from being compromised by many-to-one mappings, may, in fact, rely on them. Perkell (1996, 20) states that at least for [i] and [ɑ], "acoustic stability is achieved by virtue of a nonlinear relation between constriction *location* and vowel formants, in combination with a physiologically-based nonlinear relation between motor commands and the *degree* of constriction."

In cases of congenital and acquired physical abnormalities, speakers might explore these nonlinear relations to discover ways of producing the right acoustic/auditory results. Ferrier, Johnston, and Bashir (1991) describe auditorily acceptable realizations of /i/ by a child with insufficient tongue length to attain a high front articulation in the region of the hard palate. Morrish (1984; 1988), reporting on adult speakers following glossectomy, describes subtle adjustments of the jaw and pharynx that facilitate auditory vowel distinctions.

Temporary changes to the vocal tract also have been shown to bring about compensatory articulatory changes aimed, apparently, at maintaining the auditory qualities of vowels. Hamlet and Stone (1976), for example, identified patterns of apparently unconscious compensatory behavior in normal adult speakers after the insertion of dental prostheses. In comparison, a study by Daniloff, Bishop, and Ringel (1977) demonstrated a lack of compensatory features in children's vowel articulations under conditions of oral anaesthesia. Vowels became less well-differentiated and typically were more centralized, a pattern which has also been reported in vowel articulations in a number of speech disorders. These include speech associated with hearing impairment (Angelocci, Kopp, and Holbrook, 1964; Dagenais and Critz-Crosby, 1992), stammering (Blomgren, Robb, and Chen, 1998), and long-term tracheostomy (Kamen and Watson, 1991).

In the light, then, of research into articulatory-acoustic-auditory relationships, and the observation that vowels only have linguistic value when heard by a listener, it would seem prudent and appropriate to use vowel symbols primarily to denote auditory qualities. In normal vocal tracts, the articulatory correlates can be recovered approximately through application of the acoustic theory of speech production, and, if necessary, more precisely through the use of instrumentation.

If we have good reason to believe that a speaker's vocal tract is structurally or functionally incapable of assuming typical articulatory configurations for certain vowels, then instrumental investigation of the articulatory domain is essential if we are to have any useful information about his or her vowel productions. We need to recognize those conditions under which inferences about vocal tract configurations based on auditory impressions and acoustic measurements are less reliable. If there is little or no tongue, then any symbol used to denote a vowel quality obviously cannot be interpreted in terms of tongue position (Barry and Timmerman, 1985).

Taking a developmental perspective, the acquisition of vowels and vowel oppositions will be affected if the articulatory-acoustic-auditory relationships do not remain balanced over the normal course of anatomical growth from birth through the language acquisition period. In abnormal patterns of growth, any effect of this kind might be amplified, making it more difficult for stable representations of vowel sounds to become established. Any model of the development of an infant's articulatory-auditory feedback loop (Locke and Pearson, 1992) has to take into account the relationship between the auditory and vocal motor systems in terms of anatomy, physiology, and neurology. We know that vocal tract architecture changes quite extensively over the first 4 or 5 years of life (Beck, 1997; Buhr, 1980; Kent, 1992).

Lieberman, Crelin, and Klatt (1972) anticipate many later researchers in observing that the vocal tracts of human neonates more closely resemble those of other primates, such as apes and chimpanzees, than those of adult humans. Buhr (1980) lists the main differences between the vocal tracts of newborns and adults. The human neonate has a relatively high larynx, so high, in fact, that for the first 6 months of life the epiglottis makes contact with the soft palate (Mackenzie Beck, 1997), and, consequently, a reduced pharyngeal space. Typically the tongue is also relatively large and thus fills the oral cavity quite extensively; and, significantly, the right-angle configuration of the adult vocal tract, where the lip-to-velum area is on a horizontal plane relative to the vertical velum-to-larynx area, is not present in the neonate or infant vocal tract where there is a much more continuous, horizontal configuration of the tract from lips to larynx.

These observations led Buhr (1980) to suggest that acoustic measurements of F1 and F2 are more useful in describing infant vowel productions than articulatory categories such as high, mid, low, or front and back. As well as these anatomical differences, which resolve towards the adult geometry over the first 4 or 5 years of life, there are neuromuscular immaturities which limit the range and accuracy of independent movements of the tongue, lips, and mandible (Fletcher, 1973; Mackenzie Beck, 1997).

The infant's task, which has a profound effect on the realization of vowels, is to achieve independent but coordinated movement of the different articulators over a period when the vocal tract is undergoing continual changes in shape and dimensions. Lieberman (1980) is among those who have postulated an innate mechanism for normalization during this stage, that allows the infant to accommodate to vocal tract changes, and to master normal vowel articulations during this period of anatomical, physiological, and perceptual development.

A number of authors suggest that the patterns of typical vowel articulations in early prespeech and speech behavior can be linked to a lack of articulatory independence, particularly of the tongue and mandible. Buhr (1980) notes that the front vowels, [ɪ, e, ɛ], which seem to occur early in speech development, can be produced without independent lingual movement merely by modifications of the position of the mandible. This compares with the later developing vowel [u] which requires integration of lingual, labial, and mandibular activity.

Davis and MacNeilage (1990), Fletcher (1973), and Kent and Murray (1982) also underline the important role of the mandible in early vowel production and to the vowels found in early babbling. That this mandibular activity may not be intentionally producing differentiated vowel sounds in early output is supported by the observation by Meier, McGarvin, Zakia, and Willerman (1997) that, interspersed in early babbling sequences, are silent rhythmic mandibular movements or *jaw wags*, which seem to correspond motorically with audible babbled syllables.

Fletcher (1973) suggests that the infant tongue is limited to the thrusting and rocking movements associated with sucking and swallowing, and that neuromuscular immaturity may prevent the early development of other lingual movements necessary for the production of different vowels. Similarly, Kent (1992) suggests that early tongue movements are likely to be in a horizontal (anterior-posterior) plane, rather than in the vertical plane which would involve raising and lowering of the tongue body.

Given the large body of literature which emphasizes the significant role of vocal tract development and change on the production and development of vowels in infancy, it is useful to also weigh conflicting evidence. Clement and Wijnen (1994), studying Dutch speech development, found very similar patterns in the limitations on vowel productions in normal 2 year olds and in 4 year olds with developmentally delayed sound systems. These, in turn, were different from both normal 4 year olds and from adults. As the authors surmised that significant vocal tract maturation would have taken place by age 4 years, they argued that the immature speech output patterns in these children could not be accounted for by anatomical factors. Nittrouer, Studdert-Kennedy, and Neely (1996) similarly argue that the acoustic patterns of consonant-vowel interaction observed in children of different ages could not be explained by differences in vocal tract anatomy or dimensions. We can only conclude that the significant anatomical differences between the infant and the adult vocal tracts pose a real problem for the perceptual analysis of early vocalization and early vowel productions.

At the other end of the loop, the outer and middle ear are affected by changes during infancy and childhood. In the outer ear, compared to adults, infants have a much shorter external canal leading to a smaller tympanic membrane set at a more oblique angle (Lowry, 1978). The shorter canal has a higher natural resonance frequency and will impose a different transfer function on incoming acoustic stimuli (Keefe, Burns, Bulen, and Campbell, 1994). No one knows exactly when the transfer function becomes fully mature, but it may be as late as age 7 or 8 years (Werner and Marean, 1996).

Similarly, regarding the middle ear, no one knows when the impedence characteristics of the ossicular chain reach mature levels, but research shows differences of up to 8dB in conduction in parts of the frequency spectrum at age two years (Werner and Marean, 1996).

In the inner ear, the third of the three rows of outer hair cells in the organ of Corti is not present at birth (Atkinson, Barlow, and Braddick, 1982). The function of outer hair cells is to increase the sensitivity of the inner hair cells (Stach, 1998). Norton and Widen (1990) report age-related differences in otoacoustic emissions persisting to age 13 years. Myelination of the auditory nerve fibers is not complete until age 4 years (Tanner, 1989), which may mean that transmission of information to the auditory cortex is relatively less efficient. Although these immaturities of the auditory system are minor by comparison with those of the vocal tract and motor abilities, they do introduce variables into the articulatory-auditory relationship from the auditory end such that we, perhaps, cannot regard an infant or child's auditory capacity as homeostatic, nor regard as constants the constraints it exerts on the less consistent behaviors of the articulators.

On the other hand, perhaps we should not make too much of these auditory immaturaties. A study by Bertoncini, Bijeljac-Babic, Jusczyk, and colleagues (1988) indicated that newborn infants can extract information from certain vowel stimuli accurately enough to recognize them on subsequent presentations. Findings of this nature corroborate other research evidence that infants are particularly tuned in to vocalic contrasts (Kuhl and Miller, 1982).

The fact that there are developmental variables at both ends of the articulatory-auditory loop raises the question as to what extent there might be a significant mismatch between an infant's auditory impressions of his or her own vowel sounds at age 1 year and at age 2 years. Of course, this will not be the only mismatch the infant has to contend with. There will be gross acoustic differences between the infant's vowels and those of adults due to differences in vocal tract dimensions, with formant values being up to twice those of adult vowels (Kent and Murray, 1982). This particular difficulty may be avoided by a normalization process (Kent, 1992). However, normalization would not so easily account for differences in the infant's own productions over time, and, in fact, the concept of normalization as a necessary part of speech processing has recently been questioned (Pisoni, 1997).

In addition to the effects of physical growth and development, there is the problem of knowing when we can attribute phonological intentionality to early vocalizations and start to relate them in a meaningful way to the *target* vowels in real lexical items. One problem is that early words are produced as *gestalts* which cannot justifiably be analyzed at a segmental level (Bates, Dale, and Thal, 1995). This means that the vowel is not separable from the rest of the syllable, and so cannot be seen as the intentional realization of a vowel phoneme.

Furthermore, how can we reliably distinguish between babbled syllables and gestalt words, and what problems might children have moving through this phase of development? Locke (1993, 89) has an interesting perspective on this latter point. He argues that infants might have difficulty in moving from "vowel-as-voice to vowel-as-voice-and-linguistic-unit" because of the prevalence of vowel-like articulations to express emotion and affect in early vocalizations.

A number of authors have posited a discontinuity between babbling and speech for vowels as opposed to consonants (Davis and MacNeilage. 1990), but not all evidence supports this view. Boysson-Bardies, de Hallé, Sagart, and Durand (1989) point to the early phonological differentiation of vowels in their cross-linguistic study, showing how 10-month-old infants from different language backgrounds were already showing consistent language-specific patterns in their use of vowels.

In addition, Blake and Fink (1987) used narrowly transcribed phonetic data to argue that the relation between sound and meaning emerges gradually during the transition period from babbling to speech. Generally, however, researchers have questioned the methodological validity of applying IPA transcriptional conventions to early infant vocalizations and babbling.

Cardinal Qualities or Accent-Specific Qualities?

Besides the problem of what exactly is the information value of a vowel symbol, there is the question of the relationship of the symbol to the vowel space and its quadrilateral projection.[2] The symbols for the English vowels are also used for cardinal and IPA vowels, but the vowel qualities are quite noticeably different.[3] The symbol for Cardinal 8 and the English GOOSE vowel is [u] but the latter is less peripheral and in many accents is slightly diphthongized (Wells, 1982).[4] If [u] is to be used with its cardinal value, then a transcription of a normal GOOSE vowel would have to have diacritics to denote these facts, and a transcription of a disordered GOOSE would generally require additional diacritics to show in what way it differed from the expected norm, such as being too open. The principle is represented in Table 2-4.

The advantage of using cardinal qualities as reference points in clinical transcription is that they can be interpreted by anyone trained in the system, without knowledge of the accent, or even the language, of the speaker. The disadvantage is the cumbersome nature of the diacritics. If symbols are used with their accent-specific values, there is a twofold advantage: Generally fewer diacritics are needed so transcription is easier to make and to read, and one can see more readily whether a vowel was produced normally or not. Interpretation of the accent value of the symbol needs, however, to be facilitated by a short account of the accent's vowel qualities, using the Cardinal Vowels as reference points (Table 2-5).

Of course, it will not always be the case that use of diacritics is the most appropriate way to represent a disordered vowel. If we judge the vowel quality to be normal for a different target (so-called substitutions), we would simply use the symbol for the error vowel. In this case, our judgement as to whether an error was *phonetically* deviant or not in terms of the set of normal vowel qualities of the accent would be reflected in the presence or absence, respectively, of

Table 2-4   Using Vowel Symbols with their Cardinal/IPA Values

Cardinal Vowel	Accent-specific normal	Accent-specific disordered
Symbol without diacritics, such as CV 8 [u]	Symbol with diacritics, such as [u̟]	Symbol with additional diacritics, such as [ü̟]

Table 2-5 Using Vowel Symbols with their Accent-Specific Values

Cardinal Vowel	Accent-specific normal	Accent-specific disordered
Reference point for accent-specific vowel quality, such as CV8 [u]	Symbol without diacritics, such as [u]	Symbol with diacritics, such as [u̜]

Table 2-6 Using Vowel Symbols with their Accent-Specific Values, Including the Possibility of Cross-Category Realizations

Normal target realization	Normal nontarget realization	Phonetically deviant realization
Target symbol without diacritics, such as [ɛ]	Nontarget symbol without diacritics, such as [a]	Symbol (target or non-target) with diacritics, such as [ɛ̞]

diacritics (Table 2-6). Use of a normal [a] TRAP vowel quality if the target is a DRESS vowel would be transcribed with [a], but use of a quality between TRAP and DRESS if this is a quality not typically found in the accent, could be transcribed with [ɛ̞] or [a̝].

There will, however, be cases where this approach is not appropriate. Vowel symbols for qualities present in a speech sample but not present in the normal inventory for the accent will frequently be needed. For example, in a language with only the three vowels /i/, /a/, /u/, a realization of one of them as a midcentral vowel could not really be represented accurately with the target symbol plus diacritics; or in the use of a back unrounded vowel for English GOOSE, the simplest recourse might be to use [ɯ] rather than [u̜]. Note the implication that [ɯ] represents an unrounded equivalent of GOOSE, not of Cardinal Vowel 8. This would be our suggestion: Symbols representing opposite lip postures are used with reference to accent-specific vowels, not cardinal or IPA vowels.

The basic question, then, is whether it is more useful for a clinical transcription to relate to the norms of the speaker's speech community, or to a set of fixed, absolute universal phonetic qualities, such as those of the cardinal or IPA systems. This question arises most acutely when considering vowels, but,in fact, applies to consonants too. Does IPA [ʃ] mean exactly the same to an English-speaking phonetician as it does to a French-speaking or Japanese-speaking one? Is it true that, "for the phonetician there is no universal truth independent of the observer" (Ladefoged, 1990, 335)? Is our interpretation of IPA and Cardinal Vowel symbols inevitably influenced by our own speech experience? If we accept Ladefoged's claim, it perhaps suggests that our reference point for clinical transcription should be the norms of the relevant speech community. It also reinforces the widely held view in clinical phonetics and phonology that familiarity with those norms is essential if the aim is to phonetically resettle a client's speech into its sociolinguistic context.

The Cardinal Vowel system is still, however, valuable for clinical phoneticians. It enables the vowel qualities of a particular accent, our points of clinical transcriptional reference, to be specified with a descriptive precision that allows others without familiarity with the accent to get a good idea of what they are. The English GOOSE vowel for received pronunciation (RP) can be described as a slightly midcentralized Cardinal Vowel 8, and any realization judged normal for an RP speaker can be transcribed as [u]. Any production judged to deviate from the norm can be transcribed in such a way as to show the nature of the deviation, such as [ɯ] if fully unrounded, [ʉ] if partly unrounded, [u̝] if raised. The possibility that different people may have slightly different interpretations of cardinal qualities is something we simply have to live with, for there is currently no alternative: "to abandon the Cardinal Vowel system is to abandon the only internationally known method of specifying vowels at all accurately" (Ladefoged, 1967, 142).

Plotting the normal vowel qualities of a client's accent on a vowel quadrilateral is an important first step. They can be situated in a vowel space whose limits are defined by cardinal or IPA vowel qualities, and the client's disordered or immature productions can be compared to them. Ascertaining these norms, however, is problematic because any study of the spoken form of a language is complicated by the fact that across speech communities there are sociolinguistic differences that include pronunciation differences. Vowels are particularly affected, making it imperative that before diagnosing or remediating any vowel disorder, SLTs should be well acquainted with the vowel system of the client's speech community. Of course this is no easy task, although sources are available containing useful information in this regard, such as Wells (1982) and the more recent studies in Foulkes and Docherty (1999). Ball (1992) has proposed the construction of clinical sociolinguistic checklists for use by SLTs which could include vowel data.

Vowel differences are not just found across speech communities. Sociolinguistic influences cut through speech communities along lines of gender, class, age, and ethnicity. This results in a number of vowel variants coexisting not only in the community at large, but also in the speech of individuals. Often one variant predominates, but over a period of time, another may take its place and become the new norm, and new variants may appear (Watt and Tillotson, 1999). Foulkes and Docherty (in press) provide a review of some current changes in vowel qualities in England from a sociolinguistic perspective.

One therefore has to try to distinguish between a speaker using a new variant, and one using a pathological deviant variant. Confronted by these in a pediatric SLT clinic the temptation might be to intervene without taking the time to distinguish the sociolinguistic from the pathologic.

Transcriptional Conventions

Ball (1991, 61), warning that "It is not possible to use a phonemic transcription when you do not know the phonology," advocates the use of narrow phonetic transcription in the analysis of speech development and speech disorder. This view is shared by Kelly and Local (1989, 26), who argue that, "it is not possible to have too much phonetic detail . . . we must attend to and reflect everything that we can discriminate." Using the broad vowel phoneme symbols of the target phonology for vowels that are clearly atypical and that are auditorily distant from the norms provides no greater detail than attempting to describe the auditory quality of vowels using orthographic symbols. This is typified by the following early effort of Hasluck and Hasluck (1898, 8), "In 'Cockney' pronunciation . . . the tendency is to transfer the sounds from one vowel to another. Thus the *a* in "day" is unconsciously converted into a sound resembling the *i* in "die" and when the word "die" is intended it comes out more like *doy*."

What does the present literature offer us to aid in the transcription of vowels? Over the last 10 years or so, considerable work has gone into developing extensions to the IPA specifically for the representation of disordered speech (Ball and Local, 1996; Duckworth, Allen, Hardcastle, and Ball, 1990). A number of symbols and diacritics are known as the extensions to the IPA (extIPA). These are reproduced in ICPLA News (1994).

There are several new consonant symbols for sounds that, as far as is known, only occur in disordered speech. Ball, Rahilly, and Tench (1996) provide a detailed account of the use of IPA and extIPA symbols to capture different aspects of vowel articulation. They provide a checklist of features they feel should be considered in the narrow transcription of vowels: airstream mechanism and direction of airflow; phonation and voice quality; vertical and horizontal tongue positions; lip shape; secondary articulations; length; and what they term vowel stability, which distinguishes a diphthong, such as [aĩ] from a sequence of two consecutive vowel articulations [a.i].

Recent developments to the IPA and extIPA systems have not, however, provided any new vowel symbols. The Cardinal Vowel/IPA system is assumed to define the totality of available vowel space in both articulatory and acoustic/auditory terms (Ball, 1993; Catford, 1977). No doubt this is true for all mature, structurally normal vocal tracts, but it might not always be true in the case of immature or abnormal ones.

As we have already noted, there might be significant differences in the anatomy of the vocal tracts of infants and speakers with a cleft palate or a glossectomy. These differences might make it difficult for us to use phonetic symbols with their normally assumed articulatory implications. Very young infants do not have a developed pharynx (Mackenzie Beck, 1997), and therefore their vocalic sounds do not have the same kind of formant structure as those of older children and adults. They have been termed *quasi* resonant as opposed to fully resonant by some writers (Oller, 1980) and *vocants* by others (Martin, 1981) for this reason. Oller and Lynch (1992) discuss the inappropriateness of IPA conventions for early vocalizations and draw attention to the problem of how to interpret acoustic displays without a related set of concepts.

Later studies benefited from a greater understanding of the stages of vocal development (Proctor, 1989). These provided researchers with such concepts as *squeal* and *coo* (Oller, 1980; Stark, 1980). Although these approaches have also been criticized (Bauer and Robb, 1992), the descriptors used, or their conventional abbreviations, such as SQ for squeal, can be incorporated into transcriptions and interpreted narrowly enough to function much like symbols.

Regarding IPA conventions, whereas some researchers use IPA transcription conventions for vowel data in children as young as 15 months (Selby, Robb, and Gilbert, 2000), many researchers have chosen to avoid phonetic transcriptions based on linear strings of segments for vowel production during the early stages of speech development. Instead, they have attempted to categorize sounds in terms of broader physiological parameters. These are often linked to the mandibular cycle of opening and closing that features so strongly in early output. This also relates to the gradual emergence of vowel-like and consonant-like sounds (Bauer and Robb, 1992; Koopmans-van Beinum and van der Stelt, 1986; Oller, 1980).

A further challenge for the accurate transcription of vowels is noted by Goldstein and Pollock (2000), who observe that the number of vowels in the sound system of a particular language might affect transcription. They note that in comparison with the relatively large and complex vowel system of English, Spanish has a small and simple vowel inventory. Goldstein and Pollock (2000, 231) question whether this "less crowded vowel space" might cause small, but potentially significant, variations in the production of individual vowels in speech development and speech disorder to go unnoticed in perceptual analysis, because they do not cross the relatively large vowel spaces occupied by each of the small number of vowels in the system.

Certain peculiarities of vowel resonance can be transcribed using the voice quality symbols (VoQS) as shown in Ball, Esling, and Dickson (1995). Nuances of timbre that characterize individual voice qualities can be captured, that is, a speaker's habitual *articulatory setting* (Laver, 1980) such as palatalized or pharyngealized voice. Conventions are also provided for electrolarynx speech, esophageal speech, diplophonia, harsh voice, and other phenomena affecting the phonatory component of vowels. This might have consequences for resonance definition and the perception of vowel quality.

Speakers with anatomically highly deviant vocal tracts, for example, those who have had large amounts of tongue removed, might produce resonances that even VoQS conventions cannot adequately represent. This highlights a methodological problem that might easily be overlooked. Articulatory settings are judged against a speaker-specific neutral setting in which the vocal tract approximates to uniform cross section and the tongue has "a regularly curved convex shape" (Laver, 1994, 403). Deviant anatomy, whether congenital or resulting from surgical intervention, might prevent approximation to these conditions: If a large part of the anterior section of the tongue has been removed, then it cannot assume a curved convex shape. It therefore becomes difficult to heed Wirz and Beck's (1995, 49) otherwise justifiable warning that "neutral should not be confused with any notion of normality."

The possibility of a neutral setting, as defined by Laver, might not be a reality for speakers with grossly atypical vocal tract architecture. If a speaker has an abnormally high larynx or a tongue that protrudes because it is oversized, then to use the VoQS symbols L (raised larynx), or Θ (protruded tongue voice), is not really describing a deviation from that speaker's neutral setting, but rather his or her neutral setting itself. They need to be represented because they deviate from some notional norms, however imprecisely defined, of larynx height or tongue size; otherwise, we wouldn't be drawing attention to them. At present, there are no conventions for distinguishing between abnormal neutral settings and deviations from normal neutral settings. What should we do in the case of a speaker with an abnormal neutral setting deviating from it by raising his or her larynx yet higher, or pushing the tongue even further out? This kind of problem highlights the need to make a clear decision about whether one's transcription is aiming to represent the listener's auditory experience, or the speaker's articulatory behavior (Hewlett, 1985).

The availability of instrumental information to supplement perceptual analysis introduces greater delicacy into our potential representations of speech. Finer distinctions are now possible in a number of phonetic parameters than was previously the case. Transcriptional conventions, such as those offered by the IPA, extIPA, and VoQS, are not always able to represent such fine distinctions. The retracted tongue root diacritic [̪], often used with vowel symbols, cannot indicate the *degree* of retraction. Therefore measurements of that parameter from x-ray or other sources cannot be represented in transcriptions using that convention, neither can dynamic data, such as articulator velocity.

Vowel duration is another example of instrumentation usefully supplementing transcription. We know that young children take time learning to control the durational aspects of vowel production (Clement and Wijnen, 1994; Stoel-Gammon and Herrington, 1990), and that vowel durations are vulnerable across a range of speech impairments, but identifying subtle durational differences might be difficult using perceptual analysis alone. Ball, Rahilly, and Tench (1996) demonstrate how vowel length can be differentiated using phonetic symbols and diacritics: shorter than normal vowel length [ă]; normal length [a]; half-long vowel [aˑ]; long vowel [aː]. These distinctions are to be understood as relative rather than absolute.

For precise quantitative information, however, spectrographic analysis has proved a very fruitful method of investigation, although as Blomgren and Robb (1998, 406) note, "determining the duration of a vowel segment is no simple matter." There is perhaps a widening gulf between what a segmentally conceived transcription can represent and what increasingly sophisticated instrumentation can reveal. Historically, this gulf can be traced to the fact that IPA-type transcription conventions are based on classification of sounds, whereas instrumental data are by nature more richly descriptive, that is, they include much more than just the location and degree of those strictures that phonetic theory identifies as the salient ones and on which classifications are based.

Attempts have been made to develop forms of transcription with a more descriptive rather than classificatory orientation by analyzing speech *horizontally* into separate parameters instead of *vertically* into separate segments (Abercrombie, 1965). Dynamic properties can be represented by lines that move up and down as one follows them from left to right, and degrees of a property can also be iconically represented (Ball and Rahilly, 1999; Tench, 1978). A major disadvantage, however, is that parametric transcriptions are cumbersome to make and difficult to read, although the latter objection can be overcome by combining parametric and IPA-type transcriptions together.

A possible reason why parametric transcriptions are not widely employed is that, if no instrumental information were available, they would have to be derived from segmental transcriptions anyway by applying phonetic theory. In the case of vowels under these conditions, a parametric transcription showing the movements of the tongue, lips, and velum through time is only going to show what we infer those movements to have been, not necessarily what they actually were. For the parametric approach to be useful, it has to use reliable information about the vocal tract's movements, and this has to come from instrumental sources. An alternative to converting instrumental data into parametric form is simply to show them in graphic form. An EPG print, an EMA trace, a spectrum envelope, or combinations of these, could be indexed to the relevant vowel symbol in a transcription of a particular utterance.

Vowels and Prosody

So far, attention has been restricted to vowels without reference to the larger units in which vowels occur. The minimum quantum of speech is the syllable and the structural role of a vowel is to function as the nucleus of a syllable. One can approach this function from two angles: the relations vowels have in syllables with consonants, and their role in larger multisyllabic rhythmic structures.

Relations with Consonants

As syllable nuclei, vowels have intimate spectral and temporal relations with tautosyllabic consonants to the extent that they encode acoustic information about them in formant transitions and duration values (Fry, 1979; Kent and Read, 1992). Acquisition of vowels must entail some sorting of this information, and the recognition of which properties are intrinsic to the vowel and which are coarticulatory. At least, this must be the case if the notion *acquisition of vowels* is to be interpreted as acquiring a stock of vowel segments abstracted away from contextual influences (Kuhl, 1980). Research shows that some children may find this kind of processing of vocalic information difficult (Tallal and Stark, 1980).

Many phonologists view vowels as having a key organizational role in syllables. They explain the sequencing of consonants in syllable margins with reference to their resemblance to vowels in terms of sonority. They claim that syllables can be conceptualized as a sonority profile, with the unmarked syllable types exhibiting low sonority onsets rising to a high plateau. Vowels provide this high plateau. The predominance of consonant-vowel (CV) structures in immature speech has been noted for a long time (Jakobson, 1968; Kent and Bauer, 1985), while in mature speech, sonorant consonants occur adjacent to vowels with the extreme margins being occupied by obstruents.

The sonority profile view of the syllable is based on the principle of syntagmatic contrast, that consonants with low sonority followed by vowels with high sonority provide a perceptual aid to the listener, who can more easily keep track of events through time if successive elements are maximally different. It also rather neatly correlates with the *frame and content* view of syllable production based on the mandibular cycle of an alternating closed and open buccal chamber (MacNeilage and Davis, 1990). Lindblom's (1986, 502) conception of the syllable as, "a gestalt trajectory coursing through the phonetic (articulatory/acoustic/perceptual) space" accommodates both the sonority and frame-and-content characterizations.

It might be, however, that sonority itself is not the heart of the matter. Ohala (1984) has suggested that signal modulation, in general, might be the important factor; in which case, obstruent-vowel sequences, with their rapid modulation of several acoustic parameters at once, can be seen as particularly good exemplars. Other contrasts occur that are not explainable in terms of sonority, such as the sequences [ju] and [wi], which Ohala points out are much more common than [ji] and [wu]. This is also discussed in Christman (1992).

Furthermore, Heselwood (1999) has discussed problems with defining sonority adequately, and has argued that some oral stops seem sometimes to function both as sonorants and as obstruents (1998), which obscures the match between sonority and an open vocal tract.

We have seen earlier how, for purposes of general phonetic taxonomy, different classificatory frameworks have been used for consonants and vowels, but, recently, there has been some discussion in nonlinear approaches to phonology as to whether a single set of features can account for the internal structure of both classes (Gierut, Cho, and Dinnsen, 1993). This would be particularly useful for investigating and describing cases of consonant-vowel interaction (see Chapter 5; also Bates and Watson, 1996). Reports of individual cases have noted consistent patterns of consonant-vowel interaction (Braine, 1974; Camarata and Gandour, 1984; Oller, 1973; Wolfe and Blocker, 1990), with the co-occurrence of front vowels with coronal consonants and round vowels with labial consonants being repeatedly observed (Davis and MacNeilage, 1995; Gierut, Cho, and Dinnsen, 1993). In a study of 23 young children reported in Vihman (1992), however, the statistical significance of consonant-vowel associations of this kind was not clear for the sample as a whole, with a large amount of intersubject variability. Similar results for a group of 9 children studied by Tyler and Langsdale (1996) suggest that these interactions might not be common generally across children's sound systems.

Some more striking examples of CV interaction have been noted when long vowels and diphthongs have been realized as short vowel plus consonant (Bates and Watson, 1996), and vice versa (Reynolds, 1990). The locus for these realizations that cross the vowel-consonant divide seems to be the second mora of the syllable. This is precisely the one syllabic position in English with a paradigm comprising almost all the vowel and consonant phonemes of the language, that is, the content of the second mora in English varies across the whole sonority hierarchy (Zec, 1995), and across the whole range of articulatory stricture. These behaviors might indicate a problem sorting out the phonotactics that some children simplify by disallowing certain consonantal features, such as [stop] or [obstruent], while others disallow vowels in that position. It would be interesting to see if such developmental behaviors occur where the ambient language does not have postvocalic consonants.

Bernhardt and Stemberger (1998, 101) cite research by Öhman indicating that, in speech production, vowels and consonants are programmed separately, yet they also acknowledge that "vowels can interact with consonants," which suggests that any separation in programming cannot be total. There might even be a developmental progression from integration in infancy toward separation in maturity. This could account for high levels of CV interactional constraints in babbling and early speech in, at least, some children (Davis and

MacNeilage, 1990; 1995; MacNeilage, 1997; Tyler and Langsdale, 1996) that are not evident later.

Rhythmic Structures

Natural speech is inherently rhythmic. An important aspect of the rhythm of English is the succession of syllables of contrasting degrees of stress. These can be seen in the same terms as the contrasts between successive segments within syllables, that is, as another instance of signal modulation which may aid the listener's perception. The perceptually most prominent syllables typically occur in words of high semantic content, and these can be expected to often have high imageability, particularly in child-directed speech. Insofar as this is the case, the occurrence of maximally differentiated vowel qualities in stressed syllables correlates with the visual prominence of the word's referent. For example, *It's on the table by the window* produced as [ɪts ɒ̃n ðə tʰeɪbɫ baɪ ðə wĩndəʊ], or in a more reduced and syncopated form such as [tsp̃ ðə̃ tʰeɪbɫ bə ðə wĩndə] where the syncopations affect those items that already have low perceptual prominence.

In early speech development, children are generally much more accurate in vowel production in target stressed syllables, and often appear uncertain as to the phonetic content of unstressed ones (Peters, 1995). This affects weak forms of modal and auxilliary verbs, prepositions, pronouns, conjunctions, and copulas, and might also affect children's ability to recognize stems that take part in vowel alternations (Clark, 1995). Allen and Hawkins (1980) discuss 2 year olds whose speech was more towards the syllable-timed end of the syllable-stress timing continuum. They also observed deletion of unstressed syllables when word-initial or when adjacent to another unstressed syllable. Grabe, Post, and Watson (1999) suggest that rhythmic patterns resulting from the wide variation in vowel duration associated with stress-timing are harder for children to acquire than patterns with less variation.

It is important when assessing a vowel disorder, to realize that rhythm might be the problem, not the vowels as such. Children's acquisition of speech rhythm has a developmental path (Young, 1991), and poor, nonlinguistic rhythmic skills have been noted in children with speech disorders (Henry, 1990).

Processing capacity might also be relevant in assessing vowel disorders. Vowels are the principal carriers of perceptually prominent pitch movements and durational values associated with stress and tonicity, which encode information about grammatical class, information focus, discourse structure, and speaker affect (Cruttenden, 1986). Attention to these factors might be at the expense of target vowel quality in speakers with restricted linguistic processing capacity (Crystal, 1987).

Conclusion

Our examination of the various instrumental and perceptual approaches to vowel description showed what a rich range of information they can provide, and highlighted the care with which they must be used and interpreted. We perceived how anatomically atypical vocal tracts offer particular challenges for vowel description, both in perceptual and instrumental analysis. In terms of phonetic transcription, we saw how the IPA, extIPA, and VoQS systems provide a rich range of symbols for the detailed description of normal and atypical vowel productions.

We showed how important it is to be clear about the implications of vowel symbols in phonetic transcription. Is a particular symbol to be interpreted as having specific articulatory values in relation to a speaker's tongue and jaw movements, or is it meant to have a purely auditory value? Given Perkell's theory of *motor equivalence* and given the anatomical differences found in some speakers with speech impairments, it could have been produced by somewhat different vocal tract configurations. We suggest that it is important to adopt a listener perspective on vowels where phonetic symbols imply particular auditory qualities that are not associated with invariant articulatory values. Aspects of articulation might, of course, be recovered via different types of instrumental analysis, if required.

Our examination of vowel description and classification also showed how the Cardinal Vowel system provides us with an important framework for plotting an individual speaker's vowel system against a known set of reference vowels. At the same time, we argued that our reference point for the transcription of vowels, whether normal or atypical, should be the accent of the speech community of the individual speaker.

Although it is unlikely that we would ever actually combine all the different perceptual and instrumental methods available in the analysis of any single set of vowel data, we must be aware of them and have an understanding of their relative strengths and weaknesses and of the potential pitfalls associated with their use. In this way, we are aware of what our chosen analytical methods show, and what they do not show. We noted that a perceptual analysis of vowel durations does not provide the quantitative accuracy of a spectrographic analysis. A spectrographic analysis, meanwhile, is unable to provide the detailed qualitative information about type of lip-rounding that a visual perceptual analysis can.

An understanding of the opportunities and the limitations of different analytic techniques allows us to select the most suitable ones for investigating our data, depending on our specific aims. These aims might range from clinical assessment and the assessment of developmental appropriateness, to the investigation of intraspeaker or interspeaker variability or the disentangling of sociolinguistic from pathologic variation. What is most important is spending time on selecting appropriate methods and carrying them out with care, in order to gain detailed qualititative and quantitative insights into the rich domain of vowel production.

Notes

1. Unfortunately, Maurer, Gröne, Landis, and colleagues (1993, 130), do not provide information on the durations of the sustained vowels in their data, and state that, "There were no restrictions on the duration of the vocalizations."
2. In light of the discussion in the preceding section concerning the articulatory basis of vowel classification, the terms *Cardinal Vowels* and *IPA vowels* will be used more or less interchangeably. They are both presented as fixed universal qualities independent of particular languages, although the IPA set contains more nonperipheral vowels. The International Phonetic Association fully endorsed the principles of the Cardinal Vowel system (Pullum and Ladusaw, 1986).
3. Ladefoged's (1975) suggestion that Cardinal Vowels be identified by underlining is perhaps not a good one to follow, given the standard IPA retracted articulation diacritic.
4. For the *lexical set* approach to naming vowels, see Wells (1982, 127–168).

References

Abberton, E., Howard, D., and Fourcin, A. J. (1989). Laryngographic assessment of normal voice. Clinical Linguistics and Phonetics, 3, 281–296.

Abercrombie, D. (1965). Parameters and phonemes. Chapter 12 in Studies in phonetics and linguistics. Oxford: Oxford University Press, 120–124.

Abercrombie, D. (1967). Elements of general phonetics. Edinburgh, Scotland: Edinburgh University Press.

Alfonso, P. J., and Baer, T. (1982). Dynamics of vowel articulation. Language and Speech, 25, 159–173.

Allen, G. D., and Hawkins, S. (1980). Phonological rhythm: Definition and development. In G. H. Yeni-Komshian, J. F. Kavanagh, and C. A. Ferguson (Eds.), Child phonology, Vol. 1: Production (pp. 227–256). New York: Academic.

Amorosa, H., von Benda, U., Wagner, E., and Keck, A. (1985). Transcribing detail in the speech of unintelligible children: A comparison of procedures. British Journal of Disorders of Communication, 20, 281–287.

Angelocci, A. A., Kopp, G. A., and Holbrook, A. (1964). The vowel formants of deaf and normal-hearing eleven- to fourteen-year-old boys. Journal of Speech and Hearing Disorders, 29, 156–170.

Atkinson, J., Barlow, H. B., and Braddick, O. (1982). The development of sensory systems and their modification by experience. In H. B. Barlow and J. D. Mollon (Eds.), The senses. Cambridge, England: Cambridge University Press.

Baer, T., Alfonso, P., and Honda, K. (1988). Electromyography of the tongue muscles during vowels in /pVp/ environment. Annual Bulletin of the Research Institute of Logopedics and Phoniatrics, Tokyo: University of Tokyo, 22, 7–19.

Baken, R. J. (1987). Clinical measurement of speech and voice. London: Taylor and Francis.

Ball, M. J. (1988). The contribution of speech pathology to the development of phonetic transcription. In M. J. Ball (Ed.), Theoretical linguistics and disordered language. London: Croom Helm.

Ball, M. J. (1991). Recent developments in the transcription of non-normal speech. Journal of Communication Disorders, 25, 59–78.

Ball, M. J. (1992). Is a clinical sociolinguistics possible? Clinical Linguistics and Phonetics, 6, 155–160.

Ball, M. J. (1993). Phonetics for speech pathology (2nd ed.). London: Whurr.

Ball, M. J., and Code, C. (Eds.) (1997). Instrumental clinical phonetics. London: Whurr.

Ball, M. J., Esling, J., and Dickson, G. (1995). The VoQS system for the transcription of voice quality. Journal of the International Phonetic Association, 25, 61–70.

Ball, M. J., and Gröne, B. (1997). Imaging techniques. In M. J. Ball, and C. Code (Eds.), Instrumental Clinical Phonetics. London: Whurr.

Ball, M. J., and Local, J. (1996). Current developments in transcription. In M. J. Ball and M. Duckworth (Eds.), Advances in clinical phonetics. Amsterdam: John Benjamins, 51–89.

Ball, M. J., and Rahilly, J. (1999). Phonetics: The science of speech. London: Arnold.

Ball, M. J., Rahilly, J., and Tench, P. (1996). The phonetic transcription of disordered speech. San Diego: Singular.

Barry, W. J., and Timmerman, G. (1985). Mispronunciations and compensatory movements of tongue operated patients. British Journal of Disorders of Communication, 20, 81–90.

Bates, E., Dale, P. S., and Thal, D. (1995). Individual differences and their implications for theories of language development. In P. Fletcher and B. MacWhinney (Eds.), The handbook of child language (pp. 96–151). Oxford: Blackwell.

Bates, S., and Watson, J. (1996). Consonant-vowel interactions in developmental phonological disorder. In Proceedings of the Golden Jubilee Conference of the RCSLT. Royal College of Speech and Language Therapists, 274–279.

Bauer, H. R., and Robb, M. P. (1992). The ethologic model of phonetic development: III. The phonetic product. Clinical Linguistics and Phonetics, 317–327.

Bernhardt, B. H., and Stemberger, J. P. (1998). Handbook of phonological development. New York: Academic.

Bertoncini, J., Bijeljac-Babic, R., Jusczyk, P. W., et al. (1988). An investigation of young infants' perceptual representations of speech sounds. Journal of Experimental Psychology: General, 117, 21–33.

Bladon, A. (1983). 2-formant models of vowel perception: Shortcomings and enhancements. Speech Communication, 2.

Blake, J., and Fink, R. (1987). Sound-meaning correspondences in babbling. Journal of Child Language, 14, 229–253.

Blomgren, M., and Robb, M. (1998). How steady are vowel steady-states? Clinical Linguistics and Phonetics, 12, 405–415.

Blomgren, M., Robb, M., and Chen, Y. (1998). A note on vowel centralisation in stuttering and non-stuttering individuals, Journal of Speech and Hearing Research, 41, 1042–1051.

Boysson-Bardies, B., de Hallé, P., Sagart, L., and Durand, C. (1989). A cross-linguistic investigation of vowel formants in babbling. Journal of Child Language, 16, 1–17.

Braine, M. D. S. (1974). On what might constitute a learnable phonology. Language, 50, 270–300.

Buckingham, H. W., and Yule, G. (1987). Phonemic false evaluation: Theoretical and clinical aspects. Clinical Linguistics and Phonetics, 1, 113–125.

Buhr, R. (1980). The emergence of vowels in an infant. Journal of Speech and Hearing Research, 23, 56–72

Butcher, A. (1982). Cardinal vowels and other problems. In D. Crystal (Ed.), Linguistic controversies. London: Arnold.

Butcher, A. (1989). The uses and abuses of phonological assessment. Child Language Teaching and Therapy, 5, 262–276.

Byrd, D. (1995). Palatogram reading a a phonetic skill: A short tutorial. Journal of the International Phonetic Association, 24, 21–34.

Camarata, S., and Gandour, J. (1984). On describing idiosyncratic phonologic systems. Journal of Speech and Hearing Disorders, 49, 262–266.

Carrell, T., Smith, L., and Pisoni, D. (1981). Some perceptual dependencies in speeded classification of vowel color and pitch. Perception and Psychophysics, 29, 1–10.

Catford, J. C. (1977). Fundamental problems in phonetics. Edinburgh, Scotland: Edinburgh University Press.

Catford, J. C. (1988). A practical introduction to phonetics. Oxford: Oxford University Press.

Chistovich, L. A., Sheikin, R. L., and Lublinskaja, V. V. (1979). Centers of gravity and spectral peaks as the determinants of vowel quality. In B. Lindblom and S. Öhman (Eds.), Frontiers of speech communication research (pp. 143–158). London: Academic.

Christman, S. S. (1992). Uncovering phonological regularity in neologisms: Contributions of sonority theory. Clinical Linguistics and Phonetics, 6, 219–247.

Clark, E. V. (1995). Later lexical development and word formation. In P. Fletcher and B. MacWhinney (Eds.), The handbook of child language (pp. 393–412). London: Blackwell.

Clark, J., and C. Yallop (1995). An introduction to phonetics and phonology (2nd ed.). London: Blackwell.

Clement, C. J., and Wijnen, F. (1994). Acquisition of vowel contrasts in Dutch. Journal of Speech and Hearing Research, 37, 69–82.

Cruttenden, A. (1986). Intonation. Cambridge, England: Cambridge University Press.

Crystal, D. (1982). Terms, time and teeth. British Journal of Disorders of Communication, 17, 3–19.

Crystal, D. (1987). Towards a "bucket" theory of language disability: Taking account of interaction between linguistic levels. Clinical Linguistics and Phonetics, 1, 7–22.

Dagenais, P., and Critz-Crosby, P. (1992). Comparing tongue positioning by normal-hearing and hearing-impaired children during vowel production. Journal of Speech and Hearing Research, 35, 35–44.

Daniloff, R., Bishop, M., and Ringel, R. (1977). Alteration of children's articulation by application of oral anesthesia. Journal of Phonetics, 5, 285–298.

Davis, B. L., and MacNeilage, P. F. (1990). Acquisition of correct vowel production: A quantitative case study. Journal of Speech and Hearing Research, 33, 16–27.

Davis, B. L., and MacNeilage, P. F. (1995). The articulatory basis of babbling. Journal of Speech and Hearing Research, 38, 1199–1211.

Delgutte, B. (1997). Auditory neural processing of speech. In W. J. Hardcastle and J. Laver (Eds.), Handbook of phonetic sciences (pp. 507–538). London: Blackwell.

Duckworth, M., Allen, G., Hardcastle, W., and Ball, M. J. (1990). Extensions to the International Phonetic Alphabet for the transcription of atypical speech. Clinical Linguistics and Phonetics, 4, 273–280.

Fant, C. G. M. (1956). On the predictability of formant levels and spectrum envelopes from formant frequencies. In M. Halle, H. Lunt, and H. MacLean (Eds.), For Roman Jakobson (pp. 109–120). The Hague:

Mouton. Reprinted in I. Lehiste (Ed.), Readings in acoustic phonetics (pp. 44–56). Cambridge, Mass.: MIT Press.

Fant, C. G. M. (1960). The acoustic theory of speech production. The Hague: Mouton.

Farmer, A. (1997). Spectrography. In M. J. Ball and C. Code (Eds.), Instrumental clinical phonetics. London: Whurr.

Ferrier, L. J., Johnston, J. J., and Bashir, A. S. (1991). A longitudinal study of the babbling and phonological development of a child with hypoglossia. Clinical Linguistics and Phonetics, 5, 187–206.

Fletcher, S. (1973). Maturation of the speech mechanism. Folia Phoniatrica, 25, 161–172.

Fletcher, S., McCutcheon, M., and Wolf, M. (1975). Dynamic palatometry. Journal of Speech and Hearing Research, 18, 812–819.

Foulkes, P., and Docherty, G. J. (1999). Urban voices. London: Arnold.

Foulkes, P., and Docherty, G. J. (in press). Phonological variation in the English of England. To appear in D. Britain (Ed.), Language in the British Isles (2nd ed.). Cambridge, England: Cambridge University Press.

Fry, D. B. (1979). The physics of speech. Cambridge, England: Cambridge University Press.

Fujimura, O., Tatsumi, I. F., and Kayaga, R. (1973). Computational processing of palatographic patterns. Journal of Phonetics, 1, 47–54.

Gentil, M., and Moore, W. H. (1997). Electromyography. In M. J. Ball and C. Code (Eds.), Instrumental clinical phonetics. London: Whurr.

Gierut, J. A., Cho, M-H., and Dinnsen, D. A. (1993). Geometric accounts of consonant-vowel interaction in developing systems. Clinical Linguistics and Phonetics, 7, 219–236.

Goldstein, B. A., and Pollock, K. E. (2000). Vowel errors in Spanish-speaking children with phonological disorders: A retrospective, comparative study. Clinical Linguistics and Phonetics, 14, 217–234.

Grabe, E., Post, B., and Watson, I. (1999). The acquisition of rhythmic patterns in English and French. Proceedings of the 14th International Congress of Phonetic Sciences, 1201–1204.

Grunwell, P. (1987). Clinical Phonology (2nd ed.) London: Croom Helm.

Hamlet, S., and Stone, M. (1976). Compensatory vowel characteristics resulting from the presence of different types of experimental dental prostheses. Journal of Phonetics, 4, 199–218.

Hardcastle, W. J., and Gibbon, F. (1997). Electropalatography and its clinical applications. In M. J. Ball and C. Code (Eds.), Instrumental clinical phonetics. London: Whurr.

Hasluck, S., and Hasluck, A. (1898). Elements of pronunciation and articulation. London: Simpkin, Marshall, Hamilton, Kent.

Hayward, K. (2000). Experimental phonetics. London: Longman.

Henry, C. E. (1990). The development of oral diadochokinesia and non-linguistic rhythmic skills in normal and speech-disordered young children. Clinical Linguistics and Phonetics, 4, 121–137.

Heselwood, B. (1998). An unusual kind of sonority and its implications for phonetic theory. Leeds Working Papers in Linguistics and Phonetics, 6, 68–80.

Heselwood, B. (1999). Sonority, glottals, and the characterisation of [sonorant]. In B. Maassen and P. Groenen (Eds.), Pathologies of speech and language (pp. 18–24). London: Whurr.

Hewlett, N. (1985). Phonological versus phonetic disorders: Some suggested modifications to the current use of the distinction. British Journal of Disorders of Communication, 20, 155–164.

Honda, K. (1996). Organization of tongue articulation for vowels. Journal of Phonetics, 24(1), 39–52.

Howard, S. J. (2001). Compensatory articulatory behavior in cleft palate speech: Comparing the perceptual and instrumental evidence. Paper presented at the 9th Conference on Cleft Palate and Related Craniofacial Anomalies, June 25th–29th, Göteborg, Sweden.

ICPLA (1994). ICPLA News. Clinical Linguistics and Phonetics, 8, 259–265.

Iivonen, A. (1994). A psychoacoustical explanation for the number of major IPA vowels. Journal of the International Phonetic Association, 24, 73–90.

Ingrisano, D., Klee, T., and Binger, C. (1996). Linguistic context effects on transcription. In T. W. Powell (Ed.), Pathologies of speech and language: Contributions of clinical phonetics and linguistics. New Orleans: International Clinical Phonetics and Linguistics Association.

Jakobson, R. (1968). Child language, aphasia, and phonological universals. The Hague: Mouton.

Johnson, K. (1997). Acoustic and auditory phonetics. Cambridge, Mass.: Blackwell.

Jones, D. (1972). An outline of English phonetics (9th ed.). Cambridge, England: Cambridge University Press.

Kamen, R. S., and Watson, B. C. (1991). Effects of long-term tracheostomy on spectral characteristics of vowel production. Journal of Speech and Hearing Research, 34, 1057–1065.

Keating. P. (1983). Comments on the jaw and syllable structure. Journal of Phonetics, 11, 401–406.

Keefe, D. H., Burns, E. M., Bulen, J. C., and Campbell, S. L. (1994). Pressure transfer function from the diffuse field to the human infant ear canal. Journal of the Acoustical Society of America, 95, 355–371.

Kelly, J., and Local, J. (1989). Doing phonology. Manchester, England: Manchester University Press.

Kent, R. D. (1992). The biology of phonological development. In C. Ferguson, L. Menn, and C. Stoel-Gammon (Eds.), Phonological development: Models, research, implications (pp. 65–90). Timonium, Md.: York Press.

Kent, R. D., and Bauer, H. R. (1985). Vocalisations of one-year-olds. Journal of Child Language, 13, 491–526.

Kent, R. D., and Miolo, G. (1995). Phonetic abilities in the first year of life. In P. Fletcher and B. MacWhinney, (Eds.), Handbook of child language. London: Blackwell.

Kent, R. D., and Moll, K. L. (1972). Tongue body articulation during vowel and diphthong gestures. Folia Phoniatrica, 24, 278–300.

Kent, R. D., and Murray, A. (1982). Acoustic features of infant vocalic utterances at 3, 6, and 9 months. Journal of the Acoustical Society of America, 72, 353–365.

Kent, R. D., and Read, C. (1992). The acoustic analysis of speech. San Diego: Singular.

Koopmans-van Beinum, F. J., and van der Stelt, J. M. (1986). Early stages in the development of speech movements. In B. Lindblom and R. Zetterström (Eds.), Precursors of early speech. Basingstoke, England: Macmillan.

Kuhl, P. (1980). Perceptual constancy for speech-sound categories in early infancy. In G. H. Yeni-Komshian, J. F. Kavanagh, and C. A. Ferguson (Eds.), Child phonology, Vol. 2: Perception (pp. 41–66). New York: Academic.

Kuhl, P., and Miller, J. (1982). Discrimination of auditory target dimensions in the presence or absence of variation in a second dimension by infants. Perception and Psychophysics, 31, 279–292.

Ladefoged, P. (1967). The nature of vowel quality. Chapter 2 in Three areas of experimental phonetics, 50–142. Oxford: Oxford University Press.

Ladefoged, P. (1975). A course in phonetics. New York: Harcourt, Brace, Jovanovich.

Ladefoged, P. (1990). Some reflections on the IPA. Journal of Phonetics, 18, 335–346.

Ladefoged, P. (1993). A course in phonetics (3rd ed.). Fort Worth: Harcourt, Brace, Jovanovich.

Ladefoged, P. (2000). Vowels and consonants: An introduction to the sounds of the world's languages. London: Blackwell.

Ladefoged, P., Harshman, R., Goldstein, L., and Rice, L. (1978). Generating vocal tract shapes from formant frequencies. Journal of the Acoustical Society of America, 64, 1027–1035.

Ladefoged, P., and Maddieson, I. (1996). Sounds of the world's languages. London: Blackwell.

Laver, J. (1980). The phonetic basis of voice quality. Cambridge, England: Cambridge University Press.

Laver, J. (1994). Principles of phonetics. Cambridge, England: Cambridge University Press.

Lieberman, P. (1980). On the development of vowel production in young children. In G. Yeni-Komshian, J. F. Kavanagh, and C. J. Ferguson (Eds.), Child phonology, Vol. 1: Production. New York: Academic.

Lieberman, P., Crelin, E. S., and Klatt, D. H. (1972). Phonetic ability and related anatomy of the new-born, adult human, Neanderthal man, and the chimpanzee. American Anthropologist, 74, 287–307.

Lindblom, B. (1986). On the origin and purpose of discreteness and invariance in sound patterns. In J. Perkell and D. H. Klatt (Eds.), Invariance and variability in speech processes. Hillsdale, N.J.: Erlbaum.

Lisker, L. (1989). On the interpretation of vowel "quality": The dimension of rounding. Journal of the International Phonetic Association, 19(1), 24–30.

Local, J. (1983). How many vowels in a vowel? Journal of Child Language, 10, 449–453.

Locke, J. L. (1993). The child's path to spoken language. Cambridge, Mass.: Harvard University Press.

Locke, J. L., and Pearson, D. M. (1992). Vocal learning and the emergence of phonological capacity. In C. A. Ferguson, L. Menn, and C. Stoel-Gammon (Eds.), Phonological development: Models, research, implications (pp. 91–129). Timonium, Md.: York Press.

Lotto, A. J., Holt, L. L., and Kluender, K. R. (1997). Effect of voice quality on perceived height of English vowels. Phonetica, 54, 76–93.

Lowry, G. H. (1978). Growth and development of children (7th ed.). Chicago: Year Book Medical.

Maassen, B., Offeringa, S., Vieregge, W., and Thoonen, G. (1996). Transcription of pathological speech in children by means of extIPA: Agreement and relevance. In T. W. Powell (Ed.), Pathologies of speech and language: Contributions of clinical phonetics and linguistics. New Orleans: International Clinical Phonetics and Linguistics Association.

Mackenzie Beck, J. (1997). Organic variation of the vocal apparatus. In W. Hardcastle and J. Laver (Eds.), The handbook of phonetic sciences (pp. 256–297). Oxford: Blackwell.

MacNeilage, P. F. (1997). Acquisition of speech. In W. J. Hardcastle and J. Laver (Eds.), Handbook of phonetic sciences (pp. 301–332). London: Blackwell.

MacNeilage, P. F., and Davis, B. L. (1990). Acquisition of speech production: Frames, then content. In M. Jeannerod (Ed.), Attention and performance XIII: Motor representation and control. Hillsdale, N.J.: Erlbaum.

Maeda, S., and Honda, K. (1994). From EMG to formant patterns of vowels: The implication of vowel system spaces. Paper presented at the ACCOR workshop on lingual data and modeling in speech production. Barcelona, 20–22 December, 1994. Cited in Perkell, J. S. (1997).

Martin, J. A. M. (1981). Voice, speech and language in the child: Development and disorder. New York: Springer.

Maurer, D., Gröne, B., Landis, T., et al. (1993). Re-examination of the relation between the vocal tract and the vowel sound with electromagnetic articulography (EMA) in vocalizations. Clinical Linguistics and Phonetics, 7(2), 129–143.

McGarr, N. S., and Harris, K. S. (1983). Articulatory control in a deaf speaker. In I. Hochberg, H. Levitt, and M. J. Osberger (Eds.), Speech of the hearing impaired: Research, training, personnel preparation. Baltimore: University Park Press.

Meier, R. P., McGarvin, L., Zakia, R. A. E., and Willerman, R. (1997). Silent mandibular oscillations in vocal babbling. Phonetica, 54, 153–171.

Moore, B. C. J. (1997). An introduction to the psychology of hearing. Cambridge, England: Cambridge University Press.

Moore, B. C. J., and Glasberg, B. R. (1983). Suggested formulae for calculating auditory-filter bandwidths and excitation patterns. Journal of the Acoustical Society of America, 74, 750–753.

Morrish, E. (1984). Compensatory vowel articulation of the glossectomee: Acoustic and videoflourocopic evidence. British Journal of Disorders of Communication, 19, 125–134.

Morrish, E. (1988). Compensatory articulation in a subject with total glossectomy. British Journal of Disorders of Communication, 23, 13–22.

Nittrouer, S., Studdert-Kennedy, M., and Neely, S. (1996). How children learn to organise their speech gestures: Further evidence from fricative-vowel syllables. Journal of Speech and Hearing Research, 39, 379–389.

Norris, M., Harden, J.R., and Bell, D. M. (1980). Listener agreement on articulation errors of four- and five-year-old children. Journal of Speech and Hearing Disorders, 45, 378–389.

Norton, S. J., and Widen, J. E. (1990). Evoked otoacoustic emission in normal-hearing infants and children: Emerging data and issues. Ear and Hearing, 11, 121–127.

Ohala, J. J. (1984). Prosodic phonology and phonetics. Phonology Yearbook, 113–127.

Öhman, S. (1966). Coarticulation in CVC utterances: Spectrographic measurements. Journal of the Acoustical Society of America, 66, 1691–1702.

Oller, D. K. (1973). Regularities in abnormal child phonology. Journal of Speech and Hearing Disorders, 38, 36–47.

Oller, D. K. (1980). The emergence of the sounds of speech in infancy. In H. Yeni-Komshian, J. F. Kavanagh, and C. A. Ferguson (Eds.), Child phonology, Vol. 1: Production. New York: Academic.

Oller, D. K., and Eilers, R. E. (1975). Phonetic expectation and transcription validity. Phonetica, 31, 288–304.

Oller, D. K., and Lynch, M. P. (1992). Infant vocalisations and innovations in infraphonology: Toward a broader theory of development and disorders. In C. A. Ferguson, L. Menn, and C. Stoel-Gammon (Eds.), Phonological development: Models, research, implications, (pp. 509–536). Timonium, Md.: York Press.

Perkell, J. S. (1996). Properties of the tongue help to define vowel categories: Hypotheses based on physiologically-oriented modeling. Journal of Phonetics, 24(1), 3–22.

Perkell, J. S. (1997). Articulatory processes. In W. J. Hardcastle and J. Laver (Eds.), The handbook of phonetic sciences (pp. 333–370). London: Blackwell.

Perkell, J. S., Cohen, M., Svirsky, et al. (1992). Electro-magnetic midsagittal articulometer (EMMA) systems for transducing speech articulatory movements. Journal of the Acoustical Society of America, 92, 3078–3096.

Peters, A. M. (1995). Strategies in the acquisition of syntax. In P. Fletcher and B. MacWhinney (Eds.), The handbook of child language (pp. 462–482). London: Blackwell.

Peterson, G., and Barney, H. E. (1952). Control methods used in a study of vowels. Journal of the Acoustical Society of America, 24, 175–184.

Pike, K. L. (1947). Phonemics: A technique for reducing languages to writing. Ann Arbor: University of Michigan Press.

Pisoni, D. (1997). Some thoughts on "normalization" in speech perception. In K. Johnson and J. W. Mullenix (Eds.), Talker variability in speech processing. San Diego: Academic.

Proctor, A. (1989). Stages of normal non-cry vocal development in infancy: A protocol for assessment. Topics in Language Disorders, 10, 26–42.

Pullum, G. K., and Ladusaw, W. (1986). Phonetic symbol guide. Chicago: University of Chicago Press.

Pye, C., Wilcox, K., and Siren, K. A. (1988). Refining transcriptions—the significance of transcriber "errors." Journal of Child Language, 15, 17–37.

Reynolds, J. (1990). Abnormal vowel patterns in phonological disorder: Some data and a hypothesis. British Journal of Disorders of Communication, 25, 115–148.

Rippmann, W. (1911). English sounds. London: Dent.

Schönle, P., Grabe, K., Wenig, P., et al. (1987). Electromagnetic articulography: Use of alternating magnetic fields for tracking movements of multiple points inside and outside the vocal tract. Brain and Language, 31, 26–35.

Schwartz, J. L., Boë, L. J., Valée, N., and Abry, C. (1997). Major trends in vowel system inventories. Journal of Phonetics, 25, 233–253.

Selby, J. C., Robb, M. P., and Gilbert, H. R. (2000). Normal vowel articulations between 15 and 36 months of age. Clinical Linguistics and Phonetics, 14, 255–265.

Shankweiler, D., Harris, K. S., and Taylor, M. L. (1968). Electromyographic studies of articulation in aphasia. Archives of Physical Medicine and Rehabilitation, 49, 1–8.

Shriberg, L. D., and Lof, G. L. (1991). Reliability studies in broad and narrow phonetic transcription. Clinical Linguistics and Phonetics, 5, 225–279.

Stach, B. A. (1998). Clinical audiology. San Diego: Singular.

Stark, R. (1980). Stages of speech development in the first years of life. In H. Yeni-Komshian, J. F. Kavanagh, and C. A. Ferguson (Eds.), Child phonology, Vol. 1: Production. New York: Academic.

Stevens, K. N. (1989). On the quantal nature of speech. Journal of Phonetics, 17(1), 3–46.

Stevens, K. N. (1997). Articulatory–acoustic–auditory relationships. In W. J. Hardcastle and J. Laver (Eds.), The handbook of phonetic sciences (pp. 462–506). London: Blackwell.

Stevens, K. N. (1998). Acoustic phonetics. Cambridge, Mass.: MIT Press.

Stevens, K. N., and House, A. S. (1955). Development of a quantitative model of vowel articulation. Journal of the Acoustical Society of America, 27, 484–493.

Stevens, K. N., and House, A. S. (1961). An acoustical theory of vowel production and some of its implications. Journal of Speech and Hearing Research, 4, 303–320. Reprinted in I. Lehiste (Ed.), (1967). Readings in acoustic phonetics (pp.75–92). Cambridge, Mass.: MIT Press.

Stoel-Gammon, C. (1985). Phonetic inventories 15–24 months: A longitudinal study. Journal of Speech and Hearing Research, 28, 505–512.

Stoel-Gammon, C., and Herrington, P. (1990). Vowel systems of normally-developing and phonologically-disordered children. Clinical Linguistics and Phonetics, 4, 145–160.

Stone, M. (1997). Laboratory techniques for investigating speech articulation. In W. J. Hardcastle and J. Laver (Eds.), The handbook of phonetic sciences (pp. 11–32). London: Blackwell.

Stone, M., Shawker, T., Talbot, T., and Rich, A. (1988). Cross-sectional tongue shape during vowels. Journal of the Acoustical Society of America, 83, 1586–1596.

Stone, M., and Vatikiotis-Bateson, E. (1995). Trade-offs in tongue, jaw, and palate contributions to speech production. Journal of Phonetics, 23, 81–100.

Strange, W. (1989). Dynamic specification of coarticulated vowels spoken in sentence context. Journal of the Acoustical Society of America, 85, 2135–2153.

Sundberg, J., and Gauffin, J. (1979). Amplitude of the voice source fundamental and the intelligibility of super-pitch vowels. In R. Carlson and B. Granström (Eds.), The representation of speech in the peripheral auditory system (pp. 223–228). Amsterdam: Elsevier.

Tallal, P., and Stark, R. (1980). Speech perception of language-delayed children. In G. H. Yeni-Komshian, J. F. Kavanagh, and C. A. Ferguson (Eds.), Child phonology, Vol. 2: Perception (pp. 155–171). New York: Academic.

Tanner, J. M. (1989). Foetus into man. Ware, England: Castlemead.

Tench, P. (1978). On introducing parametric phonetics. Journal of the International Phonetic Association, 8, 34–46.

Tyler, A., and Langsdale, T. E. (1996). Consonant-vowel interactions in early phonological development. First Language, 16, 159–191.

Vieregge, W., and Maassen, B. (1999). ExtIPA transcriptions of consonants and vowels spoken by dyspractic children: Agreement and validity. In B. Maassen and P. Groenen, (Eds.), Pathologies of speech and language: Advances in clinical phonetics and linguistics. London: Whurr.

Vihman, M. M. (1992). Early syllables and the construction of phonology. In C. A. Ferguson, L. Menn, and C. Stoel-Gammon (Eds.), Phonological development: Models, research, implications (pp. 393–422). Timonium, Md.: York Press.

Watt, D., and Tillotson, J. (1999). A spectrographic study of vowel-fronting in Bradford English. Leeds Working Papers in Linguistics and Phonetics, 7.

Wells, J. C. (1982). Accents of English (3 vols). Cambridge, England: Cambridge University Press.

Werner, L. A., and Marean, G. C. (1996). Human auditory development. Oxford: Westview Press.

Wirz, S. L., and Beck, J. (1995). Assessment of voice quality: The vocal profiles analysis scheme. In S. L. Wirz (Ed.), Perceptual approaches to communication disorders. London: Whurr.

Wolfe, V., and Blocker, S. (1990). Consonant-vowel interaction in an unusual phonological system. Journal of Speech and Hearing Disorder, 55, 561–566.

Wood, S. (1979). A radiographic analysis of constriction locations for vowels. Journal of Phonetics, 7, 25–43.

Yamashita, Y., Michi, K.-I., Imai, S., et al. (1992). Electropalatographic investigation of abnormal lingual-palatal contact patterns in cleft palate patients. Clinical Linguistics and Phonetics, 6, 201–217.

Young, E. C. (1991). An analysis of young children's ability to produce multisyllabic English nouns. Clinical Linguistics and Phonetics, 5, 297–316.

Zec, D. (1995). Sonority constraints on syllable structure. Phonology, 12, 85–129.

Zwicker, E., and Terhardt, E. (1980). Analytical expressions for critical-band rate and critical bandwidth as a function of frequency. Journal of the Acoustical Society of America, 68, 1523–1525.

3

Identification of Vowel Errors: Methodological Issues and Preliminary Data from the Memphis Vowel Project

Karen E. Pollock

Vowel errors attracted the attention of several researchers and practicing clinicians working in the area of child phonology in the 1980s and 1990s (Davis and MacNeilage, 1990; Gibbon, Shockey, and Reid, 1992; Hargrove, 1982; Pollock and Keiser, 1990; Pollock and Swanson, 1986; Reynolds, 1990; Stoel-Gammon and Herrington, 1990). They provided detailed descriptions of the vowel errors produced by a variety of individual children and small groups of children. However, although there has been increased awareness of vowel errors, many important theoretical and practical questions concerning vowel errors remain unanswered. It is not known how frequently vowel errors occur in children with phonological disorders or which, if any, types of vowel errors are most common. In addition, to date there have been no reports of a large group study of vowel errors in children. The purpose of this chapter is to present preliminary data from such a study of American English-speaking children and to discuss some of the complex methodological issues encountered in the identification of vowel errors in children.

The Memphis Vowel Project

The experiences recounted and data presented are from a recent study of American children from Memphis, Tennessee, and surrounding communities. The study was designed to address the nature and significance of vowel errors in children. Primary goals were to determine the incidence of vowel errors in phonologically disordered children, to provide detailed descriptions of vowel errors observed, and to investigate the relationship between vowel errors and consonant errors. In addition, the study sought to address the clinical significance of vowel errors through experimental investigations of the effects of vowel errors on intelligibility and to determine the need for direct intervention for vowel errors through longitudinal observations of children with vowel errors.

Although transcription and analyses are still under way, preliminary data on vowel production accuracy are available for 283 children. Of these children, 162 had normal phonological development (hereafter referred to as the NP group) and 121 had delayed or disordered phonological development (the DP group). Children in the NP group were recruited from local preschools, elementary schools, and Headstart centers. Those in the DP group were recruited from the caseloads of speech-language pathologists working in local preschools, elementary schools, Headstart centers, and private practice. Children with gross sensory (such as hearing impairment), motor (such as cerebral palsy), or oral structural (such as cleft palate) involvement were not included.

The NP children were evenly distributed with respect to gender (85 boys, 77 girls). However, there were twice as many boys (81) as girls (40) in the DP group. All children were born and raised within 100 miles of Memphis, Tennessee. Consistent with the demographics of the Memphis area, roughly half of the NP children were African American (76) and the other half European American (86). However, in the DP group, only one fourth (30 out of 121) were African American. This imbalance is partially due to a variety of complex sociological factors, such as a lower tendency among African Americans to seek speech-language services or to volunteer to participate in research studies.

In addition, it was more difficult to find African American children who met the selection criteria for the DP group (normal receptive language and nonverbal IQ, expressive language within 1 year of chronological age, primary difficulty with expressive phonology). It appeared that many of the African American children enrolled in speech-language intervention showed more widespread disorders of receptive and expressive language. However, this may reflect test bias in the standardized instruments used to assess language and cognitive skills, such as the Columbia Mental Maturity Scale (Burgemeister, Blum, and Lorge, 1972), the Leiter International Performance Scale (Arthur, 1969), and the Preschool Language Scale–3 (Zimmerman, Steiner, and Pond, 1992).

Children in the NP group ranged from 18 to 82 months of age and those in the DP group ranged from 30 to 81 months of age. Younger children were included in the NP group in order to compare the vowel errors of DP children to younger NP children. Preliminary group assignment (NP or DP) was determined by the percentage of consonants correct (PCC) on a single-word elicitation task. All NP children over 36 months of age had PCC scores greater than 85%. For NP children under 36 months of age, the cutoff was lower and greater reliance placed on parent or teacher report of normal speech-language development. Table 3-1 shows the mean PCC scores by age group (in 6-month intervals) for the NP and DP children.

The majority of children in the DP group had PCC scores under 85%. However, 29 children with borderline scores between 85% and 95% were also included in the disordered group because they were currently enrolled in therapy for a phonological disorder. Many of these children had primarily distortion errors on sibilants or /r/. Some of them had been in therapy for several months and had remediated many of their earlier, more severe consonant errors. Thus, this group is best thought of as having borderline/normal or resolved consonant production errors. Of the remaining DP children, 44 were mild/moderate (PCC 66–84%), 34 were moderate/severe (PCC 50–65%), and 14 were severe (PCC < 50%) (Shriberg and Kwiatkowski, 1982).

Before presenting preliminary group data on vowel production accuracy, it is important to provide some methodological background. Because the study of vowel errors is relatively new, different investigators have developed their own protocols for data collection and analysis. The following section will focus on a variety of methodological issues that were encountered in our attempts to

Table 3-1   Mean Percent Consonants Correct (PCC) by Age for Both NP and DP Groups

Age (in months)		NP Group				DP Group	
	(n)	Mean PCC	SD		(n)	Mean PCC	SD
18–23	(10)	53.21	10.00				
24–29	(18)	70.37	9.47				
30–35	(21)	80.90	10.39		(1)	34.92	—
36–41	(17)	91.47	4.90		(2)	58.70	14.43
42–47	(16)	92.56	4.11		(16)	58.44	22.29
48–53	(18)	92.94	5.14		(19)	66.05	16.60
54–59	(25)	94.24	4.01		(29)	72.91	14.07
60–65	(19)	93.32	4.10		(23)	74.38	14.41
66–71	(13)	95.92	3.88		(21)	72.25	14.67
72–77	(4)	97.17	2.00		(8)	74.34	15.94
78–83	(1)	93.09	—		(2)	89.83	4.86

identify vowel errors and describe error patterns. Throughout the discussion, data from one child, referred to as K25, will be used as illustration. The appendix contains background information, data, and analysis forms for K25. The procedures presented are not being proposed as an ideal clinical or research protocol, but, rather, as a way of illustrating some of the challenges inherent in any study of vowel errors in children. It is hoped that this discussion will facilitate further development of improved clinical and research protocols for the study of vowel errors.

Methodological Issues

Description of Target Vowel System

Not everyone agrees on the best system for describing English vowels. In addition, there is considerable variation in vowel production across regional dialects of American English. Therefore, it is necessary to first describe the terminology and classification system used in the current study. Our descriptive framework primarily follows those of Ladefoged (1993; 2000) and Mackay (1987), and has been described in more detail elsewhere (Pollock, 1994; Pollock and Berni, 2001).

Briefly, we consider four broad categories of American English vowels: (1) *nonrhotic monophthongs* (/i, ɪ, e, ɛ, æ, ʌ, u, ʊ, o, ɔ, ɑ/); (2) *nonrhotic diphthongs* (/aɪ, aʊ, ɔɪ/); (3) the *rhotic monophthong* (/ɝ/); and (4) *rhotic diphthongs* (/ɪɚ, ɛɚ, ɔɚ, ɑɚ/). The rhotic monophthong is also frequently referred to as vocalic or syllabic /r/. Similarly, the rhotic diphthongs are often described as vowels plus postvocalic /r/ (such as /ɪɚ/ = /ɪr/). The vowels /e/ and /o/ are considered to be monophthongs at a phonemic or abstract level, but are typically produced as diphthongs (that is, at a phonetic or allophonic level).

Each vowel can be described with the four dimensions of *height, frontness, tenseness,* and *rounding*. The two left-most columns of Table 3-2 provide the standard International Phonetic Alphabet symbols and four-term descriptions of American English vowels according to this framework. Two symbols are given for the central vowels (/ʌ, ə/ and /ɝ, ɚ/), with the first used in stressed syllables and the second in unstressed syllables. This usage departs from the IPA (where /ʌ/ and /ə/ represent different vowel qualities), but represents their most common usage in speech-language pathology in the United States (Edwards, 1997; Mackay, 1987; Shriberg and Kent, 1995; Small, 1999).

Vowel Variation in Memphis

Table 3-2 also illustrates some of the most common phonetic representations for each vowel in the three major dialects observed in our children, namely Informal Standard English (ISE), Southern White Vernacular English

Table 3-2 Vowel Phonemes of American English and Some Common Phonetic Representation(s) in Informal Standard English (ISE), Southern White Vernacular English (SWVE), and African American Vernacular English (AAVE) Speech in Memphis

Phoneme	Description	Example	ISE	SWVE	AAVE
Monophthongs:					
/i/	highfront tense (spread)[a]	*bead*	[i]	[i, ᵉi]	[i, ɪ]
/ɪ/	highfront lax (unrnd)	*bid*	[ɪ]	[ɪ, ɪ̣, i, ɪ³, i³]	[ɪ, ɪ̣, i ,ɪ³, i³˒ɝ]
/e/	midfront tense (unrnd)	*bade*	[eɪ]	[eɪ, ȩ-ɪ, aɪ]	[eɪ]
/ɛ/	midfront lax (unrnd)	*bed*	[ɛ]	[ɛ, ȩ-, eᴵ, ejə, ɪ]	[ɛ, ȩ-, eᴵ, ejə, ɪ]
/æ/	lowfront (lax) (unrnd)	*bad*	[æ]	[æ, æ³]	[æ, æ³, ɛ]
/ʌ, ə/[b]	midcentral (lax) (unrnd)	*bud*	[ʌ, ə]	[ʌ, ə]	[ʌ-, ə]
/u/	highback tense (rnd)	*boot*	[u]	[u, u̜, ʉ, y]	[u]
/ʊ/	highback lax (rnd)	*book*	[ʊ]	[ʊ, ʊᴵ, ʋ]	[ʊ, ʊᴵ]
/o/	upper midback (tense) (rnd)	*boat*	[o͜u]	[o͜u, ǫ͜u, ə͜u]	[o͜u]
/ɔ/	lower midback (tense) (rnd)	*bought*	[ɔ,a]	[ɔ, ɔ°, o͜u]	[ɔ, ɔ°, o͜u]
/ɑ/	lowback (tense) (unrnd)	*dot*	[ɑ]	[ɑ]	[ɑ]
/ɝ, ɚ/[b]	(midcentral) rhotic (part. rnd)	*bird*	[ɝ, ɚ]	[ɝ,ɚ]	[ɝ, ɚ, ə, ʊ]
Diphthongs:[c]					
/a͜ɪ/	lowback to highfront	*bye*	[a͜ɪ]	[aː]	[aː, a͜ɪ]
/a͜ʊ/	lowback to highback	*how*	[a͜ʊ]	[a͜ʊ, æ͜ʊ, ajʊ]	[a͜ʊ, a]
/ɔ͜ɪ/	midback to highfront	*boy*	[ɔ͜ɪ]	[ɔ͜ɪ, ɔ͜ə, ɔ, owi]	[ɔ͜ɪ, ɔ͜ə, ɔ]
/ɪ͜ɚ/	highfront to rhotic	*ear*	[ɪ͜ɚ]	[ɪ͜ɚ, i͜ɚ, ijɚ]	[ɪ͜ɚ, i͜ɚ, ɝ, ɪ͜ɚ³, ɝ³]
/ɛ͜ɚ/	midfront to rhotic	*air*	[ɛ͜ɚ]	[ɛ͜ɚ, e͜ɚ, ejɚ]	[ɛ͜ɚ, e͜ɚ, ɝ, ɛ͜ɚ³, ɝ³]
/o͜ɚ/	midback to rhotic	*oar*	[o͜ɚ, ɔ͜ɚ]	[o͜ɚ, ɔ͜ɚ, ɑ͜ɚ]	[o͜ɚ, o͜ə, o͜u, ɔ͜ɚ, ɑ͜ɚ]
/ɑ͜ɚ/	lowback to rhotic	*are*	[ɑ͜ɚ]	[ɑ͜ɚ]	[ɑ͜ɚ, ɑ, ɔ]

Notes: [a]Terms in parentheses are redundant for a unique description of a phoneme (that is, a description distinguishing that phoneme from all other vowel phonemes in the language). [b]Where two phonemic symbols are given, the first is used in stressed syllables and the second in unstressed syllables. [c]Only phonemic diphthongs (which contrast phonemically with nondipthongized counterparts) are included here.

(SWVE), and African American Vernacular English (AAVE) (Pollock and Berni, 2001; Pollock and Meredith, in press; Wolfram and Shilling-Estes, 1998).

It is important to note that not all of the variants listed in Table 3-2 are acceptable in all instances. In some cases the variants are contextually conditioned. [ɪ] for /ɛ/, [ɛ] for /æ/, and [oʊ] for /ɔ/ are only acceptable when they precede nasal consonants (such as [pɪn] for *pen*, [hɛm] for *ham*, [oʊn] for *on*). Similarly, [ɔ] for /ɔɪ/ is allowed only before /l/ (such as [ɔl] for *oil*). In addition, individual speakers may not use all the features characteristic of their dialect, and frequently vary their usage according to factors such as the formality of the situation and the speech patterns of the listener (Wolfram and Schilling-Estes, 1998).

Many of the productions in the SWVE column are the result of what Labov (1991; 1994) has termed the southern vowel shift. In this shift, peripheral (or tense) vowels are moving lower and more central in the vowel space, while nonperipheral (or lax) vowels are rising. The onset of /eɪ/ may be lower than that of /ɛ/, and in extreme cases lower than [æ]. However, because the offglide of /eɪ/ is still a highfront vowel, the resulting vowel is perceptually close to ISE /aɪ/. At the same time, the lax vowels /ɪ/ and /ɛ/ are often raised toward [i] and [e], respectively.

In addition, back tense vowels are shifting forward in SWVE (such as /u/ is [ʉ] or [ʉ], and in extreme cases, [y]). As a result of these shifts, the same number of vowel contrasts is maintained (/e/ and /ɛ/ do not merge, but their nuclei trade places; /u/ is still distinct from /i/ by lip rounding). However, the traditional categorization of vowels according to height and frontness dimensions may not be appropriate for SWVE speakers.

As can be seen in Table 3-2, AAVE shares many of the same vowel representations as SWVE. In both dialects, some front lax vowels tend to be raised and some produced with an offglide. These productions are typically referred to as the *southern drawl* (Feagin, 1987). Similarly, /ɔ/ is produced with an upglide, typically transcribed as [ɔ°]. Diphthongs, especially /aɪ/, tend to be monophthongized but maintain length ([aː]).

However, AAVE also differs from SWVE in many important ways. Some differences are in the extent to which a feature is applied. AAVE does not monophthongize /aɪ/ before voiceless consonants (such as [raːd] for *ride*, but [raɪt] for *right*), but many varieties of SWVE do so in all contexts (Bailey and Thomas, 1998; Wolfram, 1994). It has also been suggested (Bailey and Thomas, 1998; Labov, 1994) that southern AAVE speakers are not participating in some aspects of the southern vowel shift, just as African Americans in northern regions are not participating in the northern cities vowel shift. Front tense vowels are not lowered, and most AAVE speakers produce fully backed back vowels as in ISE.

Finally, there are some vowel changes in AAVE that are not apparent in either SWVE or ISE. These include raised /æ/ before nasals (such as [hɛm] for *ham*) and raised and backed /ʌ/ (such as [mʌd] for *mud*) (Bailey and Thomas, 1998).

In addition, although historically both SWVE and AAVE were *r-less* (that is, lacking rhotic vowels and diphthongs), there has been a dramatic increase in the use of vocalic and postvocalic /r/ in both dialects since the 1940s (Bailey, 1993; Feagin, 1990). In the Memphis area, the change to an *r-full* dialect is essentially complete for SWVE speakers (that is, vocalic and postvocalic /r/ are produced in all contexts). However, in Memphis AAVE, the use of rhotic vowels and diphthongs is still highly variable (Pollock and Berni, 1996). This variability is reflected in Table 3-2 in productions such as [ɔə] or [oʊ] for /oɚ/, [ɑ] for /ɑɚ/, and [ə] for /ɚ/, but [ɪɚ] for /ɪɚ/, [ɛɚ] for /ɛɚ/, and [ɝ] for /ɝ/.

We also observed some variations of rhotic vowels and diphthongs in Memphis AAVE that had not been described previously, including the use of a schwa offglide following /ɪɚ/ and /ɛɚ/ (such as [hɪɚᵊ] for *here*, [t͡ʃɛɚᵊ] for *chair*); the reduction or loss of the front vowel in /ɪɚ/ and /ɛɚ/ (such as [ɝ] for *ear*, [hɝ] for *hair*), and combinations of these two features (such as [ɝᵊz] for *ears*, [t͡ʃɝᵊ] for *chair*) (Pollock and Berni, 1996; 1997a).

In addition, /ɪ/ was rhotacized in words with following postvocalic or syllabic /l/ (such as [mɝk] for *milk*, [pɝkl̩] for *pickle*) by many Memphis AAVE speakers (Pollock, Bailey, Berni, et al., 1998).

In summary, there was considerable dialectal variation in the vowels produced by children in the Memphis Vowel Project. Initially, it was important to identify the full range of possible dialect variants for each vowel. The implications of this variation for identifying vowel errors are discussed later. However, first we present a description of our data collection protocol.

Data Collection Protocol

Vowel productions in children's speech have been analyzed using various sources of data, including (but not limited to) continuous speech from a conversational language sample (Gibbon, Shockey, and Reid, 1992), single-word productions elicited from pictures (Penney, Fee, and Dowdle, 1994; Pollock and Keiser, 1990), and imitative productions of vowels in isolation, syllables, or carrier phrases (Peterson and Barney, 1952).

Each method has advantages and disadvantages. Spontaneous language samples provide the best view of the child's typical production patterns, and allow for additional assessment of intelligibility and interaction with other components of the language system. However, certain low frequency vowels (such as /ʊ/ and /ɔɪ/) may not occur a sufficient number of times unless the sample is very large and it is not possible to control factors such as syllable structure, stress, or phonetic environment.

Elicited single-word productions, although not as natural as conversational speech, show what the child is capable of doing on his or her own (that is, without a direct model). A single-word list can be constructed to provide sufficient opportunities to produce each vowel, and, at the same time, control the surrounding phonetic context, syllable structure, and stress pattern. However, a list that controlled all of these factors would be unwieldy, and increases the likelihood that many of the words would be unfamiliar to young children.

Finally, imitative productions in highly controlled contexts provide an opportunity to observe what the child can do under near optimal conditions (that is, directly following an adult model), and allow for the greatest control over contextual factors. Such data offer certain advantages when performing acoustic analyses (such as consistent phonetic environment, reduced influence due to consonant transitions, and other coarticulatory phenomena), but are the least representative of their typical production patterns.

Our protocol attempted to combine a variety of data collection methods, including single-word elicitation, a story-retelling task, and a controlled imitation task. First, 140 single words were elicited from a set of color photographs. In many instances, a single photograph elicited multiple words. For example, one picture showed a set of four colored blocks. This picture was used to elicit the words *blocks, four, blue, red, orange,* and *green.* As a result, many children produced the words in short phrases ("a *glass* with *ice* in it") rather than in isolated citation forms. The stimulus words were selected to provide six to nine opportunities to produce each vowel and diphthong in both monosyllabic and multisyllabic words.

Monosyllabic words included both open syllables (if permissible in English) and closed syllables with a variety of different following consonant types. Words with postvocalic /l/ were avoided, as earlier work (Pollock and Keiser, 1990; Reynolds, 1990) showed that vowels were frequently altered in this context.

Multisyllabic words included opportunities for each vowel to occur in syllables with and without primary stress. For each vowel, at least one word was elicited on two separate occasions to look at intraword variability. Table A-1 in the appendix shows K25's score form for the single-word elicitation task, and includes the complete list of stimulus words arranged by vowel and context (monosyllabic versus multisyllabic, open versus closed syllable).

With the younger children, word familiarity was often problematic. A shorter list of 66 stimulus words (providing three to four opportunities for each vowel), elicited using toys and objects, was used with children under 3 years of age. When a child did not produce a stimulus word spontaneously or following verbal cues (such as "It has stripes and lives in a zoo."), attempts were made to elicit the word through delayed imitation (such as "Look, the *zebra* and the tiger both have stripes. Which one is this?"). Direct imitations were only used as a last resort, and all imitative responses were coded for later analysis.

A story-retelling task was used to obtain vowel productions in connected speech, while still exerting some control over vowel frequency of occurrence. The story was constructed to also provide multiple opportunities for each vowel and diphthong, using many of the same words that were contained in the single-word elicitation task. The story was illustrated with four line drawings, and read to the child by the examiner. The child was then asked to retell the story with the aid of the pictures.

The transcription of K25's story retelling is included in Table A-2. Many children had difficulty with the story-retelling task, and needed repeated prompts to "tell me more." Although K25 produced several short sentences (such as "Tiger's blowing up a balloon." and "Pig ate all of the cake."), further prompting tended to elicit primarily naming or listing responses (such as "a zebra and a cow, " "Deer and Pig," "candles"). As a result, the data collected with this task were not all that different from those obtained in the single-word elicitation task.

Finally, each vowel and diphthong was elicited imitatively in the carrier phrase, "Say [bəh_d] again." This placed each vowel in a relatively neutral context, reducing the influence of consonant transitions, and with a schwa vowel in the preceding and following syllable. A female speaker of Standard American English recorded all target productions using a natural rate and intonation. Children were asked to *copy* what the woman said on the tape.

If children had difficulty imitating the taped productions, the same female speaker provided live models of target productions. Some children had difficulty with the sequencing of syllables within the carrier phrase or with the iambic pattern of [bəh_d]. In these situations, the targets were simplified to, "Say [h_d]." Other children were simply confused by the task, and tended to perseverate on the same vowel over several different target presentations.

Table A-3 shows K25's transcribed productions on the imitation task. In many instances, his vowel errors were the same as those on the single-word elicitation task (such as /eɪ/ → [aɪ], /aʊ/ → [ɔ], /ɝ/ → [ʊ]). But in other cases, the errors were slightly different. For example, /ɔɪ/ was consistently produced as [aɪ] or [ɑɪ] on the word task, but quite differently here. In fact, K25 struggled with the imitation of /bəhɔɪd/, and appeared to be aware that his production was not accurate.

This problem was not unique to K25. Other children also demonstrated different vowel errors on the imitation task. For example, K26 (3 years, 7 months) produced [ɑ] for /eɪ/ consistently on the single-word elicitation and story-retelling tasks. But on the imitative task, /eɪ/ was produced as [ɑɪ]. Apparently, when presented with a direct model, he attended to the diphthongal nature of the target, and did his best to replicate it. Examples such as these (although interesting from the standpoint of children's perceptual and productive abilities) validate concerns about imitative responses. We had initially intended to use these data for acoustic analysis, but decided against it because the productions frequently did not represent the children's typical production patterns.

Definition of Correct Response

One of the most difficult aspects of the present study was developing an objective criterion for determining which productions were correct and which were not. How different from the expected production could a vowel be and still be considered correct? Some vowel errors produced by the children were readily identified as substitutions of one vowel sound for another (such as [aɪ] for /ɔɪ/ in K25's production of *boy*). However, it was less clear how to handle productions transcribed with diacritics (such as K25's production of [bɛ̞-d][1] for *bed*). We considered establishing two categories of errors, minor and major. Minor errors (transcribed with diacritics) would involve slight shifts in vowel productions, similar to what are often referred to as *distortions* in consonant errors. Major errors (transcribed with different base symbols) would include substitutions of one vowel for another or a loss of contrast between two or more vowels.

However, given the fact that diacritics and offglides were used to transcribe both normal dialect variation and minor errors, this was not a reasonable choice. For example, [bɛ̞-d] for *bed* might represent a dialectal production for a SWVE-speaking or AAVE-speaking child, but a minor error for an ISE-speaking child. If all dialect productions were transcribed with diacritics, then another possibility would be to establish a conservative definition of vowel errors. In this definition, the base symbol used to transcribe the child's response must differ from the base symbol in the target. This would exclude both normal dialect variation and minor vowel shifts from the definition of error. However, some dialect variations were also transcribed with different base symbols (such as [oʊn] for *on* or [pɪnsl] for *pencil* in SWVE or AAVE; [ɝ] for *ear* or [foʊ] for *four* in AAVE). As a result, it was necessary for the transcriber to code each vowel as correct [+] or incorrect [-] on an individual (word by word) basis for each child.

In order to do this, first one must identify the dialect spoken by each child. This is not an easy task. You cannot rely on race or ethnicity alone. Not all African Americans speak AAVE, and some non-African Americans do. You also cannot make assumptions about a child's dialect based on their parents' speech patterns. The parents might be ISE speakers, but the children have learned SWVE or AAVE from their peers. Or the parents might be bidialectal (ISE/SWVE or ISE/AAVE) speakers, using ISE in their conversations with the investigator, but speaking primarily SWVE or AAVE with their children at home. Therefore, we found that it was necessary to make this determination based on the overall patterns found in the child's own speech.

Some dialect patterns involved productions that are not similar to common vowel errors in ISE speakers (such as [ɔ°] for /ɔ/ in SWVE and AAVE, [ɝ·ə] for /ɛɚ/ in AAVE). The presence of these types of productions in a child's sample increased the likelihood that they spoke either SWVE or AAVE. However, many of the dialect productions are highly similar in nature to common vowel error patterns, such as lowering and backing of midfront vowels (such as [e̞-ɪ] or [aɪ] for /eɪ/). In such cases, we would also look to see how the child produced /aɪ/ targets. If these were produced as [aː], then most likely the productions were dialectal. However, if the child used [aɪ] for both /eɪ/ and /aɪ/ (that is, with a loss of contrast between the two target sounds), credit was not given for dialect.

Another southern dialect feature, monophthongization of /aɪ/, was also sometimes difficult to differentiate from the common child error pattern of diphthong reduction. In SWVE, monophthongization of /aɪ/ can occur in any phonetic environment. However, /aʊ/ is rarely reduced, and /ɔɪ/ is typically reduced to [ɔ] only before /l/ (although it may be [ɔə] in words such as *boy*).

As mentioned earlier, in AAVE, monophthongization of /aɪ/ does not occur before voiceless consonants. Therefore, across-the-board reduction of /aɪ/ is not typical AAVE. In addition, when /aɪ/ is reduced in either SWVE or AAVE, it is produced as [aː], with a lengthened lowcentral vowel. Productions of [a] (that is, without length maintained) or [ɑː] (that is, fully back low vowel) are not characteristic of either dialect, and were considered errors.

Types of Analyses

Several different types of descriptive analyses were conducted, including measures of vowel production accuracy, inventories of vowels produced, correspondence charts, and error pattern analyses. All of these analyses were based on perceptual phonetic transcriptions. Additional plans have been made for listener ratings of intelligibility and severity and for acoustic analyses. However, the focus of this chapter is on the transcription-based analyses.

Vowel Accuracy Measures

Each vowel was coded by the transcribers as correct or incorrect, after accounting for dialect variation as described previously in the text. From these codes, percent correct values (PVC) were calculated for each individual vowel, for all nonrhotic vowels (PVC-NR), and for all rhotic vowels (PVC-R). The calculations of these measures for K25 are shown in Table A-1. Because the frequency of occurrence of vowels in our elicited word sample was controlled, their distribution was not representative of conversational speech. Therefore, the PVC scores may not provide a good estimate of the impact of a child's vowel errors on their overall intelligibility or severity. A child with errors on primarily low frequency vowels would not be as disadvantaged as a child with the same percentage of errors on high frequency vowels.

Therefore, we have also experimented with a weighted score (PVC-WS), which takes into account each nonrhotic vowel's frequency of occurrence in conversational speech. As an illustration, K25's PVC-WS calculation is included in Table A-1. His PVC-WS of 76% is slightly higher than his PVC-NR of 71%, primarily because of his errors on the lower frequency diphthongs /aʊ/ and /ɔɪ/. In the group data analyzed thus far, 85% of the children's PVC-NR and PVC-WS values were within three points of each other. Only five children (2% of the total sample) had PVC-NR and PVC-WS values that differed by 10 or more points. The greatest difference observed between the two types of scores was 12 points.

Vowel Inventories

Another basic analysis is an inventory of the vowels produced, regardless of whether they are produced correctly or not. Such inventories show the range of vowels produced, and allow for easy identification of vowel errors due to restricted use of the vowel space. In addition to providing basic information about a child's range and frequency of vowel productions, the vowel inventory might have prognostic significance. It has been hypothesized that the presence of a vowel in the phonetic inventory, even if it is not produced correctly, is an indication that the child will show improvement in vowel production without direct intervention (Pollock, 1994).

K25's vowel inventory is shown in Table A-4. He had a full inventory of American English back and central vowels (plus non-American [ɒ]), but with an unusually high proportion of [ɔ] and [ɑ] productions. However, his inventory of front vowels was more limited. Both highfront vowels [i] and [ɪ] were produced, along with a vowel transcribed as [ɪ]. He produced some midfront vowels, but they were frequently modified with lowered or retracted diacritics. There were no occurrences of [æ]. Several diphthongs were produced, including [aɪ], [ɑɪ], [ɑɪ], [eɪ], [ḛ-ɪ], [ɑo], [oʊ], and [ɔə], but not [aʊ] or [ɔɪ]. K25 did not produce any rhotic vowels or diphthongs.

Correspondence Charts

Two types of error analyses were completed for each child. The first was a correspondence chart, which shows each target vowel phoneme and how it was produced. Each target vowel is in a separate box, arranged according to vowel height and frontness, with correct productions (including allophonic and dialectal variations) in the shaded areas and error productions in the non-shaded areas. This form provides a visual representation of the child's vowel system, and works well for substitution errors. It also provides a format for viewing minor shifts in production, which can be placed in the shaded or non-shaded areas depending on the definition of correct response being used.

The vowel correspondence chart for K25 is in Table A-5. There were some minor shifts in vowel production, such as [ɪ] for /ɪ/, [e̞-ɪ] for /eɪ/, and [ɛ̞-] for /ɛ/. They are included in the shaded area here, indicating that for this analysis, such minor shifts were considered "correct". However, there were also numerous substitutions that resulted in an apparent loss of contrast among phonemes. For example, [ɔ] is the predominant vowel produced for the targets /ɔ/, /aʊ/, /ɝ/, /ɪɚ/, /ɛɚ/, /ɔɚ/, and /ɑɚ/, and was also used as an occasional substitution for /ʌ/ and /ʊ/. Similarly, [aɪ] (or [ɑɪ]) is the most frequent production for /aɪ/ and /ɔɪ/ targets, and also used sometimes for /eɪ/ targets. Finally, /ɛ/, /æ/, and /ɑ/ targets are most often produced as [ɑ].

Error Pattern Analyses

Error pattern analyses attempt to provide descriptions of common trends in feature errors (such as lowering, tensing), complexity errors (such as diphthong reduction), or assimilation errors (such as complete or partial vowel harmony) across vowel phonemes. These error pattern categories can often provide a common description for several different errors. A child who produces [i] for /ɪ/ and [u] for /ʊ/ could be said to have an error pattern of tensing that affected high vowels. This would be a more succinct (and more accurate) description than a list of two independent substitution errors. A fairly well defined set of vowel error patterns has been provided in many previous sources (Pollock, 1994; Pollock and Keiser, 1990; Reynolds, 1990; Watson, Bates, Sinclair, and Hewlett, 1994). Although some children show idiosyncratic error patterns, it is becoming clear that some patterns are more common than others. Lowering and backing appear to be much more frequent overall than raising and fronting (Pollock, 1994; Reynolds, 1990). Data from our large group study should help to confirm these trends.

K25's vowel error patterns are described in Table A-6. The assignment of errors to pattern categories was not always straightforward. The [ɪ] for /ɪ/ and [eɪ] for /ɛ/ could be considered instances of either raising or tensing. However, the [ɛ] for /æ/ could only be considered raising. Because the affected vowels were all lax front vowels, the errors might be related. Therefore, they were all assigned to the raising pattern category. The most common error patterns involved lowering, backing, or a combination of lowering and backing. Some of K25's error patterns affected only one target vowel (rounding of /ʌ/, diphthong reduction of /ɔɪ/), making it questionable whether such errors represent underlying error patterns or isolated substitution errors.

Although there appears to be a well-recognized set of vowel error patterns affecting nonrhotic vowels, no comparable set of error patterns is yet available to describe rhotic vowel errors. In our data, we have most frequently observed patterns such as derhotacization (replacement of a rhotic vowel with a nonrhotic vowel, usually a schwa or a back rounded vowel) and rhotic diphthong reduction (loss of the rhotic element of a rhotic diphthong). Another interesting pattern observed was coalescence (replacement of a rhotic diphthong with a single vowel, usually a back rounded vowel). For example, K3 (4 years, 10 months) produced [u] for /ɪɚ/ and [oʊ] for /ɛɚ/, /ɝ/, and /ɔɚ/, maintaining the height of the nonrhotic element and the rounding of the rhotic element. K25's production of [ɔ] for all rhotic vowels and diphthongs might also be viewed as a type of coalescence.

Preliminary Findings

In the following section, preliminary findings from the Memphis Vowel Project are presented. Vowel accuracy data are available for the 283 children described earlier. Because there are still some questions and concerns about the story-retelling tasks and imitation tasks (discussed earlier in the text), the data presented are limited to responses to the single-word elicitation task.

Incidence of Vowel Errors

One of the questions that has not been satisfactorily answered in previous research concerns the incidence of vowel errors, both in children with phonological disorders and in children with normally developing phonology. Given the lack of attention to vowels in child phonology research, it has been suggested (Hargrove, 1982) that vowel errors may be more common than we think, but that clinicians are generally insensitive to them. However, to date there is no large group study designed to address this important question. Previous group studies have often included relatively small groups of children (15 in Pollock and Keiser, 1990; 20 in Reynolds, 1990; 13 in Watson, Bates, Sinclair, and Hewlett, 1994), and sometimes preselected children who exhibited vowel errors (Stoel-Gammon and Herrington, 1990; Watson, Bates, Sinclair, and Hewlett, 1994). In the present study, children in the DP (disordered phonology) group were identified on the basis of their consonant errors alone, and represented a range of severity levels. This was shown in Table 3-1.

Nonrhotic Vowel Errors

In the first set of results, the PVC-NR (percentage of nonrhotic vowels correctly produced) measure was compared across groups according to age and severity level. In these analyses, a conservative definition of *correct* was used in which minor shifts in production (transcribed with diacritics) were considered correct. Generous credit was also given for possible dialect variation in these data. Therefore, it is probable that the current data slightly underestimate the incidence of vowel errors.

Table 3-3 Mean Percent Nonrhotic Vowels Correct (PVC-NR) for NP and DP Groups by Age

Age (in months)	(n)	NP Group PVC-NR Mean	SD	Range	(n)	DP Group PVC-NR Mean	SD	Range
18–23	(10)	82.19	8.30	69–96				
24–29	(18)	92.39	5.49	78–100				
30–35	(21)	93.90	6.39	78–100	(1)	77.78	—	—
36–41	(17)	97.29	3.02	89–100	(2)	97.65	2.21	96–99
42–47	(16)	97.19	2.23	91–100	(16)	88.63	10.75	64–100
48–53	(18)	98.06	2.21	91–100	(19)	93.79	6.72	80–100
54–59	(25)	98.20	1.78	93–100	(29)	95.21	7.63	61–100
60–65	(19)	99.21	0.85	98–100	(23)	96.91	4.11	81–100
66–71	(13)	99.38	0.77	98–100	(21)	97.05	2.75	88–100
72–77	(4)	98.5	1.29	97–100	(8)	97.41	2.72	92–99
78–83	(1)	99.19	—	—	(2)	96.43	5.05	93–100

Table 3-3 shows the mean PVC-NR scores for the NP and DP children by age range. The mean scores for the NP children increased with age, although they hit a ceiling around 36 months of age. However, from 3 to 5 years of age the standard deviations continued to decrease and the low end of the range rose from 89% to 98%. The means for the DP group were consistently lower than those of the NP group at each age level (except at 36 to 41 months, with only two children in the DP group). However, the standard deviations and ranges were much larger, reflecting the fact that many of the DP children had high PVC-NR scores. Age did not appear to be related to vowel accuracy for the DP group.

Looking at the data from another perspective, Table 3-4 shows the number and percentage of children exhibiting nonrhotic vowel errors. Three arbitrary cutoff levels for PVC-NR were used: less than 95%, less than 90%, and less than 85%. NP children were divided into a younger and an older group. One third of those under 3 years of age had PVC-NR scores under 90%, and nearly two thirds had scores under 95%. These data are consistent with previous research indicating that children under 3 years of age have not yet mastered the vowel system (Davis and MacNeilage, 1990; Otomo and Stoel-Gammon, 1992). However, very few of the NP children over 3 years of age exhibited vowel errors. More of the DP children had vowel errors, with 30% having PVC-NR scores under 95%, but only 9% having scores under 85%.

Table 3-4   Percentage of Children Exhibiting Nonrhotic Vowel Errors

PVC-NR	NP Group (< 3 years)	NP Group (≥ 3 years)	DP Group
< 95	31/49 (63%)	5/113 (4%)	37/121 (30%)
< 90	16/49 (33%)	1/113 (1%)	15/121 (12%)
< 85	12/49 (29%)	0/113 (0%)	11/121 (9%)

Table 3-5   Number and Percentage of DP Children with Nonrhotic Vowel Errors by Severity Level (Estimated by PCC)

Severity Level	PVC-NR < 95 #	%	PVC-NR < 90 #	%	PVC-NR < 85 #	%
Borderline/Normal (PCC ≥ 85%)	2/29	7%	0/29	0%	0/29	0%
Mild/Moderate (PCC 66–84%)	12/44	27%	4/44	9%	2/44	5%
Moderate/Severe (PCC 50–65%)	13/34	38%	4/34	12%	2/34	6%
Severe (PCC < 50%)	9/14	64%	7/14	50%	7/14	50%

The most interesting data, however, are shown in Table 3-5. These data demonstrate an increased incidence of vowel errors (measured by PVC-NR) with increased severity of consonant errors (estimated by PCC). Using the highest cutoff (PVC-NR < 95%), only two (or 7%) of the children in the borderline/normal subgroup had vowel errors, as compared to 64% of the children in the severe subgroup. Even in the mild/moderate and moderate/severe groups, a substantial proportion of children exhibited vowel errors (27% and 38%, respectively). However, as the PVC-NR cutoff is lowered to less than 85%, the percentage of children with vowel errors drops dramatically (from 0% to 6%) for all the but the most severe group. Half (50%) of the children in the severe group had PVC-NR scores under 85%.

Two words of caution are necessary in interpreting these findings. First, it is important to note that although a large percentage of children with severe consonant errors had substantial vowel errors, there are still many children with severe consonant errors (36%) who do not exhibit vowel errors (that is, PVC-NR > 95%). In other words, having a severe phonological disorder does not automatically mean that a child will have vowel errors. However, there does appear to be a much greater incidence of vowel errors in this group. Second, these preliminary data should be viewed cautiously given the relatively smaller number of children in the severe group (14) as compared to the other groups. When the complete set of data are available, there will be a more even distribution of DP children across severity levels.

Rhotic Vowel Errors

As might be expected given the age of the children in this study, rhotic vowels and diphthongs were produced with low accuracy by children in both the NP and DP groups. Table 3-6 shows the mean percent correct for rhotic vowels (PVC-R) by age range for both groups. Although there was an increase in mean scores for the NP children from 18 to 36 months of age, the means fluctuated between 79% and 90% for children over 3 years of age. Standard deviations were large (13–42%), and the ranges of scores extreme (0–100% at many age levels). Children in the DP group also showed considerable variation in their PVC-R scores, with means consistently lower than those of the NP group, but fluctuating between 29% and 68% with no apparent relationship to age. As with the NP children, the standard deviations were very large and the ranges extreme.

Considerable dialect variation was seen in the use of rhotic vowels and diphthongs. Using a subset of data from the NP children, Pollock and Berni (1997b) compared the productions of rhotic vowels and diphthongs of 34 African American and 34 European American children from age 3 years, 6 months to 6 years to those of adult speakers. The African American children showed variable usage consistent with adult AAVE speakers from Memphis. Rhotic vowels were most often produced in the stressed vocalic context (/ɝ/) and following front vowels (/ɪɚ/ and /ɛɚ/). They were most likely to be absent in unstressed syllables (/ɚ/) and following back rounded vowels (/ɔɚ/).

Table 3-6   Mean Percent Rhotic Vowels Correct (PVC-R) for NP and DP Groups by Age

Age (in months)	(n)	NP Group PVC-R Mean	SD	Range	(n)	DP Group PVC-R Mean	SD	Range
18–23	(10)	23.52	24.14	0–70				
24–29	(18)	37.54	30.65	0–87				
30–35	(21)	62.52	30.02	0–100	(1)	0.00	—	—
36–41	(17)	79.24	22.38	4–100	(2)	68.00	1.41	67–69
42–47	(16)	76.50	29.84	4–100	(16)	39.94	40.14	0–86
48–53	(18)	90.11	13.91	37–100	(19)	66.68	37.64	0–100
54–59	(25)	86.80	26.27	0–100	(29)	38.79	39.25	0–100
60–65	(19)	88.21	22.27	0–100	(23)	29.17	39.56	0–100
66–71	(13)	80.31	35.11	0–100	(21)	54.10	43.35	0–100
72–83	(5)	77.20	42.20	2–100	(10)	36.90	47.12	0–100

The absence of rhotic vowels in these environments was considered dialectal and counted as correct in the PVC-R analyses. As a result, the African American children had relatively high PVC-R scores. In contrast, the European American children exhibited an all-or-none pattern of rhotic vowel usage. Many had very high PVC-R scores (80–100%), but approximately 30% had PVC-R scores under 20%. Very few European American children had scores between 20% and 80%.

Specific Vowels in Error

Another question addressed in the present study was the extent to which the vowel errors of phonologically disordered children resembled those of younger, normally developing children. As an initial step towards answering this question, Table 3-7 compares the specific vowels in error for DP children who had PVC scores of less than 95% and NP children under age 3 years. These subgroups were selected because they exhibited the most vowel errors. For each group, the number and percentage of children who showed difficulty (that is, <80% correct) with individual vowel targets are displayed.

Table 3-7   Number (and Percentage) of Children with Less Than 80% Correct on Individual Vowel Targets for Two Subgroups of Children

Vowel	PD Group (with PVC-NR < 95) n = 37	NP Group (< 3 years) (n = 49)
/i/	0 (0%)	6 (12%)
/ɪ/	2 (5%)	4 (8%)
/eɪ/	5 (14%)	14 (29%)
/ɛ/	8 (22%)	8 (16%)
/æ/	9 (24%)	14 (29%)
/u/	1 (3%)	1 (2%)
/ʊ/	10 (27%)	15 (31%)
/oʊ/	3 (8%)	8 (16%)
/ɔ/	4 (11%)	4 (8%)
/ɑ/	7 (19%)	7 (14%)
/ʌ, ə/	12 (32%)	6 (12%)
/aɪ/	1 (3%)	3 (6%)
/aʊ/	8 (22%)	14 (29%)
/ɔɪ/	7 (19%)	21 (43%)

For the most part, both groups had difficulty with the same vowel targets. These included the midfront and lowfront vowels (/eɪ/, /ɛ/, and /æ/), diphthongs (/aʊ/ and /ɔɪ/), high back lax /ʊ/, low back /ɑ/, and central /ʌ, ə/. Lowering and backing errors on mid and front low vowels have been noted in many previous studies, as have diphthong reduction errors (Pollock and Keiser, 1990; Reynolds, 1990; Watson, Bates, Sinclair, and Hewlett, 1994). In the present study, however, the diphthong /aɪ/ was rarely in error, presumably because monophthongization of /aɪ/ is an acceptable variant in the two major dialects spoken by the participants.

The relatively high number of children with errors on /ɑ/ was somewhat unexpected. The majority of errors on /ɑ/ involved rounding (such as [ɔ] or [ɒ]). It is possible that the choice of stimulus words contributed to the high rate of rounding on /ɑ/. Although attempts were made to provide a variety of different following consonant contexts, no serious attempts were made to control preceding consonant environment. In retrospect, it was noted that five of the seven /ɑ/ target words contain a preceding labial consonant. It is possible that rounding of /ɑ/ following labials is dialectally appropriate in Memphis and that we have incorrectly categorized these productions as errors. However, we did not observe frequent instances of [ɔ] for /ɑ/ in our NP children or in adult participants in related studies. It is more likely that the preceding bilabial environment created a facilitative context for rounding, and that the accidental *loading* of preceding labial consonants elevated the percentage of errors on this vowel.

Although there are some differences between the two groups in terms of specific vowels in error (such as the NP children also had errors on /i/ and /oʊ/), there are many similarities. Additional analyses are planned to compare the types of substitutions and vowel error patterns observed in these two subgroups.

Conclusion

The identification of vowel errors in children is complicated by many factors, including substantial dialect variation and methodological issues, some of which were discussed in this chapter. However, there is a growing body of literature (including the other chapters in this book) suggesting that vowel errors are of great theoretical and clinical interest. Although the data presented were preliminary in nature, they do allow us to draw some conclusions about the nature and significance of vowel errors. The finding that vowel errors are most likely to occur in children with severe phonological disorders should not be surprising. However, the implications for clinical practice are that all children with severe phonological disorders should be screened for vowel errors.

Much work still needs to be done to complete the original goals of the Memphis Vowel Project. First, analyses of error types (substitutions and error patterns) must be completed. Further investigation of the relationship between consonant errors and vowel errors is also necessary. Many questions concerning the clinical significance of vowel errors still remain unanswered, including the need for direct intervention for vowel errors. Eight of the PD children with vowel errors were followed longitudinally and retested approximately every 6 months. Although most improved in their vowel production accuracy over time (with direct intervention for consonant errors only), several continued to exhibit vowel errors as many as 18 months after their initial testing. Further analysis of these longitudinal data is necessary to see if it is possible to predict which children are most likely to improve without direct intervention.

Acknowledgments

The author wishes to thank the numerous research associates and graduate assistants who participated in the data collection phase of this project, and to acknowledge the substantial contributions of Kristi Estes and Mary Berni in the development and implementation of data transcription and analysis procedures. The research presented in this chapter was supported by the National Institute on Deafness and other Communication Disorders Grant No. DC-01424.

Note

1. Instances where symbols need either a raising or lowering diacritic and a retraction diacritic, the latter is placed after the symbol to avoid a clutter of unreadable signs.

APPENDIX

Case Example: K25

K25 was a European American boy with a mild/moderate phonological disorder, including vowel errors. His receptive and expressive language and nonverbal cognitive skills were at or above age level. At the time of his first participation in the Memphis Vowel Project, he was 3 years, 10 months of age. He came from a working-class family. Both parents were born and raised in the Memphis area and had completed high school. When first tested, he had been receiving speech therapy (30 minutes per week) for 2 months at a local public school. His percent consonants correct (PCC) on the single-word elicitation task was 75%. His primary consonant problems involved sibilants, liquids, and glides. His clinician also noted that he had many vowel errors, which she believed significantly reduced his intelligibility.

Table A-1 shows K25's scores (PVC-NR, PVC-WS, and PVC-R) on the single-word elicitation task. Table A-2 and Table A-3 include phonetic transcriptions of his responses to the story-retelling task and the imitation task, respectively. His vowel errors were consistent across all three tasks. The analyses in the following figures are based on productions from the single-word task only.

K25's vowel inventory, vowel correspondence chart, and error pattern analysis are included in Table A-4, Table A-5, and Table A-6, respectively. Although some of K25's vowel productions could represent SWVE dialect features (such as the lowering and backing of /eɪ/, raising of /ɪ/), the majority of errors do not reflect dialectal variation (such as [ɑ] for /ɛ/ and /æ/, [ɔ] for /ʌ/ and /aʊ/, [aɪ] for /ɔɪ/). In addition, his productions show little evidence of other anticipated SWVE features (such as monophthongal /aɪ/, fronted /u/, lengthened lax vowels with offglides). Therefore, we concluded that he was not a typical SWVE speaker, and that all of these productions represented vowel errors.

K25 continued to receive speech therapy at the public school, where his primary intervention targets were consonants. K25 was re-evaluated three times at approximately 5-month intervals. At the time of his last evaluation at 5 years, 3 months, his percent consonants correct (PCC) was 92%, percent nonrhotic vowels correct (PVC-NR) was 99%, weighted score (PVC-WS) was 100%, and percent rhotic vowels correct (PVC-R) was 2%. His remaining errors, as reflected in his PCC and PVC-R scores, were predominantly on /r/ and rhotic vowels and diphthongs.

Table A-1 Score Form for Single-Word Elicitation Task
Name: K25 (3 years, 10 months)

Nonrhotic Vowels and Diphthongs

	Monosyllabic		Multisyllabic		Number Correct/Total	Percent Correct	X Freq	Weighted Score
	Open Syllable	Closed Syllable	Primary Stress	Nonprimary Stress				
/i/	three [+] [+] key [+] [+]	green [+] [+] eat [+] [+]	zebra [+] peanuts [+]	cookies [+] Ernie [+] party [+]	9/9	100	.0951	9.51
/ɪ/		in [+] [+] pig [+] ~~drink~~ [ɪ]	pickle [+] zipper [+]	sandwich [+] pudding [+] earring [+]	~~8~~ 7/7	100	.1113	11.13
/e/	play [+] [+] sleigh [+]	cake [ɑɪ] [ɑɪ] vase [+]	table [ɑɪ] radio [aɪ] reindeer [+]	birthday [+] airplane [+]	6/9	67	.0415	2.77
/ɛ/		red [ɑ] [ɑ] nest [+] bed [ɑ]	teddy bear [eɪ] feather [+] pencil [+]		3/6	50	.0734	3.67
/æ/		cat [ɑ] glass [ɑ] hat [ɑ] [ɑ]	apple [ɑ] bathroom [ɛ] sandwich [ɑ] valentine [ɑ] Santa Claus [ɑ]	snowman [ɑ]	0/9	0	.0809	0.00
/u/	two [+] [+] blue [+] shoe [+]	juice [+] spoon [+]	balloons [+] Rudolph [+]	bathroom [+]	8/8	100	.0303	3.03

Vowel						Accuracy	%		
/ʊ/		book [ɔ] good [+] foot [+]	football [+] cookies [+] pudding [+]			5/6	83	.0104	0.87
/o/	bow [+] blow [+] [+]	coke [aʊ] nose [+] [+]	donut [+] snowman [+]	radio [+] Cheerios [+]		7/8	88	.0509	4.45
/ɔ/	straw [+] [+] saw [+]	dog [+] on [+] off [+]	strawberries [+]	football [+] Santa Claus [+]		8/8	100	.0359	3.59
/a/		box [+] blocks [+] sock [+]	popcorn [+] Poptart [+]	toy box [+] Rudolph [+]		7/7	100	.0383	3.83
/ʌ,ə/		one [ɔ] [+] brush [+] thumb [+] (suck) [ɔ] [ɔ]	bubbles [+] under [+]	zebra [+] peanuts [+] donut [+] balloons [∅]		~~9~~ 7.5/10.0	75	.3186	23.90
/aɪ/	pie [+] fly [+]	knife [+] ice [+] eyes [+]	tiger [+] outside [+]	valentine [+]		8/8	100	.0927	9.27
/aʊ/	cow [ɔ]	couch [ɔ] mouth [ʌ] [ɔ]	cowboy [a] flowers [ɔ]	outside [ɔ]		0/6	0	.0192	0.00
/ɔɪ/	boy [aɪ] [aʊ] toy [aɪ] [aɪ]	toys [aɪ] ~~drink~~ [I]	toy box [aɪ]	cowboy [aʊ]		~~6~~ 0.5	0	.0015	0.00
				PVC-NR		75.5/107.0	=70.56	**PVC-WS**	=76.02

Table A-1   *Continued*

Rhotic Vowels and Diphthongs

	Monosyllabic		Multisyllabic		Number Correct/Total	Percent Correct
	Open Syllable	Closed Syllable	Primary Stress	Nonprimary Stress		
/ɝ,ɚ/	her [ɔ] stir [ʊ]	bird [ʊ] [ɔ] Bert [ɔ]	birthday [ɔ] Ernie [ɔ]	feather [ɔ] farmer [ɔ] tiger [ɔ] under [ɔ] zipper [ɔ] flowers [ʊ] quarter [ʊ]	0/13	0
/ɪɚ/	ear [ɔ] [ɔ] deer [ɔ]	ears [ɔ] beard [ɔ]	earring [ɔ] Cheerios [ʌ]	reindeer [ɔ]	0/7	0
/ɛɚ/	chair [ɔ] hair [ɔ] [ɔ]	stairs [ɔ] scared [ɔ]	carrot [ɔ] airplane [ɔ]	teddy bear [oʊ] strawberries [ʊ]	0/8	0
/ɔɚ/	four [ɔɚ] [ɔ] door [ɔ]	horse [ɔɚ] fork [ɔ]	orange [ɔɚ] [ɔ] quarter [ɔ]	popcorn [ɔ]	0/7	0
/ɑɚ/	star [ɔ] car [ɒ] [ɒ]	barn [ɑɚ] heart [ɔ] [ɔ]	farmer [ɔ] party [ɑɚ]	Poptart [ɔ]	0/7	0
			PVC-R		0/42	0

Note: Table A-1 shows all intended stimulus words. Words not produced by the child in this example are crossed out. Additional words produced by the child and included for scoring are shown in parentheses in the appropriate row and column. In both cases, the total number of opportunities is adjusted accordingly. The null symbol [Ø] indicates that the vowel was omitted and could only occur in multisyllabic words.

Table A2 Transcription   of   Story-Retelling   Task
Name: K25 (3 years, 10 months)

Tiger's Birthday Party

Picture 1

Model: It was *__Tiger__*'s *__birthday__*. He was **four years** old. **Zebra** and **Cow** were **blow**ing up **balloons** for the *__party__*.

Child: Tiger is having a balloon. Tiger's blowing up a balloon. A zebra and a cow.

[taɪgʊ ɪz havn̩ ə buːn | taɪgʊz boʊin əpə buːn | ə ʑibə anə kɔː]

Picture 2

Model: **Dog** *brought* a **toy box** with **presents in** it. **One box** had a **big green bow** *on* top. **Tiger** got a **teddy bear**, **football**, **bubbles**, and a **blue car**.

Child: Doggy brought a XX box. Yeah, and one box had a big bow on. Bubbles…a football(?)…, blue car…, and a…a teddy bear.

[dɔgi bɔ ə fa baks | jʌ | an jʌn baks hadə buːɪg bɔːn | bʌboʊz | ə jʌf | bʊ kɔ | anʌ | ə teɪbʊ]

Picture 3

Model: *__Tiger__* **heard** someone **knock**ing *on* the **door**. It was **Deer** and *__Pig__*. They *brought* a *__birthday__* *__cake__*. It had **candles** *on* it for *__Tiger__* to *__blow__* out.

Child: Uh…, a knock on the door. Deer (?) and Pig. Candles.

[ʌː | ə nak ɔn də dɔː | dɔhɔ an piː | kalonəz]

Picture 4

Model: While the others **play**ed **outside**, *__Pig__* ate up the leftover *__cake__*. And he found some **apple juice** to **drink**. It was a **good** *__party__*.

Child: Pig. Yeah. Everybody…uh…played outside. He ate…, Pig ate all of the cake. XXXX good.

[pɪʔg | jaɪʔ | ʌvibəi ʌ pe̞ɪ ətsaɪd | hi e̞ɪt | pɪg e̞ɪt ɔʔɔ də ke̞ɪk | an nəmɔ | guːd]

Note: Keyword targets are in bold. Underlined keywords are also included on the single-word elicitation task. Keywords elicited more than once are italicized.

Table A-3 Transcription of Imitation Task
Name: K25 (3 years, 10 months)

Model:	Child:
"Say /bəheɪd/ again."	[haɪ]
"Say /bəhʌd/ again."	[bəhɑːd]
"Say /bəhiːd/ again."	[bəhiːd]
"Say /bəhɝd/ again."	[bəhʊːn]
"Say /bəhaɪd/ again."	[bəhaɪn]
"Say /bəhɑd/ again."	[bəhɑːn]
"Say /bəhoʊd/ again."	[bəhoʊn]
"Say /bəhɪd/ again."	[bəhɪd]
"Say /bəhʊd/ again."	[bəhʊːn]
"Say /bəhɔɪd/ again."	[bəhaʊd], [bəhəɛod]
"Say /bəhɛd/ again."	[bəhʌd]
"Say /bəhuːd/ again."	[bəhuːd]
"Say /bəhɔd/ again."	[bəhɔːd]
"Say /bəhaʊd/ again."	[bəhɔːd], [bɪhəɔn]
"Say /bəhæd/ again."	[bəhɔːd]

Table A-4 Vowel Inventory
Name: K25 (3 years, 10 months)

Monophthongs:

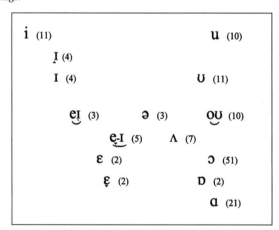

Diphthongs (in addition to [eɪ] and [oʊ], whose onsets are shown above):

aɪ (12)	ɔə (5)
ɑɪ (6)	ɑo (1)
ɑi (1)	ɑə (1)

Table A-5   Vowel Correspondence Chart
               Name: K25 (3 years, 10 months)

Nonrhotic Monophthongs:

i-11		u-10
ɪ-4 ḭ-4		ʊ-6
		ɔ-1
eɪ-2 e̞-ɪ-5	ʌ-5 ə-3	oʊ-9
ɑɪ-3 ɑ̯i-1	ɔ-3	ɑo-1
ɛ-1 ɛ̞-2		ɔ-9
ɑ-3 eɪ-1		
æ-0		ɑ-8
ɑ-9 ɛ-1		

Nonrhotic Diphthongs:

aɪ-9	aʊ-0 ɔ-5 ʌ-1 ɑ-1	ɔɪ-0 aɪ-3 ɑɪ-3

Rhotic Vowel and Diphthongs:

ɪɚ-0 ɔ-7 ʌ-1		
ɛɚ-0 ɔ-7 oʊ-1 ʊ-1	ɝ-0 ɚ-0 ɔ-10 ʊ-4	ɔɚ-0 ɔ-5 oə-4
		ɑɚ-0 ɔ-4 ɒ-2 ɔə-1 ɑə-1

Table A-6   Vowel Error Pattern Analysis
Name: K25 (3 years, 10 months)

Error Pattern	Examples	No. Occ.	Summary
Raising	/ɪ/ → [ɪ]	4	Affects lax front vowels (6/25 times)
	/ɛ/ → [eɪ]	1	
	/æ/ → [ɛ]	1	
Lowering	/eɪ/ → [e̞-ɪ], [ɑɪ], [ɑi]	9	Affects mostly midfront vowels, where it is always accompanied by backing (14/17 times)
	/ɛ/ → [ɛ̞-], [ɑ]	5	
	/ʊ/ → [ɔ]	1	
	/oʊ/ → [ɑo]	1	Affects diphthongs with rounded first element, accompanied by unrounding (7/16 times)
	/ɔɪ/ → [ɑɪ], [ɑɪ]	6	
Fronting	none		
Backing	/eɪ/ → [e̞-ɪ], [ɑɪ], [ɑi]	9	Affects all midfront and lowfront vowels (24/27 times); in midfront vowels, always accompanied by lowering
	/ɛ/ → [ɛ̞-], [ɑ]	5	
	/æ/ → [ɑ]	10	
Centralization	none		
Tensing	none		But some raising errors might also be considered tensing
Laxing	none		
Rounding	/ʌ/ → [ɔ]	3	Only affects /ʌ/ (3/5 times)
Unrounding	/ɔɪ/ → [ɑɪ], [ɑɪ]	6	
	/oʊ/ → [ɑo]	1	
Diphthong Reduction	/aʊ/ → [ɔ], [ɑ], [ʌ]	7	Only affects /aʊ/ (7/7 times); often results in coalescence of [a] and [ʊ] into [ɔ]
Diphthongization	none		
Derhotacization	/ɝ/ → [ɔ], [ʊ]	48	Affects all rhotic vowels and diphthongs (48/48 times); in addition to loss of rhotic vowel, initial non-rhotic element also modified by various error types (such as lowering, coalescence)
	/ɪɚ/ → [ɔ], [ʌ]		
	/ɛɚ/ → [ɔ], [ʊ], [oʊ]		
	/ɔɚ/ → [ɔ], [ɔə]		
	/ɑɚ/ → [ɔ], [ɒ], [ɔə], [ɑə]		

References

Arthur, G. (1969). The Arthur adaptation of the Leiter International Performance Scale. Washington, D.C.: Psychological Service Center.

Bailey, G. (1993). A perspective on African American English. In D. Preston (Ed.), American dialect research (pp. 287–318). Amsterdam: John Benjamins.

Bailey, G., and Thomas, E. (1998). Some aspects of African American Vernacular English phonology. In S. Mufwene, J. Rickford, G. Bailey, and J. Baugh (Eds.), African American English: Structure, history, and use (pp. 85–109). London: Routledge.

Burgemeister, B., Blum, L., and Lorge, I. (1972). Columbia Mental Maturity Scale (3rd ed.). New York: Psychological Corporation.

Davis, B., and MacNeilage, P. (1990). Acquisition of correct vowel production: A quantitative case study. Journal of Speech and Hearing Research, 33, 16–27.

Edwards, H. (1997). Applied phonetics: The sounds of American English. San Diego: Singular.

Feagin, C. (1987). A closer look at the southern drawl: Variation taken to extremes. In K. M. Denning, S. Inkelas, F. C. McNair-Knox, and J. R. Rickford (Eds.), Variation in language: NWAVE-XV at Stanford (Proceedings of the Fifteenth Annual Conference on New Ways of Analyzing Variation) (pp. 137–150). Stanford: Stanford University.

Feagin, C. (1990). The dynamics of a sound change in southern states English: From r-less to r-full in three generations. In J. A. Edmondson, C. Feagin, and P. Mühläusler (Eds.), Development and diversity: Language variation across time and space. A Festschrift for Charles-James N. Bailey (pp. 129–146). Arlington, Tex.: SIL and University of Texas.

Gibbon, F., Shockey, L., and Reid, J. (1992). Description and treatment of abnormal vowels in a phonologically disordered child. Child Language Teaching and Therapy, 8, 30–59.

Hargrove, P. (1982). Misarticulated vowels: A case study. Language, Speech, and Hearing Services in Schools, 13, 86–95.

Labov, W. (1991). The three dialects of English. In P. Eckert (Ed.), New ways of analyzing sound change (pp.1–44). New York: Academic.

Labov, W. (1994). Principles of linguistic change: Internal factors. Cambridge, Mass.: Blackwell.

Ladefoged, P. (1993). A course in phonetics (3rd ed.). New York: Harcourt, Brace, Jovanovich.

Ladefoged, P. (2000). Vowels and consonants. Malden, Mass.: Blackwell.

Mackay, I. (1987). Phonetics: The science of speech production (2nd ed.). Boston: Little, Brown.

Otomo, K., and Stoel-Gammon, C. (1992). The acquisition of unrounded vowels in English. Journal of Speech and Hearing Research, 35, 604–616.

Penney, G., Fee, E. J., and Dowdle, C. (1994). Vowel assessment and remediation: A case study. Child Language Teaching and Therapy, 10, 47–66.

Peterson, G., and Barney, H. (1952). Control methods used in a study of the vowels. Journal of the Acoustical Society of America, 24, 175–184.

Pollock, K. E. (1994). Assessment and remediation of vowel misarticulations. Clinics in Communication Disorders, 4, 23–37.

Pollock, K. E., Bailey, G., Berni, M. C., et al. (1998). Phonological characteristics of African American Vernacular English: An updated checklist. Poster presentation at the annual convention of the American Speech-Language-Hearing Association, San Antonio, Tex. (Also available at http://www.ausp.memphis.edu/phonology)

Pollock, K. E., and Berni, M. C. (1996). Vocalic and postvocalic /r/ in African American Memphians. Paper presented at the New Ways of Analyzing Variation in English (NWAVE) meeting, Las Vegas, Nev.

Pollock, K. E., and Berni, M. C. (1997a). Variation in vocalic and postvocalic /r/ in AAVE. Presented at the annual convention of the American Speech-Language-Hearing Association, Boston, Mass.

Pollock, K. E., and Berni, M. C. (1997b). Acquisition of /r/ by African American and European American children. Presented at the annual convention of the American Speech-Language-Hearing Association, Boston, Mass.

Pollock, K. E., and Berni, M. C. (2001). Transcription of vowels. Topics in Language Disorders, 21(4), 22–40.

Pollock, K. E, and Keiser, N. (1990). An examination of vowel errors in phonologically disordered children. Clinical Linguistics and Phonetics, 4, 161–178.

Pollock, K. E., and Meredith, L. H. (in press). Phonetic transcription of African American Vernacular English. Communication Disorders Quarterly.

Pollock, K. E., and Swanson, L. (1986). Analysis of vowel errors in a disordered child during training. Presented to the American Speech-Language-Hearing Association, Detroit, Mich.

Reynolds, J. (1990). Abnormal vowel patterns in phonological disorder: Some data and a hypothesis. British Journal of Disorders of Communication, 25, 115–148.

Shriberg, L. D., and Kent, R. D. (1995). Clinical phonetics (2nd ed.). Boston: Allyn and Bacon.

Shriberg, L., and Kwiatkowski, J. (1982). Phonological disorders III: A procedure for assessing severity of involvement. Journal of Speech and Hearing Disorders, 47, 256–270.

Small, L. (1999). Fundamentals of phonetics: A practical guide for students. Boston: Allyn and Bacon.

Stoel-Gammon, C., and Herrington, P. (1990). Vowel systems of normally developing and phonologically disordered children. Clinical Linguistics and Phonetics, 4, 145–160.

Watson, J. M. M., Bates, S. A. R., Sinclair, A. E., and Hewlett, N. R. F. (1994). Unusual vowel systems in some Edinburgh children with phonological disorder. Poster presentation at the annual convention of the American Speech-Language-Hearing Association, New Orleans.

Wolfram, W. (1994). The phonology of a sociocultural variety: The case of African American Vernacular English. In J. Bernthal and N. Bankson (Eds.), Child phonology: Characteristics, assessment, and intervention with special populations (pp. 227–244). New York: Thieme.

Wolfram, W., and Schilling-Estes, N. (1998). American English: Dialects and variation. Oxford: Blackwell.

Zimmerman, I. L., Steiner, V., and Pond, R. (1992). Preschool Language Scale–3. San Antonio, Tex.: Psychological Corporation.

4

Recurring Patterns and Idiosyncratic Systems in Some English Children with Vowel Disorders

Joseph Reynolds

This chapter presents some of the data and analyses from a study originally undertaken in the 1980s, and summarized previously elsewhere (Reynolds, 1990). Some proposals are also made regarding how this data might be reconsidered in the light of more recent approaches to phonological analysis.

The original project arose from difficulties encountered by the writer in clinical work with phonologically disordered children. Development and disorder of consonant phonology had been extensively described and investigated, and analytic frameworks had been proposed by, among others, Ingram (1989) and Grunwell (1987). Children with any abnormality of vowel production, on the other hand, had not received much attention, and the writer could find no clear guidance on how to proceed, either in assessment or in intervention. Once hearing loss and abnormality of the articulators and their movements had been ruled out, colleagues advised the writer to leave well alone. This did not fit in well with the idea that vowel abnormalities probably constituted disordered development, rather than delay (Renfrew, 1966). Received wisdom suggested that disordered development in the consonant system was a high priority for intervention, so why were we not applying the same principle to disorder in other aspects of phonology? Information about normal development was similarly hard to find.

The study started with the gathering of audio recordings of children receiving speech and language therapy showing vowel abnormalities. The intention was to produce more detailed and considered transcriptions than were possible within routine clinical settings, to analyze the data, and to look for patterns. The working hypothesis was that the analysis would reveal linguistic regularities relevant to speech therapy intervention. It was hoped that this would lead to a more refined view of the delay and disorder question in this area, and of whether there were patterns also occurring in normal development. This would then be relevant to assessment and diagnosis, as well as to planning intervention.

As part of the original project, efforts were made to draw together the available information on normal development of vowel systems (Reynolds, 1990). An up-to-date account of this area is provided elsewhere in this volume. The original project looked particularly at whether emerging vowel systems conformed with any linguistic frameworks predicting earlier or later acquisition of vowel subsystems. Limited evidence suggested that *marked* sound-types were acquired later than *unmarked* ones, but some of the sources described patterns of development not fitting into any obvious hierarchical approach (such as Jakobsonian oppositions, markedness, sonorance scales). Limited material from languages other than English was identified. This only hinted at possible regularities. The project also considered links to recent work on phonological universals (Maddieson, 1984). Again, cross-language patterns in adult systems were not always comparable to the features of early phonological development, whether normal or disordered.

The Target Adult System

The majority of the children studied lived in West Yorkshire, United Kingdom, and the local vowel system can thus be summarized (Wells, 1982).

Inventory

short vowels	ɪ	ɛ a	ɒ	ʊ	(ə)	
long vowels	iː	eː/ɛɪ	aɪ	ɒɪ		
	uː	ɔː/oʊ	aʊ			
	ɪə	ɛː aː	ɜː	ɒː	ɔə	ʊə

Realization

short vowels	similar to Received Pronunciation (RP) corresponding vowels, generally slightly greater opening and more lax articulation; /ɒ/ a little more front than RP
long vowels	laxer than RP corresponding vowels /aɪ/, /ɒɪ/ starting points similar to /a/, /ɒ/

/iː/ sometimes noticeably diphthongized [ɪi]
/ɛɪ/ either [eː] or [ɛɪ] with starting point like /ɛ/
/aʊ/ front starting point
/uː/ sometimes diphthongal [ʏy̯] [ʉy̯]
/oʊ/ either [oː] or [oy̯] with back starting point
/ɪə/ often more closed [ɪə] or disyllabic [ɪːə]
/ɜː/ more back and high than RP
/ɒː/ more open and less lip-rounded than RP; can sometimes approximate to RP /ɑː/

Distribution

short vowels — as in RP (all RP /ʌ/-class assigned to /ʊ/-class)
/a/ distributed for RP words in /ɑː/ followed by voiceless fricative (*glass, bath, laugh* etc.)
RP words in /-ʊk/ (*look, book, cook* etc.) may be realized in /-uːk/; probably less common in younger speakers

long vowels — /iː, aɪ, ɒɪ, uː, aʊ, ɪə, ɜː/ similar to RP
/eː ~ ɛɪ/ generally in free variation; possibly two contrasting phonemes for some speakers in words with historical velar fricative (*weight ~ wait* /ɛɪ ~ eː/)
/oː ~ oʊ/ similar possible distinctive potential as in *owt ~ oat* [oy̯t ~ oːt]
/ɛː/, RP /ɛə/; /aː/ RP /ɑː/; marginal distinctions with historical postvocalic 'r' in /ɒː ~ ɔə ~ ʊə/ *shaw ~ shore ~ sure*

Without much more extensive data collection and analysis involving children from different geographical areas, it is impossible to be sure how much the general conclusions of this study reflect specific factors about the system being acquired. It is argued, nonetheless, that the patterns involved have broad applicability, and that the evidence from children not living in West Yorkshire might confirm this. Furthermore, there were inevitably variations between parents, and some children were exposed to less uniform modelling of some or all features of the local accent than were others. Certain features of accent mixture and variability were identified in the case studies (Reynolds, 1987), but the disordered features are too extensive to be accounted for by potential confusion of accents.

Data and Analysis

The data for this study were collected from 25 children under the care of speech and language therapists. Recordings were made in a setting familiar to the children, usually school, home, or speech clinic. High-quality equipment was used. It was considered essential to use an everyday setting, in spite of the potential for background noise interference, to obtain the most natural and spontaneous samples from the children. Some transcription was done at the time, but detailed records were subsequently made (see Reynolds, 1987).

Recurring Patterns and Context-Free Processes

Which Adult Phonemes Are Implicated?

The children studied in the project showed instances of abnormal realizations in all areas of vowel space, and in all parts of the vowel system except the long /aː/ (front in West Yorkshire systems: *farm*, and so on). The short /a/ was less prone than most other vowels to be implicated in disorders of the system. This would fit in with the Jakobsonian view that it is a term in the basic closed-open contrast "p ~ a." However, there were some cases where /a/ itself has anomalous realizations.

Most other elements of the adult vowel system were implicated in some part of the data. These include most commonly the group of midfront vowels /ɛ, ɛː, ɛɪ/, the set of diphthongs and triphthongs, and the central vowel /ɜː/. Less frequently occurring areas have been the high vowels, the lowback vowels, and the unstressed vowels.

Within each of these basic groups, the patterns of difficulty have varied, so that the treatments of particular parts of the system by different children are not necessarily identical, although common patterns occurred.

Common Context-Free Processes

The three common processes or tendencies occurring in the data are lowering, fronting and diphthong reduction. A possible fourth case is the treatment of the central vowel. They tended largely to produce reduced and simplified phonological systems; a section of the adult vowel system was realized in such a way as to neutralize a distinctive opposition or set of oppositions.

Lowering:

Lowering typically affected the group /ɛ, ɛː, ɛɪ/. It virtually always affected the /ɛ/, in the familiar neutralization *bed ~ bad* → [bad], and affected /ɛː/ and /ɛɪ/ in many cases. Thus, the following types of subsystems came about, with major loss of contrastivity, and simplification.

1. $\begin{array}{l}/ɛ/\\/a/\end{array} \to$ [a]

   $\begin{array}{l}/ɛː/\\/aː/\end{array} \to$ [aː]

   $\begin{array}{l}/ɛɪ/\\/aɪ/\end{array} \to$ [aɪ]

2. $\begin{array}{l}/ɛ/\\/a/\end{array} \to$ [a]

   /ɛː/ → [ɛː]

   /aː/ → [aː]

   $\begin{array}{l}/ɛɪ/\\/aɪ/\end{array} \to$ [aɪ]

3. $\begin{array}{l}/ɛ/\\/a/\end{array} \to$ [a]

Lowering also affected the high vowels in some cases, and the phonological results were more varied and less tidy or systematic.

Case P (age 5 years, 3 months)

beard	ba	pig	ba̠ˑk beːk bək pag
leaf	ʔaːpʰ ɛp	zip	ap ɛp
tree	tʃaː	ring	bʷaː bʷe̞a we̞
sweep	wɪp	fish	wa̠ʃ we̞ʔʃ weʃ
sweetie	ʈ-ːtɪ	fishes	wɪtʃas
shoe	tsɔː ɒː		
soup	sǫ̈ːp tʊp sɛp ʃɒːs		

The variability and apparent randomness usually operate by lowering to some degree, but maintaining the frontness or backness of the target adult form, while contrastivity and system are severely compromised.

Another less common form of this difficulty was a neutralization of the /iː ~ ɪ/ contrast. In one case (Child B in Reynolds, 1987), this applied only in the context of a following nasal, and in another (Child A), the overuse of diphthongs and triphthongs led to loss of this contrast. The clearest case is Child C, who showed a partial neutralization of the set of contrasts /iː ~ ɪ ~ ɛɪ/.

Case C

fish	tʃɛə	milk	nɛn
string	wɛə	swings	wi
pig	be̞ə bɪ	brick	wɪ
queen	d̪ɛː	three	wɛə
teeth	t̪ʰɛə	cheese	niˑ
tree	wɛə	tea	ti
train	d̪ɛəd	cage	d̪eˑᵊd
spade	bɛə	paint	be̞ᵊ
cake	d̪ɛd̪	newspaper	njubæbə

Fronting

Fronting tends to apply most often to the lowback vowels (very open for West Yorkshire speakers) /ɒ ~ ɒː ~ ɒɪ/ (*dog, fork, boy*). This case operates phonologically in parallel to the treatment of /ɛ ~ ɛː ~ ɛɪ/, although phonetically it is a different process, involving a movement from back to front vowel quality. Typical subsystems could be as follows:

1. $\dfrac{/ɒ/}{/a/} \rightarrow$ [a]   2. $\dfrac{/ɒ/}{/a/} \rightarrow$ [a]   3. $\dfrac{/ɒ/}{/a/} \rightarrow$ [a]

$$\left.\begin{array}{l}/ɒː/\\/aː/\end{array}\right\} → [aː] \qquad \begin{array}{l}/ɒː/ → [ɒː]\\/aː/ → [aː]\end{array}$$

$$\left.\begin{array}{l}/ɒɪ/\\/aɪ/\end{array}\right\} → [aɪ] \qquad \begin{array}{l}/ɒɪ/\\/aɪ/\end{array}\right\} → [aɪ]$$

One logical conclusion could be the reduction of adult phonology from nine terms to three, as follows:

$$\begin{array}{lll}/ɛ/ & /ɛː/ & /ɛɪ/\\ /a/ → [a] & /aː/ → [aː] & /aɪ/ → [aɪ]\\ /ɒ/ & /ɒː/ & /ɒɪ/\end{array}$$

This system could, of course, be further reduced by diphthong reduction.

Case S (age 10 years)
$$\left.\begin{array}{l}/ɛ/\\/a/\\/ɒ/\end{array}\right\} → [a] \text{ (all other vowels realized normally)}$$

A less common cause of fronting was the treatment of u-diphthongs and u-triphthongs. The glide element was replaced by a front glide, neutralizing the oppositions as shown in the following examples:

$$\left.\begin{array}{l}/ai/\\/au/\end{array}\right\} → [aɪ] \quad \left.\begin{array}{l}/aɪə/\\/auə/\end{array}\right\} → [aɪə] \quad \begin{array}{l}/ou/\\/aɪ/\end{array}\right\} → [aɪ] \begin{array}{l}\text{(with altered}\\\text{nucleus)}\end{array}$$

Some children showed persistent difficulty with the back rounded /uː/, and tended to maintain the phonological contrast by introducing the non-English [y].

Diphthong Reduction

Diphthong reduction most commonly operates by the loss of the offglide element, and the result is therefore a monophthong of the same quality as the original nucleus. In most cases it will retain extra length, though for some children there can be a shortening process, leading to a less systematic pattern of error and greater difficulty for the adult listener. It is also clear that diphthong reduction may interact with the processes of fronting and lowering, as the following examples indicate:

1. /ɛɪ/ → [ɛ]↘
   /aɪ/ → aː→ [aː]
   /ɒɪ/ → [ɒː]↗
2. /ou/ → [oː]
   /au/ → [aː]
3. /aɪ/ → [aː]
   /ɒɪ/ → [ɒː]

Children who have difficulty in this area tend to reduce triphthongs to monophthongs as well

$$\left.\begin{array}{l}/aɪə/\\/auə/\end{array}\right\} → [aː]$$

There is a clear loss of contrastivity in all these changes, even if the West Yorkshire speaker has monophthongal [e:], [o], *plate, boat*), because other processes reduce the number of contrastive terms. In contrast with RP, the North of England standard tends to have more definite triphthongs in *fire, flower,* and so on.

Similarly, /ɪə/ tends towards a more triphthongal version [ɪiə] [ɪjə], which is therefore more subject to monophthongization than the less definitely diphthongized RP [ɪə]. However, in these cases, the communicative impact is probably less crucial than the treatment of the noncentering diphthongs, because the triphthongs are less prominent in the lexicon. It is interesting to note that diphthong reduction, while having its own formal structure and its own possible rationale (considered later in the text), also tends (in English) to maximize open articulations. This is due to the noncentering diphthongs having close offglides. Both lowering and diphthong reduction move the system in the same direction, and produce the same systematic simplification.

Central Vowels

The treatment of the central vowel /ɜ:/ is less easy to specify. It is clear that some children with disordered speech introduce a stressed central quality into their repertoire later on in development, and that there are various possible realizations. The most common is the substitution of a midfront quality [e:], and this may occur alongside /ɛ:/ → [a:] (Case J; for more detail see Reynolds 1987). Another possibility is that /ɜ:/ is lowered to [a:], which might be seen as a combination of fronting and lowering /ɜ:/ → [e:] → [a:]. In one case, there was a progression over time as follows:

Case P

1. /ɜ:/ → [a:]	2. /ɜ:/ → [e:]	3. /ɜ:/ → [ɜ:]
/ɛ:/ → [a:]	/ɛ:/ → [a:]	/ɛ:/ → [a:]
/a:/ → [a:]	/a:/ → [a:]	/a:/ → [a:]

However, in other cases /ɜ:/ is realized with a back vowel or a front high vowel. It might be more appropriate to think of the process in terms of *avoidance of central vowel quality,* or *preference for peripheral vowel quality.* The following data from one sample illustrate this in extreme form.

Case R

girls	geːᵘ	squirt	skwaːt
purse	pʊˑs	curtains	kɜːtn̩z
circus	fɛthṣ	burn	bɪənt

Case M

girl	gɒɪ gɒɛ
purse	pɒːç
purple	pɒpy

Explanatory Frameworks

The patterns of lowering, fronting, diphthong reduction, and central vowel avoidance occurred in a variety of forms in the data, and occurred in the speech of some children showing delayed development and common types of simplification in the consonant system. This tends to support the view that there could be *simple delay* and common simplifications in the vowel system, as well as in the consonant system. Caution is, however essential; different varieties of English show widely different vowel patterns, and the specific features of different varieties could easily determine different common simplifications in phonological development. Much more evidence is needed from phonological disorder, normal development, and by looking at different languages and at different varieties of English, before broader conclusions could be drawn.

Three studies, published in the early 1990s, show interesting comparisons (Pollock and Hall, 1991; Pollock and Keiser, 1990; Stoel-Gammon and Herrington, 1990). All provide data regarding children learning American English. The studies identify a range of processes and patterns consistent with the evidence of normal early development of the vowel system. Pollock and Keiser found that lowering and backing occur commonly, but that fronting is rare. Stoel-Gammon and Herrington identify lowering, but not as a systematic phenomenon. These points might suggest that different patterns are found in different varieties of English, and that more detailed analysis is needed across varieties of English and across other languages.

All three studies identify the tense and lax contrast as an important dimension that some children fail to manipulate reliably. For the Yorkshire data, the distinction might be based mainly on length differences and associated vowel quality, making it easier to deal with such contrasts as *bid ~ bead*. This would not apply to all varieties of British English; more detailed study would be needed.

All three studies comment on the children's treatment of rhotic vowels, a further complication not present in nonrhotic British varieties.

There is, therefore, no strong support for the hypothesis that the processes of lowering, fronting, and central avoidance are natural. Diphthong reduction seems more justifiable, though the American varieties might use fewer consistent diphthongs than the Yorkshire sample.

Although we cannot prove that these observed processes are either common or natural, it is interesting to consider whether there is any phonetic plausibility to this hypothesis, and whether it can be defended in phonological terms.

Lowering of vowels, particularly front vowels, seems to maximize the articulatory contrast between the full closure or the close stricture of plosives and fricatives, and the maximally open articulatory posture of the fully open vowel. From an acoustic and perceptual standpoint, the open vowel carries the greatest amount of acoustic energy, the greatest perceptual salience, and therefore could be the preferred natural sound if the system is operating with reduced contrastivity and opposition.

Diphthong and triphthong reduction involve phonetic simplification, in the disappearance of an offglide. The offglide is a complex phonetic feature due to its requirement for precise timing, and its secondary articulatory and acoustic prominence. In phonological terms, simplification of these complex nuclei might connect with other simplifications (such as consonant cluster reduction and the omission of final consonants).

This maximizes the use of the simplest canonical form consonant-vowel-consonant-vowel (CVCV) with simple open syllables. For learners of English, there are important phonological consequences.

The reviewed data showed examples of diphthongs being replaced by relatively long monophthongs, maintaining the time slot for the offglide and also cases where the offglide was replaced by a consonant, or the vowel nucleus was short and the offglide completely lost.

A proposed process of fronting is more difficult to argue in terms of perceptual salience, or articulatory ease. A more promising approach proposes that fronting is parallel to the fronting of back sounds in consonant systems. Back sounds might be disfavored because children have less visual information about velar articulation in other speakers. Therefore, children take longer to become fully aware of the distinction between alveolar and velar contacts. This seems less likely with learning vowel production.

In the cases studied, the fronting applies most commonly to the /ɒ, ɔː, ɔɪ/ group (*dog, fork, boy*), which could be especially difficult for some young speakers dealing with tongue retraction within a fully open articulatory posture. Within this variety of English, there does seem to be a crowded space of fully open front, and near-front vowels (/a, aː, aɪ/) and back vowels (ɒ, ɔː, ɔɪ), and this might contribute to early difficulty. Within RP, a wider spread of qualities is used (/æ, aɪ, aː/ /ɔ, ɔː, ɔɪ/). Data from varieties of English with closer realizations of this group would be an interesting comparator.

We have noted in previous text the phonetic considerations around central vowel avoidance, both in the commoner processes /ɜː/ → [ɛː, aː], and in the more idiosyncratic treatments of these target forms. The local variety uses a different realization from RP, and one might consider accent mixture and conflict as a complicating factor. The simple geometry of vowel space could justify a tendency to avoid central vowels for articulatory ease and perceptual salience, and the relatively low frequency in the lexicon also might be relevant.

It is interesting to consider whether there are phonological frameworks relevant to the description and analysis of these patterns. They can be listed in a descriptive framework, identifying misarticulation and distinguishing substitutions, distortions, omissions, and additions of sounds. We can then identify particular patterns, that might be commoner or more natural than others. Reynolds (1990) proposed that natural phonological processes could be set up, analogous to consonantal simplifications. These processes would identify normal features of early development, and distinguish them from less common, more idiosyncratic systems. This approach to finding patterns and regularities within disordered phonological system remains current in a good deal of clinical work in practical field settings. It is very helpful in dealing with systems showing relatively systematic simplifications, but less helpful in dealing with more complex and unusual disordered systems.

More recently, there has been much interest in applying the framework of nonlinear phonology to disordered speech (Bernhardt and Gilbert, 1992; Bernhardt and Stoel-Gammon, 1994). This offers the possibility of more systematic descriptions of phonological phenomena, operating both in the individual sound-segment and its features, and also at the level of onset-rhyme, syllable, and word structures. Diphthong reduction lends itself well to this type of analysis, as strikingly demonstrated by Harris, Bates, and Watson (1999). They show how apparently diverse surface phenomena can be described as part of a single underlying pattern in the treatment of target diphthongs.

For other context-free patterns (fronting, lowering, central avoidance), the feature configurations of nonlinear autosegments might provide more economical justification for hypothetical natural processes, positing a simplification favoring the {A} (fully open vowel) element if the complexity of a segment is reduced. This would account for some of the simplifications of mid vowels outlined earlier in the text. A different application is necessary for analyzing the phonetic variation of Child C (mentioned previously), who neutralized /iː ~ ɪ ~ ɛɪ/ and produced a range of tokens in the [i, ɪ, ɛ, ɛɚ] region.

The system of contrasts in the target forms is lost, there is wide variation in the degree of lowering, and there is wide variation in the treatment of rhyme codas, whether or not a consonantal coda is present in the adult target. It appears that underlying forms for the child are only loosely specified, both in terms of how many segments are required in the structure, and also of what their phonetic feature complex should be. It might be appropriate to build up the word schema in terms of very general word shapes, thus permitting wide variation (Waterson, 1978).

Context–Sensitive Processes

Consonantal influences are described in detail by another contributor in this volume. Some examples occurred in the data from this project, although the data was not extensive enough to allow for fully clear analyses on this point. Fairly extensive backing and lowering occurred in the context of a following underlying lateral (preconsonantal or final). This is shown in the following examples.

Case A

milk	mewək	wool	wʌl
building	bɜʊdɪn	wolf	wʊwᵊlf

Case D

milk	bʊk dʊk	ill	ʊ
doll	dɔᵁ dɐᵁⁿ dʊⁿ		

Some following nasals in the target form provoked lowered vowel realization, even if the nasality was not manifested in the surface form. This might be justified by perceptual factors. If a vowel nasalized through anticipatory assimilation sounds more open, it might be misconstrued by children. This is shown in the following examples.

Case P

ring	wɛə	train	tsɛə
queen	kɛə	crown	kɛə
green	gɛə		

Case E

queen	kɪə
green	kɪŋ
ring	ʔɛə
drinking	ʔɒkɪ

A slightly different case of nasal influence occurred in a child showing a specific conditioned phonological simplification. Child B showed normal contrastivity of /iː ~ ɛɪ/, except before underlying nasal consonants.

queen	keɪə̃	train	tẽɪ̃
ice-cream	'aɪˀgẽɪ̃	aeroplane	ɛləpẽɪ̃
green	gẽɪ̃		

These patterns might exemplify the lowering that general phonetics would predict; there is not enough data to be sure of their phonological status. Their main feature of interest is that these contextual influences go in the same direction as the context-free processes, maximizing more open vowel nuclei and reducing close vowels. They could be built into natural process accounts of phonological disorder, and would also fit in well to a nonlinear account, which could accommodate a variety of feature spreading and feature modification phenomena.

Idiosyncratic Systems

Alongside patterns recurring in similar forms in many children, the project also identified a smaller number of children with idiosyncratic vowel systems (or broader phonological idiosyncrasies). Following established practice (Grunwell, 1987; Ingram, 1989), we can distinguish a range of idiosyncrasies. For some children, there is a chronological mismatch, in a persistent (possibly common or natural) process from an earlier stage. Child S had generally well-developed phonology, but at age 10 still neutralized /ɛ ~ a ~ ɒ/. In other instances, a common process is implemented in a more unusual or extensive way. Child P (previously discussed in text) showed lowering of high vowels.

The most unusual cases, however, are those of a child's system being structured differently from the adult system, not purely a reduced and simplified version of it. These are cases where the child has moved up a phonological blind alley to create a system with different parameters or frameworks. Three cases are briefly sketched here.

Child M

Child M had a reduced and bizarre consonant system. Her vowel system also showed neutralizations and enough variability to cause further disruption of the remaining contrastivity. The more nearly normal contrastive system is as follows:

short vowels	ɪ	a	ɒ
long vowels	iː	aː	ɒː
diphthongs	ɔɪ	aɪ	ɪə (ʔaʊ)

The most unusual feature was the realization of back high vowels /uː/ and /ʊ/, and vowels before dark l.

/ʊ/

bus	bʊsː	duck	dʊʔs
book	gɯʔ byʔ	drum	dɒn̩
wool	ʔyː	cutting	kadɪ
wolf	ʔyç ʔyːç	bubbles	bɒbɯɤ

/uː/

shoes	tsɯːz ʃʉːz	two	tyː
school	syː	boots	bɯʔs
spoon	ʃy-ː	flute	syk

lateral

| milk | [yː], [uː] |
| seal | [ʔyː] |

The forms in /ʊ/ show influence of a contrast between the /ʊ/ class and the /ʌ/ class, a contrast present in Child M's mother, though the forms *bus* and *duck* do not follow this pattern. There is, however, a separation between the /ʊ/ group and the /ʌ/ group, in that only the RP /ʊ/ group shows the secondary Cardinal Vowel types. For these items, and for all the items in /uː/, this fairly small sample reveals no clear conditioning factors determining whether [y] or [ɯ] is used. It seems likely that the two sounds are in free variation and that other intermediate forms can occur (compare *shoes*). Child M produced very few forms with a highback rounded vowel. This is consistent with other aspects of the phonology (including virtual absence of [w], and the treatment of vocalized syllabic lateral).

This suggests that Child M arrived at a hypothesis regarding vowel space in the target system, precluding back rounded vowels, but allowing realizations in the form of an unrounded back vowel, or a rounded front vowel. The possible contrastive systems might be as follows:

short vowels ɪ/a/ɒ/ʊ ~ y ~ ʌ ~ ɯ
long vowels iː/aː/ɒː/yː ~ ɯː

The two inventories are parallel in general form, and the consistency suggests a general principle being applied throughout the system. The guiding principle might be that there are no back rounded high vowels, and that target highback vowels should be realized as high vowels, and thus kept separate from any other high vowels in the system. This contrastivity is maintained at the cost of a radical distortion of vowel space. In the case of the consonant system, the matter was dealt with more simply by the deletion of /w/ in most cases. For the vowel system, this was not an option, and we see the disruptive effects of having to find some representation for a segment obligatory in the structure.

In phonological terms, this pattern maintains contrastivity within the system, but the phonetic manifestation reflects a disordered framework of vowel space. The vowel triangle [i ~ a ~ u] is inherent in the adult system that the child was exposed to. These bizarre productions might reflect the phonetic coordinates of a preferred articulation, established lexically, before or alongside the emergence of segmental phonological contrastivity. The data collection exercise did not allow for detailed assessment of the child's psycholinguistic skills or underlying representations. Informally, however, evidence suggested normal discrimination of input and age appropriate comprehension, with difficulties rooted in the phonetic planning process. This will, no doubt, affect phonological planning of output, but we cannot assess this with certainty.

Case A

This case showed a preferred articulation creating a pattern of speech not particularly unintelligible, and yet with interesting systematic consequences. The fairly mature and normally developing consonant system assisted intelligibility, but the vowel system often contributed little to the intelligibility of the utterance. The triphthong was the preferred articulation. The short vowel system was close to normal, as was the long monophthong system (apart from /iː/ and /uː/). These two phonemes and noncentering diphthongs all tended to be realized as triphthongs, as well as having certain alterations in the quality of the nucleus.

The following forms were typical.

/iː/		/uː/	
tree	tɛɪ̯ tɪj	new	nʊ̯w
sleeping	lɛ̯ɪpɪn	school	skəʊ̯l
sheep	tɪjəp sɪ̯jəp sejəp	spoon	pəʊl
sleep	l̯ɪjəp lɪjəp	moon	mɒʊn
teacher	tɛɪ̯tə	shoe	ʃɛwə
teeth	tɪ̯jəf	afternoon	apənɒʊ̯ən
peas	pɪjəd	two	tʊwᵊ tʊw
wheel	wɪjə	boot	bɔʊ̯ət

In these sets, the local form of English provided a model for diphthongal realization, but generally within the high vowel range (typically [ɪ̯ɪ], [ɪ̯ɪ]; [ʊ̯ʊ], [i̯ʊ], [ɪʊ̯].) The child has much more instability in the nucleus, as well as inconsistent introduction of a triphthongal pattern with centering offglide following a strengthened /ʊ/ or /ɪ/ offglide. No obvious factor in the data conditioned the occurrence of triphthong as opposed to diphthong.

/aɪ/		/eɪ/	
light	lajət	cake	kɛjək
slide	lajəs	painting	paɪ̯tɪn
time	tajᵊm	baby	bɛjəb bɛjbɪj
climbing	tɛ̯ɪmɪn	lady	lɛɪ̯dɪ
smiling	smaɪ̯lɪn		

/oʊ/		/aʊ/	
boat	ba̯wə bɛ̯wət	house	ʔaʊ̯əs
sew	sɛʊ̯	houses	ʔaʊ̯əsəz
stones	tɛʊ̯nd	down	daʊ̯ən
no	noʊ̯	out	awət aʊ̯t

sewing	sawɪn	cow	kau̯
golden	gɜu̯dan		
go	gau̯		

/ɒɪ/

| boy | bɑ̠ɪ bɑ̠ɪˀ bɑ̠ɪ̠ | | |
| boys | bɑ̠jəd | | |

In these cases the triphthong form can be seen, and in some cases, the modified diphthong starting point is also evident. From a phonological point of view, the occurrence of many more triphthongs than usual might not change the system very much, since there are not many oppositions between diphthong and triphthong pairs. The treatment of long high vowels could lead to neutralization of the contrasts /iː/ ~ /ɛɪ/ and /uː/ ~ /oʊ/ because of the partly overlapping realizations. Furthermore, a three-way homophony in [baɪə] (*buyer, buy, boy*) could be envisaged. From a phonetic and articulatory point of view, Child A has found an unusual way of simplifying certain aspects of the vowel system. If the strengthened [j] or [w] of the triphthong is regarded as having consonantal status, then Child A has created a CVCV pattern not by eliminating the diphthongal offglide, but by strengthening it, and adding a further syllabic.

Within a natural process approach, this might be described as a variant of diphthong reduction, or a halfway stage between diphthong reduction and normal realizations. Child A has found a way to signal the appropriate quality of offglide, but only by giving the offglide excessive strength and thereby needing a schwa glide after it. This is a parallel process to the schwa insertion seen in consonantal clusters (such as *blue* [bəluː]).

The difficulty of sequencing the relevant articulatory postures was not reflected in the segmental sound quality, but in the syllable structure of the production. A nonlinear approach could accommodate this stage of development, by excluding or disfavoring complex vowels if the offglide is different in quality from the main nucleus, or by preferring offglides with strengthened (virtually consonantal) status. This would become an onset, and require a rhyme (see Figure 4-1).

Child T

This child had a preferred articulation; he used many diphthongs. His speech contains examples of the whole range of monophthongal sounds, and of a wide range of diphthongs to [ɪ]. There are virtually no diphthongs to [ʊ]. The distribution of the diphthongs to [ɪ] is very interesting, in that they realize some monophthongal phonemes, especially short vowels as in

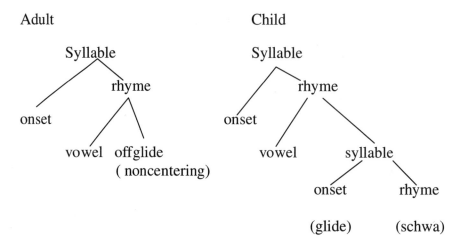

Figure 4-1   Possible Nonlinear Framework for Adult and Child A.

beds	bɛɪ̯	pram	plæɪ̯
pegs	peɪ̯	grass	ʋaɪ̯
frog	wɒɪ̯	bull	buɪ̯
dolls	dɒɪ̯	brush	bluɪ̯

This is not a consistent process, and no evidence indicates a conditioning factor at work. Although the offglide could be a reflex of the lost final consonant, forms of /uː/ suggest that there is also an independent preference for diphthongs as in

blue	bluɪ̯
new	nuɪ̯

The phonemes /ɪ/ and /iː/ appear to be merged, and to be subject to breaking to [iə]. The expected diphthongs to [ɪ] occur and the diphthongs to [ʊ] show the same preference for the [ɪ] offglide.

/aʊ/		/oʊ/	
mouth	maɪ̯	nose	nəʊ̯z
house	haɪ	snow	nəʊ̯ɪ
		throw	rəʊ̯ɪ

In phonological terms, the distinctions between long and short vowel types, between monophthongs and diphthongs, and between front and back offglides are not reliably present in the system. These tendencies could be summarized as follows.

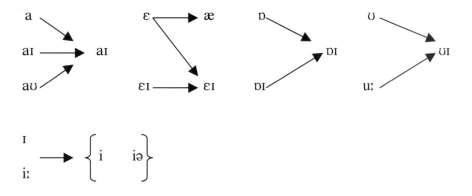

The offglide [ɪ] does not appear to be fully part of the system of contrasts, and its presence or absence appears to be a matter of free variation.

There is a striking contrast between the normal or immature realizations of word-initial consonants, and the disordered realizations of vowels and final consonants. Within a natural process approach, this would have to be handled as final consonant deletion or palatalization-cum-vocalization, with a separate process inserting a front offglide [ɪ]. The system can more conveniently be described in its own terms, rather than by reference to the adult target system. Word structure can be described as a consonantal onset (including clusters) followed by a diphthong to [ɪ]. A nonlinear approach might suggest a disorder affecting the rime section of words in particular. Child T has problems dealing with the range of vowel nuclei required and with the range of final sounds. If word-final consonants are analyzed as underlying syllables whose nucleus or rime has been deleted, it could be seen that this child has hit on a very restricted repertoire of realizations to cover the complexities of CVC and CV:C words in English.

Idiosyncratic Disorders Related to Nonsegmental Features

We have considered a number of disordered systems, where the pattern of realization of segments can be considered in phonological terms, whether in a natural process framework or a nonlinear approach. Phonetic correlates have also been noted, confirming in some respects the naturalness of the patterns, or implying that ease of articulation might be relevant, as well as ease of production of phonological output representations. A further consideration arose from the data, in cases showing both suprasegmental aspects of the target system affecting realizations, and abnormal articulatory set affecting realizations. Relevant patterns are summarized in the following text.

Child C

Child C demonstrated a discrepancy between lexical development and overall phonology. At the time of data collection, he continued to use extensive reduplication, with little evidence of contrast between stressed and unstressed syllables. He therefore showed very reduced repertoire, not only in segments and syllable structure, but also in word structure.

The treatment of bisyllables shows reliance on reduplication as well as one odd form in the case of *monkey*.

/ɪ/		/ə/	
baby	bɛbɪ	paper	bæbə
donkey	dɒʰdɪ	Christmas	wɪdə
rabbit	baba	finger	wɪwɪ
glasses	dada	water	wəwə
		mirror	ŋaŋa
monkey	mʌmwɛə		

In the case of *monkey*, Child C treated /ɪ/ as stressed, with lowering to [ɛə] and merger with /iː ~ ɛɪ/. This isolated instance reflects the intersection of difficulty with the high vowel system and difficulty with the pattern of stressed and unstressed syllables.

Child P is an example of a converse case. This child attempted to use syllable-timing to increase intelligibility.

Case P (age 5;3 years)

he got ice cream   ʔɛgɒʔaka
    ♩ ♩ ♩ ♩

and me put it on my hands   ʔamɪpɪsɪsɒmaʔa
    ♩ ♩ ♩ ♩ ♩ ♩ ♩

sweetie shop   tɪ-ː tɪː tɒp
    ♩ ♩ ♩

Clearly this strategy was not successful in producing a better segmental outcome, or a more intelligible result. It also had consequences for Child P's intonation patterns, which were similarly unnatural.

Idiosyncratic Disorder Related to Articulatory Set

Articulatory set has been analyzed in detail by Laver (1980) for its value in looking at individual differences between speakers, and in looking at voice disorders. It has not, however, been studied a great deal as a conditioning factor in developing and disordered phonology. The following cases demonstrated broad effects on both consonantal and vowel systems.

Child O

Child O (age 13 years), with normal hearing and diagnosed as having postencephalitic dyspraxia, showed a dull vocal resonance. He also displayed minimal prosodic and rhythmic variation, lower than usual tension in the articulatory organs, and a general back of the mouth quality. His consonant system showed strong velar preference.

rabbit	wagə	scissors	sɪkəz
bubbles	bɪgə	lion	laːk
sock	kak	teeth	kəf

His vowel system displayed a general retracted articulatory set, but the main effects were seen in certain segmental processes, including centralization, broadening of diphthongs, diphthong and triphthong reduction, and opening of half-open sounds. Typical cases are as follows:

Centralizations

teeth	kəf	ear	ʔɜːs
school	sjəːk	brothers	bəkəz
boy	bəːk	now	nəʸk
door	kəːk		

Diphthong broadening

wake	waɪ̞k	clothes	gaʊ̞s

Diphthong and triphthong reduction

lion	laːk	shake	kɛk
towels	kaːlz	slide	klaːd
open	ʔapɪ	boy	p⁼ɪg
cow	kaːᵈ		

Lowering

egg	ʔak	chair	kɑ̞ː

However, these processes, all tending towards low and central articulation, were partly counterbalanced by processes noticed in other children:

Fronting of lowback vowels

sock	kak

Fronting of u-diphthongs and u-triphthongs

house	ʔaɪs	hold	ʔaɪ̞k
flower	dɒɪᵊ		

It appears that the vowel system shows certain common processes of substitution, but is then biased by the particular effects of centralization, which is the one process not found normally elsewhere. Although centralization does not always constitute a form of backing or lowering (compare *door*), it sets up an unusual pattern of vowel space. This seems to revolve around the axis /ɑː/ ∼ /ɜː/, with high vowels as an offshoot of this, rather than using a fully exploited vowel space. The segmental processes interact with the nonsegmental tendencies in articulatory setting, and all should be seen as parts of one system, informed by a general principle, which in this case has both linguistic and phonetic consequences.

The identical twins S and T (11 years of age) had only just resolved their phonological difficulties with the consonant system. Their vowel system entailed some articulatory difficulties, although it is doubtful that these had phonological consequences at this stage; in certain respects, their speech could be viewed as showing a strange and idiosyncratic accent.

The general pattern was a lax and retracted set, but it differed from the case of Child O discussed previously. Twins S and T had rather lax but phonologically normal consonant articulations, and again a rather monotonous tone of voice, which, nevertheless, had some prosodic and rhythmic variation. The laxness appeared to involve the tongue and jaw muscles, and, for the vowel system, it involved shift tendencies towards central and low vowel sounds.

With experience, the listener got used to these patterns, but at first hearing, utterances were difficult to interpret. The general pattern, illustrated in the short vowels, is as follows:

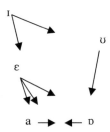

/ɪ/	fish	fɪ̣ʃ	/a/	man	man
	window	wɪ̣ndeʊ̣		back	ba̰k
	scissors	sɪ̣zəz		tractor	tʊɒktə
	milk	meɫk	/ʊ/	country	kʊntʊɪ
/ɛ/	letter	lɛ̣tə		bus	bʊ̣s
	very	vɛʊɪ vɛ̣ʊɪ	/ɒ/	sock	sɒk
	wellies	walɪz		dog	dɒ̣g
	left	lɛft			

Similar patterns occur in long vowels and diphthongs. Lowering occurs in the environment of the following lateral, but this appears to be just one part of the more general lowering occurring in Twins S and T. Although in strict phonemic terms there is no general overlap or merger, there is much indeterminacy of realization. While at this late stage Twins S and T were producing their own version of a normal phonological system, it is clear that earlier on there were much greater difficulties. The retracted and lax articulatory set was strongly related to the particular type of segmental difficulties experienced, and was part of the overall pattern that the boys found very difficult to change.

The converse case concerns two children who showed extra tension and general raising and fronting of the articulators. Whereas Child O and Twins S and T appeared to have habitually retracted tongue and perhaps jaw posture and movement, the cases of Child N and Child A show a set originating in raised tension in the larynx.

Case A is the child considered earlier as having a preference for triphthong articulations, and if the triphthong is viewed as a type of strengthened diphthong, there is some logic to the presence of general raised tension. Along with these features, Child A showed a distinctive voice quality, with slight raising of pitch and tendency to slight creak in the voice, giving an impression of a squawky quality. Child A's consonant system did not show deviations other than the common immaturities on /θ/ and /r/ and some cluster reduction and stopping. His vowel system at the point of study showed some residual features of lowering of /ɛ/ and fronting of /ɒ, ɜː, ɔː, ɒɪ, uː/.

teddy	dadɪj	boy	baɪ
dog	da̠d, dɒg	shirt	dɛ
ball	bal	shoe	ʃɛ̠wɒ

This shift of vowel quality frontwards seems to be lessening at this stage. It is easy to see why the general raising and fronting would produce fronting of back vowels. It would be more speculative, though very inviting, to suggest that the generally increased articulatory tension led to a preference for clear CV syllables, with no noncentering offglide. This necessitated schwa insertion as a stage of development. Primarily still an observation, rather than an explanation, it seems likely that there is some relationship.

In the second such case, Child N showed a similar articulatory set to Child A, with raised tension, raised larynx, and rather squawky tone of voice. But the segmental patterns were quite different. The vowel system showed a strong tendency to fronting, largely affecting /ɒ, ɔː, ɒɪ, ɜː/. In this respect Child N showed a common process, as described earlier, but its persistence can be related to nonsegmental factors. Child N is particularly interesting, because his consonant system difficulties could well have been related to the same nonsegmental patterns.

Child N showed some of the typical immature realizations of certain liquid and fricative phonemes, but he also had difficulty keeping separate the voiced and voiceless plosives. In most cases, he tended to produce a delayed voice-onset after plosion, and produced some variant of voiceless token in realization of voiced phonemes. (The opposite also happened, but to a lesser extent and less frequently.)

ball	bɑl	purse	pʰɜːs
boat	pʰɔːt	parrot	pʰajət
boy	pʰaɪ	painted	p⁼ɛɪntɪt
bucket	p⁼p⁼ʊkᵊt	piece	p⁼is
dog	tʰɑkʰ	teeth	tʰijf
doll	tʰal	tent	tʰɔnt
duck	dʊk	tin	t⁼ɪn
down	tʰaʊn		
girl	kʰɜːl	cat	kʰatʰ
going	gʊən	cow	kʰa̰ʊ

It is evident that Child N has little control over voice-onset timing, and the only evidence of a distinction between voiced and voiceless partners is the lack of fully voiced tokens representing voiceless phonemes. The voiced phonemes are represented by any point on the range from voiceless-aspirated to voiced-unaspirated. There is, therefore, some sign of appropriate distinction in the productions, although there is mainly an overlap of the two ranges of realization. The inability to control voice-onset timing might, in this case, reflect difficulty in controlling the larynx generally, and in conforming to the articulatory set of the broader speech community. It is, nonetheless, anomalous that Child N produces less vocal fold activity than expected, when he is producing a higher level of tension than expected.

An interesting postscript to this feature is its development pattern over time. Data collected 6 months later showed a major change. Instead of having difficulty initiating voicing early enough in plosives, Child N is now over-correcting. For some voiceless plosives in medial position, he has begun to produce voiced realizations.

wakened	wəːgɪnd	jumping	t̪ʊmbɪn
lookout	lʊgaʊd	water	wɑ̰də wɑtə
making	mɛgɪn		

In initial position, however, he has overcorrected the voiced stop phonemes, and produces some implosives.

| he's going | s̪ɠʊn | bed | ɓɛd |

Other forms suggest a groping around for the appropriate realization.

car	ga:	dog	dɒg at⁼ɒg

These varied attempts suggest that this is not purely a question of needing to solidify the phonological contrast between the two members of the voiced-voiceless opposition; it is more to do with the mechanics of reliably producing two quite similar sounds, making them consistently distinct. The basic difficulty is one of muscular coordination and control, and this affected nonsegmental features, and segmental aspects of vowel and consonant systems. Although in the second stage the voice quality was more normal, the segmental anomalies related to the odd articulatory setting were then resolved as a separate learning stage. The articulatory problem produced a phonological uncertainty, which had to be overcome later after articulatory control had improved.

Variability

Variability across a range of phonetic values for given target forms is a well-known aspect of phonological development and of disordered phonology. It has been viewed both as a desirable and positive phenomenon and as a problem, impeding progress in phonological development. Scholars such as Menn (1979; 1980) emphasized variability as a positive aspect of the active discovery process and the child's testing of hypotheses regarding the target phonological system.

On the other hand, Grunwell (1987) talked about the "static variable phonological system," using extreme variability as one of the indicators of deviant development.

Examples occurred in the data of both progressive and nonprogressive forms. One striking case is the occurrence of immediate self-correction, illustrating developing awareness of the target form and greater self-monitoring.

Case M	
balloons	byːz ~ buːz
book	ød ~ bʊk
beetroot	biʔyʔ ~ biʔuʔ

Case P	
shop	tʃaː ~ tʃɒᵖ
ball	bɒɪ ~ bɒː
mouse	mɒːʔs ~ maʊ̯s

Case A	
baby	bɛjɒb ~ bɛjbɪj

Case N	
falls in	fa̠lz ~ fɒlzɪn

The problematic side of variability is illustrated by some of the longitudinal data. Comparison of systems recorded over time shows clear cases with variation not assisting development, or with the child just moving slowly towards more normal realizations.

Case M
Treatment of diphthongs to -u

Stage 1: various offglides or diphthong reduction

| cow | kɒɸ | mouse | jaᵉs jaᵉs |
| house | ɒːç ʔɒɪs as | down | dau̜ |

Stage 2: more definite fronting

| house | ʔɒɪs | out | ʔʊ |
| flower | sɛjə | | |

Stage 3: front offglides (rounded or unrounded)

| cow | kɒɣ | trousers | taɪzɪs |
| house | ʔʊɪs | | |

Stage 4: some acceptable monophthongal realizations; some deviant back ones

rose	woːz	boat	boːt
cold	kɒːt	goldilocks	gʊ̜ʊ̜ʔs
broken	bʊkən		

Stage 5: mixture of monophthongal back glides

boat	bɔːt	cow	kaːʊ̜ kɒʊ̜ kəɣ
phone	sɒn	house	ʔɔys
goat	gɒːt	a house	əʊɔːs
		out	ɒːt əɯʔ ʔaːt

Realization of offglide /ʊ/ is quoted, because it provides striking examples of variability and groping towards the target sound. This development has to be seen in the context of the back vowel system as a whole, but the offglide took longer to reach the required target. It exemplifies the limited benefit this child got out of a structurally determined variability between back unrounded and front rounded high vowels.

Case P
Treatment of some front and central long phonemes (schematically)

	/aː/	/ɛː/	/ɜː/	/iː/	/aɪ/
Stage 1	aː	aː	ɜː	iː (prenasal) ɛː	aː
Stage 2	aː	aː	aː	iː/aː	aː
Stage 3	aː	aː	ɛː	iː (sometimes lowered)	aː

Stage 4	aː	aː	ɛː	iː	aː
Stage 5	aː	aː/ɛː	a/eː/eˡ/ɪ/ɪj	iː	aː
Stage 6	aˡ	aˡ	ɛː	iː	aˡ/aᵘ/aː
Stage 7	aɪ	aː	ɛʊ̯/eː/ɛɪ	iː	aɪ
Stage 8	aː/aɪ	aː	ɜː/ɪː/ɛːɪ/ɛː	iː	aː/aɪ
Stage 9	aː/aɪ	aɪ	ɪː/ệː/ɜː	iː	aː
Stage 10	aː	aː	ɜː	iː	aː/aɪ

The variation and overlap in these data indicate how difficult Child P found it to settle on consistent realizations, and suggests that he had difficulty maintaining enough distinct vowel types in his system. As one type of process (such as lowering) began to recede, another difficulty presented itself. When /ɛɪ-eː/ tended to be lowered, an open vowel [aː] resulted. However, when this lowering started to be inhibited, it initiated a partial merger with the high vowel.

The possible spelling pronunciations of postvocalic "r" (/aː/ → [aɪ], /ɛː/ → [aɪ]) might equally be explained as the result of a false start in introducing more diphthongs into his speech. But in common items such as *car*, it seems likely that Child P attempted to produce it as many children do when they first learn about postvocalic spelled "r" (for nonrhotic accents). This confused his diphthong realizations due to his difficulty with the glides and liquids required by the consonant system. The variability in his productions reflected his problems in maintaining enough distinct sound types in a crowded area of vowel space.

For some children with very disordered patterns, one asks how far lexical patterns influence the overall result. The variability in Child P's realization of /ɜː/ might reflect the relatively low frequency of this sound in the early vocabulary.

It seems likely that the child's underlying output form is not always identical to the adult target, and that the variation around [ɛː] reflects some awareness of a difference between /ɜː/ and /ɛː/, but very limited awareness of how this difference is manifested phonetically.

Discussion

This survey of the main features of the speech samples studied does not lead to a firm conclusion. In the original study, it led to a hypothesis about the existence of some natural simplification trends within developing and disordered vowel systems. Much more case analysis is needed to confirm or refute these proposals, ideally drawing from a wide range of languages and varieties.

Is there any evidence from other aspects of language to conform or disprove this hypothesis? Reynolds (1990) noted only partial confirmation from the evidence on normal developments of phonology. Historical changes in languages are also not parallel to the data considered in this chapter. Broad evidence of what is common in language systems is, however, more consistent with some of the trends shown. These are already noted as features which could be argued for on phonetic or general phonological grounds. Maddieson (1984) describes the greater prevalence of simple and often symmetrical vowel systems. These can be justified by reference to the conventional geometry of vowel space. Preference for peripheral vowels, for fully open vowels, or for monophthongs, could all be proposed on the basis of what is plausibly natural in phonetic geometry, and of what is found to be widespread in human languages.

The original study and analysis were conducted largely within a natural phonological process approach to disordered speech. Some of the phenomena identified might be ascribed to proposed natural processes, but others are not so easily accommodated. We noted at various points that a nonlinear approach to phonology might, in some cases, provide a better analytical framework. In either case, difficulties arise in describing the more unusual phenomena found in disordered speech. Natural process approaches start from the premise that one can specify what is natural, and what will put the least strain on the developing capacities of the young child learning language.

There are, however, difficulties in considering either consonantal or vowel system patterns. If fronting (as in /k/ → [t]) is natural, is more extreme fronting also natural (/t/ → [p], /k/ → [p])? It is certainly less common, and probably less easy to specify within any given model of phonological features. Analysis within a nonlinear framework might be difficult in dealing with the more unusual patterns of substitution, and might need to propose a different underlying form for a lexical item, or a separate phonological system for output forms. This has not been built into natural process analysis, though it would be more easily accommodated in the framework of prosodic analysis (Waterson, 1978), or in independent internal phonological analysis (Grunwell, 1987).

These difficulties can equally arise with vowel systems. It is easy to describe a regular /ɛ / → [a] pattern as lowering and to specify it within a segmental or feature framework. A less common pattern, operating less systematically, might be described as lowering, but would not be necessarily natural (such as instability of /i ~ ɪ ~ iə/, with variable realization as [ɛə ~ ɪ], as shown with Child C). It would also be difficult to argue that it constituted preference for {A} in nonlinear terms. These difficulties in analyzing the data in phonological terms lead to the broader question about how far these phenomena are phonological as opposed to phonetic.

Not all the children fit into the same framework. Some cases show definite difficulty in dealing with the range of phonological oppositions required in the target system, in the absence of any preferred or nonpreferred articulation (such as Child P).

In some cases, we have analyzed disordered speech as showing phonological disorder associated with some identifiable phonetic feature (such as avoidance of back rounded high vowels, preference for i-diphthongs, increased laryngeal tension and elevation). If preference or avoidance relates to particular segments or segmental features, it might be difficult deciding whether the child's evolving hypothesis about phonology conditioned the preferred phonetic form, or vice versa. In the case of nonsegmental articulatory set, it is more plausible that the phonetic tendency arose before segmental phonology began developing. In this case, the phonological disruption is at least partly related to the phonetic output system, even if other aspects of phonology are disrupted independently. We also noted at least one case in which the phonetic feature was probably not associated with phonological difficulties (the twin boys S and T).

In recent years, clinicians developed increasing understanding of the complex and varied interactions between speech praxis and phonological processing impairments. Contributions from Stackhouse and Wells (1993) and Hewlett (1985) exemplify the advances in our understanding. It is essential to consider the child's phonological system in a broad perspective, with regard to both consonant and vowel system disorders.

Conclusion

The data considered in this chapter raise various theoretical questions regarding the nature of phonological development and disorder, and about which type of phonological analysis casts the most light on the phenomena identified. These questions are considered in more detail elsewhere in this volume. The data in this present study have to be accounted for within any theoretical framework. They equally have significant consequences for providing remediation to children. They highlight the central importance of providing the best possible transcription in the prevailing circumstances. Without a narrow transcription, taking some account of nonsegmental and suprasegmental features, it is very difficult to provide more considered analysis of many complex cases. This is a continuing challenge for those supervising the theoretical and practical learning of student speech and language therapists.

All clinicians should maintain and develop these skills during their professional working lives. For researchers it will be important to learn how much influence nonsegmental and suprasegmental features have on phonological development, and how this will affect theory, assessment, and remediation.

Finally, the evidence presented in this chapter reminds us of the complexity and richness of language systems and skills, and of the challenges facing all children learning language.

References

Bernhardt, B., and Gilbert, J. (1992). Applying linguistic theory to speech-language pathology: The case for non-linear phonology. Clinical Linguistics and Phonetics, 6, 123–146.

Bernhardt, B., and Stoel-Gammon, C. (1994). Non-linear phonology: Introduction and clinical application. Journal of Speech and Hearing Research, 37, 123–143.

Grunwell, P. (1987). Clinical phonology (2nd ed.). London: Croom Helm.

Harris, J., Bates, S., and Watson, J. (1999). Prosody and melody in vowel disorder. Journal of Linguistics, 35, 489–525.

Hewlett, N. (1985). Phonological versus phonetic disorders: Some suggested modifications to the current use of the distribution. British Journal of Disorders of Communication, 20, 155–164

Ingram, D. (1989). Phonological disability in children (2nd ed.). London: Whurr.

Laver, J. (1980). The phonetic description of voice quality. Cambridge, England: Cambridge University Press.

Maddieson, I. (1984). Patterns of sounds. Cambridge, England: Cambridge University Press.

Menn, L. (1979). Transition and variation in child phonology: Modelling a developing system. In Proceedings of 9th International Congress of Phonetic Sciences, Vol. 2 (pp. 169–175). Copenhagen: International Congress of Phonetic Sciences.

Menn, L. (1980). Phonological theory and child phonology. In G. Yeni-Komshian, J. Kavanagh, and C. Ferguson (Eds.), Child phonology, Vol. 1, Production (pp. 23–41). New York: Academic.

Pollock, K., and Keiser, N. (1990). An examination of vowel errors in phonologically disordered children. Clinical Linguistics and Phonetics, 4, 161–178.

Pollock, K., and Hall, P. (1991). An analysis of the vowel misarticulation of five children with developmental apraxia of speech. Clinical Linguistics and Phonetics, 5, 207–224.

Renfrew, C. (1966). Persistence of the open syllable in defective articulation. Journal of Speech and Hearing Disorders, 31, 370–373.

Reynolds, J. (1987). The development of the vowel system in phonologically disordered children. Ph.D. thesis. Sheffield, England: University of Sheffield.

Reynolds, J. (1990). Abnormal vowel patterns in phonological disorder: Some data and a hypothesis. British Journal of Disorders of Communication, 25, 115–148.

Stackhouse, J., and Wells, B. (1993). Psycholinguistic assessment of developmental speech disorders. European Journal of Disorders of Communication, 28, 331–348.

Stampe, D. (1969). The acquisition of phonetic representation. In Papers from 5th Regional Meeting (pp. 443–454). Chicago: Chicago Linguistics Society.

Stoel-Gammon, C., and Herrington, P. (1990). Vowel systems of normally-developing and phonologically disordered children. Clinical Linguistics and Phonetics, 4, 145–160.

Waterson, N. (1971). Child phonology, a comparative study. Transactions of the Philological Society, 1971, 34–50.

Waterson, N. (1978). Growth and complexity in phonological development. In N. Waterson and C. Snow (Eds.), The development of communication (pp. 415–442). Chichester, England: Wiley.

Wells, J.C. (1982). Accents of English (3 vols.). Cambridge, England: Cambridge University Press.

5

Context-Conditioned Error Patterns in Disordered Systems

Sally A. R. Bates, Jocelynne M. M. Watson, and James M. Scobbie

This chapter reviews and expands the literature on consonant-vowel (CV) interactions in developing sound systems (normal and disordered) and explores the usefulness of current phonetic models (Davis and MacNeilage, 1995; Kent and Bauer, 1985; MacNeilage and Davis, 1990b; Studdert-Kennedy and Goodell, 1995) in accounting for and predicting the occurrence of these phenomena. The phonetic models provide a biological perspective insofar as the immature pronunciations of the normally developing child are viewed as systematic reflections of organic constraints imposed by the child's developing phonetic systems, both perceptual and motor.[1]

In the clinical setting, context conditioning manifests itself most frequently as consonantal speech errors, which only occur in specific vocalic contexts, although recent research has also uncovered evidence of vowel errors conditioned by consonantal context (Bates and Watson, 1995; Reynolds, 1990; Stoel-Gammon and Herrington, 1990). Such interdependencies accord well with current phonetically orientated models of speech acquisition and have important implications for clinical practice.

In espousing this approach, we do not intend to overlook the benefits of an analysis in terms of recent developments in phonological theory. This is an approach robustly argued in Harris, Watson, and Bates (1999), and taken up in Chapter 6. Rather, we consider the extent to which current phonetic models of speech acquisition contribute to an understanding of disordered child speech. Research into early speech production has traditionally concentrated on the order of acquisition of individual segments, especially consonants, carrying with it the assumption that vowels and consonants are under independent control. This view is strongly attacked in phonetically oriented research into acquisition and adult sound systems. We will discuss this view in the following text.

The Biological Framework

A phonetically orientated framework for linguistic description does not disregard the importance of phonological patterning, but does seek an explanation for many of these patterns from functional principles of perception and production. In this section, we will briefly describe prelinguistic[2] and adult phonetic systems, before considering the transition between the two, which corresponds to acquisition.

The prelinguistic infant generates a number of vocalization types. At approximately 7 months, the child produces canonical babble (such as [baba], [dada]). MacNeilage and Davis (1990b) suggest that the consonant in such sequences is reflective of a resting position of the velum and tongue at syllable onset, and that the identity of the vowel is the product of the extent of a simple down-up jaw movement. The execution of repeated cycles of jaw opening and closing, which MacNeilage and Davis call *frames*, therefore unavoidably results in vocalizations corresponding somewhat to CV syllables.

This view holds that the unit of speech production defined by children's holistic, and, as yet, undifferentiated groupings of articulatory gestures, corresponds to the syllable or word, not the phoneme. This is supported by evidence presented by Hodge (1989); MacNeilage and Davis (1990a); Nittrouer, Studdert-Kennedy, and McGowan (1989); Studdert-Kennedy (1987, 1991a, 1991b); Studdert-Kennedy and Goodell (1995); Wode (1994), cited by Piske (1995); and Davis and MacNeilage (1995). As the child expands its repertoire to include a number of distinct CV forms, there appears to be strong restrictions on the co-occurrence of the "C" and the "V" within these syllable-like units.

In accordance with their "frames, then content hypothesis," MacNeilage and Davis (1990b) describe the co-occurrence of both alveolar consonants and the palatal glide [j] with front vowels as *fronted* frames, and the co-occurrence of velars and back vowels as *backed* frames. Both patterns reflect the infant's restricted tongue physiology, kinematic potential and control. At the earliest stages, the tongue is thought to be pre-positioned in the horizontal plane prior to syllable onset, and is not actively moved at all during the syllable.

Thus, the association of labials and central vowels, described as pure frames, is essentially characterized by jaw movement with a neutral tongue position. Already by 9 or 10 months, some characteristics of the language spoken to the child are reflected in the relative frequency of fronted, backed, and neutral frames (de Boysson-Bardies, Sagart, Halle, and Durand 1986; de Boysson-Bardies, Vihman, Roug-Hellichius, et al., 1992).

Adult speech, on the other hand, is not similarly constrained in its inventory of syllables. This is evident from the rich possibilities for the co-occurrence of consonants and vowels. In adult language, segments are seen as crucial aspects of language (Studdert-Kennedy and Goodell, 1995), but are not taken to be the basic units of speech because they only exist as subparts of syllables and as combinations of gestures. Current gestural models of adult speech production characterize sounds indirectly as synchronized articulatory gestures, or functional groupings of gestures. The many coarticulatory effects in adult speech are a natural consequence of the literal coproduction of gestures and represent varying degrees of spatial/temporal overlap (Browman and Goldstein, 1986; 1989; Recasens, 1991). The unique contribution of the biological framework is most evident when we try to explore how the child accomplishes the transition from simple frames to the complexity of gestural scores.[3]

At first, very young children moving beyond the simplest mandibular frames produce sets of gestures in a largely synchronous manner (Kent, 1983; 1992). With the development of finer motor control and with practice, children gradually master the relative phasing of gestures, enabling more adultlike patterns of spatiotemporal overlap. This leads to a greater inventory of possible gestural routines and a greater segmental inventory (Studdert-Kennedy and Goodell, 1995).

To flesh out this characterization using the terms of the frame/content model, the child begins to reanalyze holistic fronted or backed frames as *content* corresponding to lip, tongue, velar and laryngeal gestures superimposed on top of the very simplest (mandibular) *frames*. In addition to the frame motion, undergoing refinement to allow for consonant clusters, onsetless syllables, and closed syllables, gesture patterns for the oral and laryngeal articulators are gradually refined.[4] Eventual mastery of the relative phasing of gestures produces adultlike patterns of spatiotemporal overlap in which children accomplish mature gestural patterns corresponding to segmental categories perceived on-line.

We emphasize that the path from the undifferentiated holistic syllable frame to segmentlike organization is not a simple or deterministic one. Characterizing it in detail is a major goal for current and future research in this framework. There is a great deal of intersubject variation but, in general, it seems that during acquisition children rely on syllables as organizational units. Simple syllables appear as components of a suite of relatively fixed gestural routines called *prosodic schemata* (Waterson, 1971), *word patterns* (Macken, 1979), *templates* (Menn, 1983), or *vocal motor schemes* (McCune and Vihman, 1987). Such a templatic inventory might define and limit the infant's repertoire in the early stages of lexical expansion, and the inventory itself might undergo change (Piske, 1997). Radical variation in the interrelationships of gestures is also readily observable within the word (Ferguson and Farwell, 1975).

The emergence of intergestural coordination has been examined most closely in studies of anticipatory coarticulation in vowel-vowel and consonant-vowel sequences. Interpreting this research is problematic for the reasons summarized in Kühnert and Nolan's (1999) review. Coarticulation is not a unitary phenomenon. Not all cases are alike, and they cannot be expected to develop in the same way (Repp, 1986). Thus, conflicting developmental patterns described in the literature may be attributed to intersubject variability as well as a lack of methodological agreement.

With respect to anticipatory coarticulation from vowel to consonantal onset, however, the large, well-controlled studies of Nittrouer, Studdert-Kennedy, and colleagues provide convincing evidence (Goodell and Studdert-Kennedy, 1993; Nittrouer, 1993; Nittrouer, Studdert-Kennedy, and Neely, 1996). Though they note the problem of intersubject variability, it seems clear that some children around the ages of 2 to 3 years have a great deal more intra-syllabic coproduction of consonants and vowels than older children and adults. This pattern is also maintained when looking at data averaged within these age groups. Within-syllable coarticulation (largely dependent on the control of tongue movements) may continue to mature until at least the age of 7 years (Nittrouer, Studdert-Kennedy, and McGowan, 1989; Nittrouer, 1993). These studies show, furthermore, how the organization of gestures within syllables matures at a different rate, depending upon the articulator in question and the particular sequence of segments involved.

A comparison of coarticulation in children's and adult's productions of fricative/vowel sequences *sea-she, Sue-shoe, sa-sha,* (/si-ʃi/, /su-ʃu/, /sɑ-ʃɑ/) found that only adult fricatives preceding the /u/ vowel showed modification due to anticipatory lip rounding. Children's tokens, however, showed a higher degree of tongue body fronting or backing during the fricative portion, depending on the identity of the following vowel (such as fronting for /i/ and backing for /ɑ/ and /u/), indicating greater overlap between the consonant and vowel lingual gestures. It would, therefore, appear that within syllables, young children find it more difficult to segregate or differentiate sequences sharing the same primary articulator (in this case the tongue), than sequences involving different articulators (in this case, the tongue and lips).

This difficulty in dealing with homorganicity in an adultlike way was also revealed in a study of two children (RS and AE) with phonological disorder, who reduced initial /s/ clusters to a fricative (Scobbie, Gibbon, Hardcastle, and Fletcher, 1997). Both children found the homorganic cluster /st/ more difficult to master than /sk/ or /sp/. First, one of the subjects (RS) reduced only /st/, but not /sp/ or /sk/, a pattern which was apparent to the normal listener. Second, although both children appeared, at a later date, to be producing all three clusters correctly, instrumental phonetic analysis showed that the stop in /st/ clusters was still not adult-like. It was heavily spirantized and overly short, both in absolute terms and as a proportion of the cluster duration. Catts and Kamhi (1984) report a similar pattern of reduction whereby /st/ appeared as a fricative, while /sp/ and /sk/ appeared as stops.

These observations about gestural differentiation can be interpreted as evidence for Davis and MacNeilage's "frames, then content" hypothesis and may account for the occurrence of some context-conditioned error patterns as noted in point 1 of the following list. Many of the complex articulations required by adult languages (such as to produce nonhomorganic consonant clusters and closed syllables) do not have obvious cognates with the articulatory gestalts found in the earliest babbling routines (although future research might uncover such connections). These may, however, be explained within the wider biological framework as detailed in points 2 to 4. In each case, the context of the child's error pattern is seen to be crucial.

1. The immature gestural gestalt governing a single articulator in basic syllabic frames might exert a strong repressive influence on the process of differentiation of the gestalt into a coordinated sequence of anatomically proximal, yet independent, gestures (MacNeilage and Davis, 1990b).
2. Children might have difficulty mastering some mature speech patterns, simply due to the complexity of the gestural coordination demanded (Kent, 1984; Waters, 1995).
3. Immature perceptual skills and ongoing immaturity of speech motor skills may be involved in the appearance of developmental speech errors (Nittrouer and Studdert-Kennedy, 1987; Watson, 1997).[5] "A child's phonology is grounded in both perceptual and motoric constraints" (Nittrouer, Studdert-Kennedy, and McGowan, 1989, 131).
4. Early motoric or perceptual constraints may become fossilized into simplification strategies, continuing to be manifested even once the speech production or perceptual difficulties are overcome (Bradford and Dodd, 1996; Hewlett, 1995; Nittrouer, 1983; 1992).

Given this empirical evidence, it is important, when approaching the simplifications or phonological avoidance strategies (Menn, 1983) observed for young normally developing and phonologically disordered (PD) children, to expand analyses beyond the consideration of individual segments in isolation. To illustrate, phenomena, such as alveolar backing, should not be considered without taking into account the vocalic context of the consonant, since alveolars might behave quite differently in the context of front and back vowels.

Clinical Implications

Evidence of context-conditioned error patterns in disordered systems has important implications for clinical diagnosis and management. It highlights the need for the clinician to assess a child's pronunciation beyond the production of individual sounds or classes of sounds to potentially problematic CV sequences. Failure to test a child's production of sounds in a variety of phonetic environments could result in the false impression that the child is unable to pronounce the target when, in fact, they are able to do so in a specific context or set of contexts.

Conversely, correct pronunciation in one or a few contexts might give the impression that the child has no difficulty with a given sound, although they might not be able to produce it in the full range of phonetic and phonotactic settings. Unless the clinician systematically tests for context conditioning, it might be falsely concluded that any variability noted in the child's system is random. Given the typically small number of test items in most tests and the difficulty in selecting appropriate vocabulary (such as familiar and imageable words), it is hardly surprising that the vowel context is not evenly distributed for every consonant or cluster. For example, in the Phonological Assessment of Child Speech test (Grunwell, 1985), only one probe item for word-initial /k/ has a highfront vowel context, while two are before a highback vowel, one before a mid vowel, and six before a low vowel. Evaluation of the child's progress is also likely to vary depending upon the relative frequency of the operative contexts in the words selected for production practice (Camerata and Gandour, 1984).

In addition to providing a more accurate diagnosis, identification of the operative contexts of a given error pattern or patterns narrows the focus of treatment. This minimizes time potentially wasted practising production in contexts which are unproblematic for the child (Leonard, Devescovi, and Ossella, 1987). It has also been suggested that children who do not pronounce target sounds in any contexts, or who show genuine variability (as opposed to context-conditioned variability), might be helped to achieve more accurate productions by targeting the sounds initially in maximally facilitatory contexts, and gradually progressing to more difficult contexts (Gierut, 1990; Grundy and Harding, 1995; Lancaster and Pope, 1989). In Chapter 7, Gibbon and Mackenzie Beck discuss how clinicians might utilize context to facilitate accurate vowel production.

Awareness of potential context conditioning can also assist in the prioritization of remediation targets. In the case of consonant disorders, this is generally done on the basis of whether or not the error pattern reflects delayed or deviant development, with higher priority being afforded to more atypical features. Classification of errors as either delayed or deviant has often been based on how frequent they occur in the literature or how frequent they occur in the clinician's own personal experience. This explains why clinicians tend to regard *all* vowel errors as reflecting disordered development (Reynolds, 1990). However, where vowel error patterns are phonetically principled in accordance with biological models of acquisition, these may be classified as representing delayed development. For example, while alveolar backing across all contexts is rightly regarded as more unusual, and hence more deviant, than velar fronting, alveolar backing occurring only in the context of back vowels may be seen to constitute delayed, as opposed to disordered, development.

Context-Conditioned Patterns in Normally Developing Systems

The discussion in the "Biological Framework" section of this chapter might suggest that there is an unmarked (universal) pattern for the prelexical babbling child of strong contextual conditioning of the "C" and "V" in a simple syllable.[6] In fact, the relative frequency of fronted, backed, and neutral frames in babbling can be influenced by the ambient language and the transition from babbling to early phonology is not an abrupt one (de Boysson-Bardies, Sagart, Halle, and Durand, 1986; de Boysson-Bardies and Vihman, 1991; de Boysson-Bardies, Vihman, Roug-Hellichius, et al., 1992; Davis, MacNeilage, Gildersleeve-Neumann, and Teixeira, 1999; Davis and Matyear, 1997; Vihman, Ferguson, and Elbert, 1986). It is therefore reasonable to expect some cross-linguistic variation even in the earliest recorded data, leading to differences in the apparent segmental constitution of even very highly constrained output.

Our review in this section of context-conditioned errors in normal development appears to show that variation in the set of basic frames is possible, even within a single language.

Davis and MacNeilage (1990) report, in a single case study investigating vowel acquisition (age 1 year, 2 months to 1 year, 8 months) that, almost without exception, highfront vowels occurred in the context of alveolars while highback vowels occurred in velar contexts. Midcentral and lowcentral vowels tended to co-occur with labial consonants. In a later longitudinal study of babbling and first word production by six infants, Davis and MacNeilage (1995) note a similar pattern of CV interactions (Figure 5-1).

Fudge (1969), however, reports CV patterning in his son's early system of a slightly different type (Figure 5-2). In this case, target labials and velars were realized as alveolars in the context of a following front vowel, while target alveolars were realized as labials preceding back rounded vowels, and as velars preceding back unrounded vowels (Table 5-1).[7]

If these examples indicate that more than one pattern of simple frames is available, then a simple deterministic interpretation of the biological framework is not possible. We think, however, that intersubject variation may arise at the point at which children attempt to individuate gestures, but are not yet able to recombine them so as to increase the variety of their output patterns. It is clear that more gesturally oriented research on the earliest output of normally developing children is required.

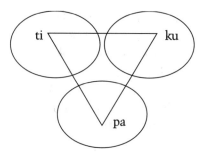

Figure 5-1   Triangular representation of the vowel space with indication of which consonantal places co-occur with different vowel regions in the "frames, then content" hypothesis.

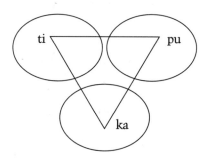

Figure 5-2   Triangular representation of the vowel space showing another possible pattern of consonant-vowel co-occurrence within different vowel regions.

Table 5-1   Fudge Junior (English, 1 year, 4 months)

Alveolar + front vowels			Labials + back rounded vowels			Velars + unrounded vowels		
Word	Target	CP	Word	Target	CP	Word	Target	CP
drink	drɪnk	ti	ball	bɔl	bo	cake	kɛik	kʌk
again	əgein	dɛn	book	bʊk	bo	truck	trʌk	kʌk
			dog	dɒg	bo bo	garden	gɑdɛn	gʌŋ
						doggie	dɒgi	gʌgɯ

Key: CP = child's pronunciation

Results from children with larger vocabularies, whose outputs are more varied and indicate more clearly a degree of gestural sophistication, are easier to interpret. Consider the major study of Dutch children undertaken by Levelt (1994; 1996). Her interest in CV interaction arises from her hypothesis that the purportedly long-distance consonant-to-consonant relationships across an intervening vowel termed *consonant harmony* are in fact *local* CV interactions. In her data, harmony was shown to be heavily influenced by the intervening vowel.

> Examination of the vowels that intervened between the consonants that were thought to be involved in the phenomenon revealed that these actually had the same articulator feature as the harmonised consonant—or as the apparent trigger consonant, for that matter. Numerous data containing consonants that were clearly affected by the adjacent vowel strengthened the hypothesis that Consonant Harmony can better be viewed as Vowel~Consonant Harmony (Levelt, 1994, 70).[8]

Several authors report systems in which only the occurrence of labial consonants is restricted. In a case study of his son J, Braine (1974) notes a general preference for alveolar consonants up until age 1 year, 9 months (Table 5-2). Between 1 year, 9 months and 2 years, Child J started to produce words with labials in initial position preceding low vowels (*mama, ball, bird*), but continued to realize target labials as alveolars where they preceded highfront vowels.

Stoel-Gammon (1983) describes the system of Child D who, at 1 year, 2 months, produced both labials and alveolars in initial position (*bottle* /bɔdl/ [babu]; *bubble* /bʌbəl/ [bʌbu]; *daddy* /dɑedi/ [dædæ]; *light* /lɑit/ [dɑɪ]). She reports a similar restriction on the occurrence of target labials, although in Child D's case the conditioning context was extended to include all front vowels and diphthongs with a front vowel offglide (*baby* /bebi/ [didi]). Child D continued to realize target labials as alveolars in this context until age 1 year, 5 months, when words containing a labial stop-front vowel sequence were produced correctly.

Table 5-2   J (English, 1 year, 9 months to 2 years)

Word	*Alveolar + highfront vowels* Target	CP
pee	pi	di
bee	bi	di
big	bɪg	di?
baby	bɛibi	didi
milk	mɪlk	ni? ni?

Ferguson and Farwell (1975) and Leonard, Newhoff, and Mesalam (1980) also observe an alternation between [b] and [d] in the early productions of their subjects. Both authors attribute this pattern to lexical variation, noting the coexistence of variant pronunciations of the same word (such as [baba] and [daɪdaɪ] for *bye-bye*). However, in each of the examples they cite, the labial target is pronounced as alveolar when followed by a front vowel or diphthong with a front vowel offglide indicating, in these cases also, that the variant pronunciation is context-conditioned although lexically variable. MacNeilage (1998) attributes the lexical variation in cases such as these to difficulty in the relative phasing of gestures. This typically results in the child producing the requisite articulatory components for a given sequence, which are gesturally scored in an incorrect way (such as *pen* /pɛn/ pronounced variably as [dɛ^{dn}], [hɪn], [mbo]) (Ferguson and Farwell, 1975). This is a good example of where the description of the child's variation in terms of indissoluble, segment-sized units fails to capture the child's success in producing appropriate gestures, albeit in inappropriate sequence and combination.

To summarize, the most common pattern to emerge from the literature on normal phonological development in English is the association of *place* of articulation in consonants and vowels. This pattern is namely alveolar consonants with front vowels, labials with round vowels, and velars with back vowels. In some cases, the distribution of either alveolars and labials or alveolars and velars is complementary, such that labials are pronounced as alveolar in the context of front vowels and alveolars are pronounced as velars and labials or just labials in the context of back vowels.

In gestural terms, each of the error patterns described above can be explained in relation to what Kent and Murray (1982) have termed the *compatibility factor*. Alveolar consonants and front vowels are both characterized by a relatively raised and fronted tongue body, while velar consonants and back vowels both involve constriction at the back of the tongue. Labials are compatible with back rounded vowels insofar as they share their specification for labiality. The co-occurrence of labials and mid or low central vowels noted by Davis and MacNeilage (1990) can also be attributed to greater articulatory compatibility between consonant and vowel gestures, in this case, with respect to jaw position since this may be lower at closure for labial than for lingual consonants (Sussman, MacNeilage, and Hanson, 1973, cited in MacNeilage, 1998).

In the normally developing child, CV interactions seem to phase out in the second year in most cases, as gestural reorganization takes hold. Tyler and Langsdale, in their cross-sectional and longitudinal study of nine children aged 18 months, 21 months, and 24 months, conclude that "CV interactions may hold for only the earliest period of lexical acquisition and with differing strengths in individual phonological systems" (Tyler and Langsdale, 1996, 159).

Consonant-Vowel Interactions in Developmental Phonological Disorder

Agreement between consonants and vowels regarding place of articulation also features predominantly in studies reporting context conditioning in PD children. However, here the effects are not confined to word initial stop consonants, but can apply across different manner classes. This can also include sounds in different word positions, reflecting the more advanced age of the children in question and, consequently, the greater overall maturity of their systems. The literature on disordered development also contains examples of error patterns not documented for normally developing children, principally involving variation in vowel quality as a function of consonantal context.

Vowel Conditioning of Consonant Error Patterns

Wolfe and Blocker (1990) report a constraint on labial consonants in the system of Child H, age 4 years, 7 months. Child H realized both labial stops (voiced and voiceless) and labiodental fricatives as [d] preceding front vowels and as [b] preceding back vowels. The bilabial nasal stop /m/ was produced as [n] in front vowel contexts. The constraint not only applied to consonants in word initial position but also in syllable-initial, word-medial position: *doorbell* [dodɛl], *baby* [dɛdi].

In the system of Child NE described by Williams and Dinnsen (1987), alveolars and velars appeared in complementary distribution depending upon the front/back specification of the following vowel. Labials were produced correctly in both environments (Table 5-3).

Table 5-3   NE (USA, 4 years, 6 months)

Word	Consonant-front vowels Alveolars maintained Velars → Alveolars Target	CP	Word	Consonant-back vowels Alveolars → Velars Velars maintained Target	CP
deer	diɚ	diʊ	soup	sup	kuʔ
leg	lɛg	dɛ	girl	gɝl	gʊ
cage	kɛiʤ	tɛ	goat	gout	goʔ, go
swim	swɪm	di			
	Labials unrestricted				
peach	petʃ	piʔ	blow	blou	bo
big	bɪg	bɪ			
page	pɛiʤ	buʔ			

Camerata and Gandour (1984) report a similar case of complementary distribution between alveolars and velars, but one conditioned by vowel height rather than frontness/backness (Table 5-4). In this case, high vowels condition alveolars whereas mid and low vowels condition velars. Labials are unrestricted. Note that Child GG reduced diphthongs to their first element and pronounced /ɛ/ as [ɑ], as shown in examples marked with * and ** in Table 5-4.

At first glance this appears to be a dissimilatory process in that velar consonants share the same height specification as high vowels, while alveolar consonants pattern with mid and low vowels (Chomsky and Halle, 1968). Notwithstanding this, Camerata and Gandour (1984) argue that this error pattern can be considered phonetically motivated insofar as it shows agreement between consonants and vowels in terms of acoustic properties, which in traditional feature terms were described as [+diffuse] (Jakobson and Halle, 1971). Diffuse sounds (that is, alveolars, labials, and high vowels) are characterized by a higher concentration of energy in a noncentral region of the spectrum, and nondiffuse sounds (that is, palatals, velars, and nonhigh vowels) by higher energy bands in a central spectral region. Diffuse sounds also have a lesser overall degree of energy than nondiffuse sounds. In contrast to previous cases described, this pattern appears to represent a perceptual as opposed to articulatory constraint on production.

Table 5-4   GG (USA, 2 years, 10 months to 3 years, 7 months)

			Consonant-high vowels					
Alveolars maintained			*Velars → Alveolars*			*Labials unrestricted*		
Word	Target	CP	Word	Target	CP	Word	Target	CP
tea	ti	di	key	ki	di	bee	bi	bi
			kick	kɪk	di	boot	but	bu
two	tu	du	cook	kʊk	du	book	buk	bu
						boat	bot	bo
			Consonant-mid and low vowels					
Alveolars → Velars			*Velars maintained*			*Labials unrestricted*		
Word	Target	CP	Word	Target	CP	Word	Target	CP
duck	dʌk	gə	cup	kʌp	gə	bus	bʌs	bə
*toe	tou	go	*goat	gout	go	bath	bath	bɑe
*tie	taɪ	gæ	*kite	kait	gæ	pan	paen	bɑeng
dog	dɒg	gɑ	*clown	klaun	gæŋ	boat	bot	bo
**train	trɛin	gæŋ	car	kɑ	gɑ	ball	bɑl	bɑ

A similar constraint on the occurrence of velars is reported by Leonard, Devescovi, and Ossella (1986) for Child E (age 3 years) (Table 5-5). Note that in this system, the distribution of labials, although not conditioned by vowel context, was not unrestricted. Child E produced a labial consonant word-initially (even in words with no initial target consonant at all) if there was a labial in medial or final position of the same word, or if a labial occurred at any position in the following word. Word-initial plosives and fricatives were replaced by a labial stop and liquids and glides by the labiovelar approximant [w] (such as *tummy* /tʌmi/ [bibi]; *jump* /dʒʌmp/ [bɛ, bʌ]; *give* /gɪv/ [bɪm]; *up* /ʌp/ [wʌ]). In words where labials did not appear, vocalic context did, however, condition the occurrence of alveolars and velars. In word-initial position, velars occurred preceding mid and low back vowels and in diphthongs with an /u/ offglide, while alveolars occurred elsewhere.

Grunwell (1981) describes a case, Child S, where the distribution of labials across three different manner classes, stops, fricatives, and approximants is conditioned by the front/back specification of the following vocalic context (Table 5-6). Target labial stops and labiodental fricatives were produced as alveolar stops and dental fricatives respectively in the context of a following front vowels. The fact that alveolar and palatal fricatives and approximants were also realized as dental fricatives in this context might suggest an earlier general preference for the dental place of articulation, which is beginning to resolve. From the biological perspective, this patterning accords with the notion of increasing refinement and differentiation of anatomically proximal gestures.

Table 5-5   E (USA, 3 years)

Consonant-high vowels					
Alveolars/Palatals maintained				*Velars → Alveolars*	
Word	Target	CP	Word	Target	CP
sit	sɪt	di	geese	gis	di
duck	dʌk	dɛ	cake	keik	dei
shoe	ʃu	du			
Consonant-mid and low vowels, diphthongs with an /u/ offglide					
Alveolars → Velars			*(Velars maintained)*		
doll	dal	gɔ			
down	dəun	gəʊ			
no	nəu	go			
nose	nəuz	go			

Table 5-6   S (English, 6 years, 3 months)

	Consonant-front vowels Labial stops → Alveolar stops	
Word	Target	CP
bee	bi	di
peg	pɛg	tɛk
men	mɛn	dɛə
Labiodental fricatives → Dental fricatives		
feet	fit	θɪ
thread	θrɛᵈ	θɛə
Alveolar/Palatal fricatives → Dental fricatives		
sea	si	θɪ
ship	ʃip	θɪʔ
Labiovelar/Alveolar approximant → Dental fricatives		
wind	wɪnd	ði
leg	lɛg	ðɛk

Table 5-7   SC (Scottish, 7 years, 2 months)

	Front vowels Velars maintained			Back rounded vowels Velars → Aveolars	
Word	Target	CP	Word	Target	CP
key	ki	ki	school	skul	stol̡
grape	grep	grep	comb'	comb	tom
curly	cʌrle	kɛle	goat	got	dot
car	car	kar	coffee	cɔfi	tɔfi

In the system described by Hezelwood (1998) the occurrence of alveolar consonants is constrained. Child JP (age 4 years, 2 months) realized all target alveolars as labials in the context of a following rounded vowel: *toy* /tɔi/ [pʷɔi]; *do* /du/ [bʷu]; *sun* (northern English /sʊn/) [pʷʊn].

The following two cases represent a departure from the typical pattern of front/back vocalic influence in that velars are fronted preceding back rounded vowels but appear as velar before front vowels (Table 5-7). In the first case reported by Bates and Watson (1995) Child SC's sound system was characterized by widespread variability with the exception of this particular context-sensitive error pattern.

In a study of consonant cluster acquisition (Scobbie, Gibbon, Hardcastle, and Fletcher 1998; 2000), unpublished data from Child DB shows that his realizations of /st/ and /sk/ are partly context-sensitive (Table 5-8). Though the materials of the study provide only partial data, it appears that Child DB's pervasive velar fronting does not occur in the context of /i/.

One hypothesis about this data is that Child DB is maintaining a covert phonetic distinction between /st/ and /sk/, which is only observable in transcription before /i/. The reason this vowel context reveals a difference between /st/ and /sk/ is that /i/ exerts a strong palatalizing influence on the gestures realizing the stops, producing a percept for /sk/ which sounds like an acceptably fronted velar and a percept for /st/ which sounds like an acceptably palatalized alveolar.

Bates and Watson (1995) also describe a system in which consonantal manner of articulation appears to be conditioned by vocalic context (Table 5-9). In this case, the labiodental fricatives /f, v/ are produced correctly preceding back rounded vowels, but as [b] in the context of a following lowcentral vowel [a], and as [sw] preceding nonlow front vowels. As in the examples of place agreement, this pattern also lends itself to an account in terms of articulatory compatibility. In the context of [ɑ], which represents maximal jaw opening, it is arguably

Table 5-8   DB (Scottish, 4 years, 1 month)

Consonant-high front vowel /i/ Velar maintained Alveolar maintained			Consonant-nonhigh front vowels (/e, a/) and /o/ Velar → Alveolar		
Word	Target	CP	Word	Target	CP
skier	skir	kia	kate	ket	det
steer	stir	tia	skate	sket	det
			sky	skai	da
			sty	staɪ	da
			score	skor	doa

Table 5-9   JC (Scottish, 6 years, 2 months)

Front vowels Labiodental fricatives linearised			Low vowels Labiodental fricatives stopped			Back vowels Labiodental fricatives maintained		
Word	Target	CP	Word	Target	CP	Word	Target	CP
feet	fit	swit	fan	fan	ban	phone	fon	fon
face	fes	swes	van	van	ban	fork	fɔrk	fork

easier to achieve a stop closure characterized by a rapid ballistic movement, than the more precise articulatory positioning required for the fricative. In the context of high- and midfront vowels, which are less antagonistic in terms of jaw position, Child JC was able to produce both a labial and fricative gesture, although not as an integrated sound. The fricative was also produced at the same place of articulation as the vowel. Correct fricative production was arguably facilitated by the back rounded vowel context, which shares the consonant's specification for labiality.

Following Lindsey and Harris (1995), Bates and Watson (1995) describe realization of /f/ as [sw] as a *linearization* of the features frication and labiality, and report a similar example in the case of a child who realized /f/ as a combination of [p] and [s] preceding the diphthong /ai/: *fence* [psains]. Again, this pattern may be interpreted as target overshoot, given the conflicting demands on jaw/lip position for the consonant and vowel gestures. (That is, it is arguably easier to attain a full stop closure in the context of a following [a], than the more precisely specified opening required for the fricative.) With the biological framework, this pattern can also be interpreted as resulting from incorrect phasing of the component gestures (Ferguson and Farwell, 1975).

Consonant Conditioning of Vowel Error Patterns

[ł] Conditioning

The most commonly reported CV effect in the literature is the lowering/backing of front vowels in the context of a following velarized lateral [ł] (Bates, Hewlett, Kaighin, et al., 1992; Bates and Watson, 1995; Gibbon, Shockey, and Reid, 1992; Pollock and Keiser, 1990; Reynolds, 1990). In their group study, Bates and Watson (1995) found examples of this process in the systems of three children (Table 5-10).

Table 5-10   RC (Scottish, 3 years, 9 months), IP (Scottish, 6 years),
SC (Scottish, 7 years, 2 months)

RC			IP			SC		
ε→[a] *preceding* /ł/			ε→[a] *preceding* /ł/			ɪ, u, ε→[o,ɔ] *preceding* /ł/		
Word	Target	CP	Word	Target	CP	Word	Target	CP
nest	nɛst	naist	vest	vɛst	vest	pencil	pɛnsɪl	pɛnsoł
egg-cup	ɛgkʌp	aig kʌp	neck	nɛk	nek	school	skul	stoḻ
melting	mɛltɪŋ	małtɪŋ	yellow	jɛlo	jawo	spell	spɛl	społᵊ
shell	ʃɛl	sał	wellie boots	wɛle buts	wawe bʉts	melting	mɛltɪŋ	mołtɪŋ
						girl	gɪrl	gɔł

With Children RC and IP, the lateral context influenced the production of a single vowel only, while in the case of Child SC there was evidence of at least three vowels being affected. Children RC and IP both had difficulty with the midlow front vowel /ɛ/. Child RC typically realized /ɛ/ as [ai]. However, in the context of [ɫ], he produced it as [a]. Child IP raised /ɛ/ to [e] in the context of velars and alveolars, and lowered it to [a] in the context of /l/, itself pronounced as [w]. These patterns also represent a natural assimilatory effect given the greater articulatory and acoustic compatibility of mid- and lowback vowels with [ɫ] or [w], rather than front vowels, high vowels, and diphthongs.

[ɹ] Conditioning

Bates and Watson (1995) also report examples of /ɹ/-conditioning. Two of their Scottish subjects, Children SC and DN, fronted, raised, or fronted and raised the midlow back vowel /ʌ/ to [ɛ], [e] or [ɪ] preceding /ɹ/ (which was itself unrealized).[9] A third subject, Child DP, realized /ʌ/ as [o] in this context (Table 5-11).

It can be argued that these error patterns represent a coalescence, or synthesis, of the vowel and consonantal properties (expressed as [+vocalic] and [+coronal] in traditional feature terms), rather than simple /ɹ/ deletion on account of the change in vowel quality. In the first two cases, the relatively raised and forward tongue position characteristic of the consonant is anticipated during the vowel gesture. In the final example, the substitution of [o] for /ʌ ɹ/, the rounded vowel might also reflect recognition of the lip-rounding quality that is associated with [ɹ] or, in the case of *purple* and *worm*, assimilation to the place of articulation of the final consonants, respectively [p] and [m]. Once again, this pattern can be explained in terms of immaturity in differentiating articulatorily compatible gestures.

Table 5-11 SC (Scottish, 7 years, 2 months), DN (Scottish, 6 years, 2 months), DP (Scottish, 5 years, 5 months)

SC ʌ→e, ɛ preceding [ɹ]			DN ʌ→e, ɛ, ɪ preceding [ɹ]			DP ʌ→o preceding [ɹ]		
Word	Target	CP	Word	Target	CP	Word	Target	CP
purple	pʌrpʌl	pepʊlə	purple	pʌrpʌl	peəpəɫ	turn	tʌrn	don
turn	tʌrn	ten	turn	tʌrn	teən	purple	pʌrpʌl	bobo
worm	wʌrm	wɛm	worm	wʌrm	weəm	worm	wʌrm	wom
curly	kʌrle	kɛli	curly	kʌrle	kɪle			
turtle	tʌrtʌl	tɛtoɫ						

Nasal Conditioning

A further pattern of CV influence noted by Reynolds (1990) is the lowering of high- and midhigh vowels preceding a nasal consonant. Reynolds suggests that this pattern may be perceptually motivated as children acquiring speech might misconstrue the tendency for nasalized vowels to sound more open. Evidence that nasalized high vowels are characterized by lower second formant frequencies than their nonnasalized counterparts is provided by Wright (1986), cited in Johnson (1997). Johnson (1997) also reports the tendency for certain vowel contrasts to be collapsed in nasal contexts in some dialects of American English.

In the children P and B reported by Reynolds (1990), vowel length associated with /iː/ is preserved in the substituted diphthong, while in his Child E, it is attached to the nasal (Table 5-12). Realization of /ɪ/ as [ɛə] and /aʊ/ as [ɛə] in Child P suggests that the pattern has extended to include all vowels preceding nasals irrespective of their high/low or long/short specification.

Vowel Devoicing

Further unpublished data from Child DB (described earlier in "Vowel Conditioning of Consonant Error Patterns") provides an example of a rather different type of context conditioning (Scobbie, Gibbon, Hardcastle, and Fletcher, 2000), which is gradient and variable. In this case, Child DB sometimes devoices vowels when they appear in closed syllables with a particular tendency for the devoicing of /i/. Table 5-13 indicates the number of tokens in which the vowel was totally voiceless (out of six attempts) for a range of words.

A phonetic explanation for this pattern given by Scobbie, Gibbon, Hardcastle, and Fletcher (2000), in keeping with the biological framework, follows from the fact that (for aerodynamic and articulatory reasons) voice onset time (VOT) tends to have a greater duration before high vowels than before low ones; that high vowels tend to be of less duration than low vowels; and that vowels in

Table 5-12   P (English, 4 years, 8 months), E (English, 4 years, 9 months), BL (English, 6 years, 6 months)

P			E			B		
ɪ, ɪ, ɛi, au→[ɛ] preceding /n/			ɪ→[ɛ]; ɪ→[ɒ] ɛi, au→[an] preceding /n/			i→[eɪ, ɛɪ] preceding /m, n/ ɛɪ→[eɪ, ɛɪ] preceding /n/		
Word	Target	CP	Word	Target	CP	Word	Target	CP
queen	kwin	gɛə	queen	kwin	kwɛnː	ice-cream	aisʁcrim	aɪʔgeɪ
green	grin	gɛə	green	grin	gwɛnː	queen	kwin	keɪə
ring	rɪŋ	wɛə	drinking	drɪɲiŋ	ʔɒkɪ	green	grin	geɪ
train	treɪn	tsɛə	train	treɪn	twanː	aeroplane	ɛərəplɛin	ɛləpeɪ
crown	kraʊn	kɛə	crown	kraʊn	kwanː	train	treɪn	teɪ

Table 5-13 DB (Scottish, 4 years,1 month)

	/6	Mean VOT	Vowel	Target	/6	Mean VOT	Vowel		/6	Mean VOT	Vowel
kate	0	43ms	71ms	pot	0	36ms	46ms	peak	5	38ms	38ms
gate	2	36ms	92ms	"Bot"	0	28ms	48ms	beak	4	6ms	50ms
skate	0	38ms	92ms	spot	0	32ms	64ms	speak	2	37ms	52ms

closed syllables tend to be of less duration than vowels in open syllables. In Child DB's case, VOT reflects vowel height to an extreme degree. (Note, however, that VOT is not a cue for the target voicing status of the initial consonant.) Scobbie and colleagues (2000) report that Child DB's mean VOT (in open syllables) before /i/ is 52 ms, appreciably longer than VOT before /o/ or /ai/ (30 ms and 22 ms, respectively). In closed syllables, vowels are so short that the VOT might therefore completely occupy the time available for the vowel (see Table 5-13, which gives the mean duration of VOT and of the voiced portion of the vowel in those cases where the vowel is not devoiced). Because the /i/ vowel is particularly short, and because it conditions the longest VOT, these factors combine to maximize the likelihood of devoicing.

Discussion

Nature of Error Patterns

The most common context-conditioned error pattern reported in studies of young normally developing children is the co-occurrence of alveolar stops and front vowels, velar stops and back vowels, and labial stops and back rounded vowels. The fact that this pattern has been observed in both the early and later stages of babbling and in early word production supports the idea that during early word acquisition children initially utilize and exploit articulatory routines already within their production capacities (MacNeilage, 1998; Piske, 1995). Where it occurs in meaningful speech, it might be understood as an assimilation by the consonant to the place of articulation of the vowel.

This error pattern is also the most common vowel-to-consonant effect reported for PD children, although in this clinical case it is not confined to stops but may extend to different manner classes (that is, nasals, fricatives, approximants). The literature on normal development also reports a relatively higher proportion of constraints on labials compared with other consonants, whereas in the case of PD children, it would appear that alveolar and velar consonants are more likely to be constrained than labial consonants. This difference between the two groups of children might be attributed to the younger age of the normally developing children and to the fact that children tend to master the spatiotemporal coordination of discrete articulators (that is, tongue and lips) earlier than the phasing of gestures involving the same articulator (such as, front and back of tongue) (Nittrouer, Studdert-Kennedy, and McGowan, 1989).

In the majority of cases, it can be argued that these error patterns reflect difficulty in the timing and coordination of adjacent articulatory gestures. There are two main factors supporting this argument. First, the sequences in question involve consonants and vowels, which are characterized by diverging or antagonistic gestures, and which involve anatomically proximal articulations (such as velars characterized by back of tongue constriction followed by front vowels characterized by front of tongue constriction). Context conditioning results in greater articulatory compatibility between segments (such as /k/ → [t] /_i).

Second, without exception, the directionality of the contextual influence observed is from right to left, that is, the target segment undergoes a quality change as a function of following context. Based on evidence from normal adult speech, right to left or anticipatory effects are believed to be timing effects reflective of articulatory preprogramming. This is in contrast to left to right or carryover effects which are thought to be largely mechano-inertial in nature (Gay, 1977), and therefore less likely to be under independent control.

The higher incidence of context-conditioned vowel errors reported in the case of the PD children, to some extent, reflects the recent increase in attention given to disordered vowel production, and in particular the group studies which have targeted this population (Bates and Watson, 1995; Reynolds, 1990). However, it can also arguably be attributed to the greater maturity and therefore more extensive segmental repertoire of the older PD children. These children have already acquired the later appearing and articulatorily more complex liquids /l/ and /r/ which, according to the literature, are the consonants most likely to condition vowel errors.[10] The consonant-conditioned vowel errors, although representing difficulties at a different stage of development (that is, beyond constraints imposed by a frames and content model), still accord with the biological framework in that they can be explained in terms of articulatory compatibility.

The majority of the context-sensitive vowel error patterns noted in this chapter involve the midvowel series (that is, /ɪ, ɛ, ʌ, ʊ/). These vowels also appear to be the most susceptible to coarticulatory effects in normal speech (Bates, 1995; Stevens and House, 1963). Within the gestural framework, degree of coarticulation is considered to be dependent on both degree of articulatory compatibility and on degree of mechanical constraint imposed on the tongue body during production (Recasens, 1984; 1991). The peripheral vowels, that is, /i, ɑ, a, u, o, ɔ/, characterized by more extreme articulations and longer inherent durations, are arguably subject to greater constraints on tongue body activity. Therefore, they show less overall compatibility with context than the mid vowels. In other words, midvowels plus consonant-midvowel sequences are more problematic because the CV gestures are more similar (that is, there is less articulatory distance between them) than is the case between consonant-peripheral vowel sequences. A similar comparison can presumably also be made between sententially stressed versus unstressed vowels (Bates, 1995). In the latter case, the vowel gestures arguably involve a greater degree of constraint on the tongue body than the consonant gestures (that is, they are characterized by more extreme articulatory configurations). In the case of the consonant plus mid vowel sequences, it could be hypothesized that the consonant gestures are more highly constrained than the midvowel gestures, thus accounting for the vowel assimilation to the consonantal place of articulation.

Phonological versus Biological Perspectives

In an earlier review of clinical CV interaction, Bernhardt and Stemberger (1998, 548) used a constraint-based phonological perspective to account for their data, and concluded that CV interactions, while not common, give rise to provocative issues for acquisition theory. For example, it must account for the fact that CV interactions are possible, but infrequent. This is a typical problem for phonological theories of symbolic representations, configurations, and constraints, which define the possible but not the probable. For those phonological theories, which also incorporate theories of markedness, the problem is that clinical phenomena are by definition marked, and so it is unclear to what extent phonological theory should explain them.

The biological framework is rather different in emphasis. Being phonetic, it attempts to cover both the very earliest structures used in babbling (which are language-specific in terms of the relative distribution of nonneutral frames) and also mature gestural systems. It also needs to provide an account of the transition between the two, drawing mainly on phonetic development in speech-motor abilities, physiology, and perception.

Aspects of linguistic development, such as phonological and morphological categorization, might be partly the result of phonetic developments in the biological framework. Thus, phonological disorders are predicted to result, in some cases, from problems in reanalyzing holistic productions into their gestural components and in relating subtle adult patterns of language-specific coarticulation to the undifferentiated and well-rehearsed infantile patterns. The apparent neutralization of contrast in the clinical cases is possible, but infrequent, because relatively few children extract the wrong lessons from CV interaction from the babbling stage and make the wrong connections between infant CV interaction and adult coarticulation.

Another problematic issue is that vowels typically influence consonantal errors, although the reverse is possible, if infrequent. A phonological theory does not easily represent this asymmetry without extra machinery being created for the purpose. Furthermore, phonological theory does not provide a nonstipulative account of why it is *place* that is involved, in the large part, in CV interactions.[11] The biological framework, on the other hand, can draw on the central concept of the frame on which content is imposed. This can account for the dominance of vowels in the majority of cases, and for the fact that it is place that is accommodated.

Conclusion

The patterns of CV interaction in disordered systems we reviewed demand explanation from theories of acquisition. It is necessary for such theories to account for the difference between the clinical cases and the much younger normally developing child. While further work needs to be done to make a really convincing case for the claim that phonological disorder will not be understood without reference to the biological framework of language, we feel this framework is useful for determining research themes and has great explanatory potential.

Endnotes

1. A phonetic system combines language-specific (and universal) "knowledge" (that is, stored schemata for patterns of behavior) which relate physical phenomena (both in perception and production) to abstract linguistic concepts, such as lexically contrastive features, sociolinguistically relevant variables, prosodic structures, and so on. A phonetic system defines the appropriate articulatory and acoustic targets for phonological features whatever prosodic, lexical, morphological, pragmatic, or other relevant context they appear in, for all the speaker's dialectal variants. Such a system also specifies the appropriate degrees of spatial and temporal coarticulation.

2. Given the language-specific perceptual knowledge of the infant (Jusczyk, 1997), and the apparent continuity between babble and early phonology in production (Davis and Matyear, 1997; Vihman, 1996; Vihman and Velleman, 2000) "pre"linguistic is an inaccurate term, but will serve our purposes here.

3. A gestural score, like an orchestral one, is a coordinated representation of a number of quasi-independent sequences, one for each articulator (or instrument).

4. We do not wish to imply that each of these physiological regions is equivalent to a single articulator. Note, though, that the tongue may act as a single unit initially, only gradually developing independent control of the tongue/tip blade (Gibbon, 1998; 1999).

5. Nittrouer and Studdert-Kennedy (1987) compared child and adult perceptual judgements of fricatives. They found that in contrast to the adults, the children relied to a greater extent on information contained in the transitional portion of the syllable between the fricative and vowel than in the steady-state portion of the fricative itself. These results sug-

gest that children's perceptual organization is less segmental than that of adults.

6. The extent to which the segment is a valid term in phonological analysis is not explicitly the topic of this chapter. Yet because our focus is primarily larger domain phenomena and because of our phonetic perspective, we should make it clear that segmental treatment of the phenomena discussed is, in part, to ensure it is relevant to current clinical practice. It should be clear, however, that the segment alone is not sufficient to capture the range of behaviors observed in normal acquisition or in the clinical population. Our data are mostly transcriptional, and therefore reflect the listener's segmentally oriented interpretation of the child's output. In most CV sequences which we discuss, either the C or the V sound is correct, while the other segment is in error. So while a nonsegmental perspective will, perhaps, be essential to a proper understanding of the underlying processes responsible for speech errors, the segment remains a highly popular means of expressing the impression a speech error induces in the child's interlocutors.

7. It is important to note that the conditioning is dependent on the child's surface realization of the vowel and not the underlying target, hence the apparently different treatment of /d/ in *dog* and *doggie* depending on realization of target /ɒ/ as [o] or [ʌ].

8. Labials are conditioned by round vowels, alveolars by front vowels, and velars are conditioned by back vowels (Levelt, 1994, 60). In addition to front unrounded vowels, Dutch has front rounded vowels, which might pattern with alveolars or labials, and the higher back rounded vowels condition both labials and velars. We are not in a position to do more than call for further data in order to enable future cross-linguistic work on C~V interaction; in particular in languages with front rounded or back unrounded vowels or both (such as Turkish).

9. The reader is reminded that Scottish English is a rhotic accent system.

10. In emerging or disordered systems acquiring a rhotic accent, the "r" itself may not be pronounced. The change in vowel quality represents a recognition of the consonant in the target system and therefore an attempt to signal its presence.

11. Bernhardt and Stemberger (1998) and Levelt (1994) exemplify the problems that arise from trying to find a feature system for phonological place which enables the appropriate generalizations to be made regarding which features might spread, the triggers and targets.

Acknowledgments

James M. Scobbie wishes to acknowledge funding by the Gannochy Trust and the ESRC (Grants R000271195 and R000237135).

APPENDIX

Summary of Consonant-Vowel Sequences Most Likely to Be Problematic and Likely Facilitatory Contexts for Remediation

A list of stimulus words is presented in Table A5-1. This is intended to form the basis of an assessment procedure designed to identify potential CV interactions, which could be administered in the form of a picture-naming response task. As far as possible, words have been selected that are most likely to be familiar to young children and that are imageable or easily stimulable through verbal prompting.

The phonetic contexts represented in the word list have been selected on the basis of the articulatory and acoustic regularities evident from the review of published reports. An attempt has also been made to target each consonant-vowel or vowel-consonant sequence at least four times, allowing for detection of inconsistency of production (following Pollock and Keiser, 1990). In general, it is important to establish patterns of variability, whether this is progressive or nonprogressive, or whether their system is static (Grunwell, 1981). Where this has proved difficult due to the relatively limited frequency of occurrence of the sequence in English words (such as /k/ + /ɛ/ sequences), it is advisable to supplement the data set either with nonsense words or repetitions of the real words that are available.

Contexts for vowel-to-consonant effects are listed separately from those designed to detect consonant-to-vowel effects. To give a more complete picture of the child's production capabilities and to ensure an accurate diagnosis of context conditioning, each of the three principal consonantal place categories are represented for each effect. For example, while it is only velars and labials that are subject to incorrect realization in front vowel contexts, alveolar consonant-front vowel sequences have also been included. It is useful to include these because they represent the contexts most likely to facilitate correct pronunciation of the target. To assist orientation, target sounds which are vulnerable to a given error process occur in the shaded sections of the word list.

A similar procedure has been adopted in the case of vowels errors. Where a vowel probe has been omitted, this indicates that no appropriate lexical items were found to illustrate that particular sequence. It is also noted that dental and palatal consonants and, in the case of vowel-to-consonant effects, liquids and glides are not represented. This reflects their apparently low incidence of involvement in context-sensitive error patterns.

The word list is designed to accommodate the nonregional or Southern British Standard accent system. However, given the potential of vowel raising, fronting, or both in Scottish English, vowel-/ɪ/ sequences have been included in the section on consonant-to-vowel effects. The question of how far error patterns vary across different accent systems and the design of a word list to encompass regional accent variations are important areas for future study.

Since all reported error patterns are conditioned by following context, examples of the target sound are restricted to syllable-initial position (CV or VC). In cases where suitable syllable-initial, word-initial words are limited, the list has been supplemented with examples of the target consonant occurring in syllable-initial, word-medial position. Target vowels occur in syllable-initial position without exception. Similarly, since there is no evidence in the literature to suggest an effect of lexical stress, no attempt has been made to systematically vary stressed and unstressed syllables. Given that the purpose of the word list is to identify CV interactions rather than vowel harmony or consonant harmony effects, the majority of words are also monosyllabic. However, a range of syllabic structures (that is, CV, CVC, CVCV) is included because children's performance may deteriorate with an increase in linguistic complexity and therefore processing load.

Table A5-1 Vowel-to-consonant effects: Front vowel contexts

Key: Individual vowel contexts are shown in the first row. The abbreviation Rz denotes realization. The shaded areas highlight the consonants that are vulnerable to incorrect realization in this context.

/i/	Rz	/ɪ/	Rz	/eɪ/	Rz	/ɛ/	Rz	/aɪ/	Rz
pea		pick		pay		pet		pie	
bee		pill		page		peck		buy	
peak		bib		paper		peg		pipe	
beak		pillow		baby		pen		pile	
peel		pigeon		pavement		bell			
piece		biscuit				bench			
beaver						better			
me		mirror		May		men		Mike	
meat		mitten		makeup		melt		marmite	
measles				mermaid		measure			
						medicine			
V		fin		veil		fence		fire	
feet		fish		vein		yest		five	
field		fist		faint		feather		file	
		finger				ferry		viking	

Labials → Alveolars

170

Alveolars realized correctly

	video / village			ferret / vegetable	fireman	
tea	Tim	day		ten	tie	
teeth	tick	tail		teddy	tile	
team	Dick	date		telly	time	
D	dig	table		desk	tidy	
teddy	dish			dentist	diet	
body	ticket			telephone		
teacher						
knee	knitting	nail		net	night	
Neil		name		neck	nine	
bunny				nest		
needle						
sea	zip	sail		settee	sign	
seat	six			tea-set		
daisy	sister			seven		
seagull	cigar			zebra		
	city			centipede		

Table A5-1 *Continued*

Velars → Alveolars

/i/	Rz	/ɪ/	Rz	/eɪ/	Rz	/ε/	Rz	/aɪ/	Rz
key		kick		Kay		get		kite	
Keith		king		cake		kettle			
geese		give		case					
goalkeeper		guitar		cage					
		kitchen		cave					
		biscuit		game					
				gate					

Vowel-to-consonant effects: Central and back unrounded vowel contexts

Key: Individual vowel contexts are shown in the first row. The abbreviation Rz denotes realization. The shaded areas highlight the consonants that are vulnerable to incorrect realisation in this context. In SBS /a/ is typically realised with a low central quality. The diphthong /au/ is also included here on account that the first element qualifies as a central vowel.

Labials → Velars

/ɜ/	Rz	/a/	Rz	/ʌ/	Rz	/ɑ/	Rz	/au/	Rz
bird		pan		bun		park			
pearl		back		bud		part			
purple		bat		bug		bark			
perfume		bang		bump		path			
		band		bucket		bath			
		badger		puddle		party			

172

	pancake		basket	
mermaid	map	mud	mars-bar	mouse
	man	mug	marmite	mouth
		mummy		mountain
fern	fan	furry	fast	
furniture	van		farmer	

Alveolars → Velars

	tap	ton	tar	town
turtle	tap	ton	tar	town
turkey	tank	tongue	tart	down
	daddy	tusks	dart	
		dustbin	dark	
		Tele-tubby	dance	
nurse	nappy	number		
	sad	sum		sound
	Sam	sun		south
	sand	Sunday		
	sandcastle	sunny		

Table A5-1   *Continued*

Velars realized correctly

/ɜ/	Rz	/a/	Rz	/ʌ/	Rz	/ɑ/	Rz	/aʊ/	Rz
girl		cat		cup		car		cow	
curl		cap		gun		card		cowboy	
curly		catch		cuddle		castle		count	
curtain		carrot		custard		garden			
		camera		cupboard					
		candle							
		garage							

Vowel-to-consonant effects: Back rounded vowel contexts

Key: Individual vowel contexts are shown in the first row. The abbreviation Rz denotes realization. The shaded areas highlight the consonants that are vulnerable to incorrect realization in this context.

/ɒ/	Rz	/ɔ/	Rz	/oʊ/	Rz	/ɔ/	Rz	/ʊ/	Rz	/u/	Rz
pot				bow				bull		boots	
pod				bowl				pull		Pooh	
bomb				bone				book			
body				boat				pudding			
bottom				pole							
bottle				post							

Labials realized correctly

Table 1:

		postman			moon
		mow			
		moat			
		mole			
		motorbike			
		foal	foot		food
four	fox		full		
fall	fog				
fort	foggy				
fork	volcano				
forty					
popcorn					

Alveolars → Labials

Table 2:

top	torn	toe	two
dog	Dawn	toad	toot
doggie	tortoise	toast	tool
dot		Tony	tooth
doll			
	naughty	nose	new
		knock	newspaper
		note	

Table A5-1 *Continued*

/ɒ/	Rz	/ɔ/	Rz	/oʊ/	Rz	/ʊ/	Rz	/u/	Rz
<u>s</u>ock		<u>s</u>aw		<u>s</u>ew		<u>S</u>ooty		<u>S</u>ue	
<u>s</u>ong		<u>s</u>auce		<u>s</u>oap				<u>s</u>uit	
		<u>s</u>word		<u>Z</u>oe				<u>s</u>oup	
		<u>s</u>alt		<u>s</u>ofa					
		<u>s</u>aucer							

Velars → Labials

/ɒ/	Rz	/ɔ/	Rz	/oʊ/	Rz	/ʊ/	Rz	/u/	Rz
<u>c</u>ot		<u>c</u>ore		<u>g</u>o		<u>c</u>ook		<u>c</u>oo	
<u>c</u>ost		<u>c</u>orn		<u>c</u>oat		<u>g</u>ood		<u>g</u>oose	
<u>c</u>otton		<u>c</u>orner		<u>g</u>oat		<u>c</u>ooker		<u>G</u>oofey	
<u>c</u>ollar		<u>c</u>ornflakes		<u>c</u>oke		<u>c</u>uckoo			
<u>c</u>offee				<u>c</u>one					
<u>c</u>ockrel				<u>c</u>omb					
<u>c</u>omputer				<u>c</u>oach					
<u>c</u>auliflower				<u>g</u>oal					
				<u>c</u>old					
				<u>g</u>old					

Consonant-to-Vowel Effects

Key: The shaded areas highlight the vowels that are vulnerable to incorrect realization in this context.

Lowering and/or backing of nonlow and/or front vowels preceding [ł]

/i/	Rz	/ɪ/	Rz	/ei/	Rz	/ɛ/	Rz	/ai/	Rz
eel		ill		whale		bell		pile	
wheel		Bill		tail		well		tile	
seal		Will		rail		shell		smile	
meal		mill		snail		sell			
peel		hill				smell			
steal		drill							
real									

/ou/	Rz	/ʊ/	Rz	/u/	Rz	/ɔ/	Rz	/au/	Rz
pole		pull		pool		call		towel	
bowl		bull		cool		Paul		owl	
goal		full		stool		wall			
hole						small			
foal						tall			
coal						ball			
whole									

Table A5-1 *Continued*

Fronting and/or raising of midback and lowback vowels preceding /ɹ/ (rhotic accents)

/ɝ/	Rz	/ɔ/	Rz				
purple		shorts					
turn		door					
worm		fork					
turtle		four					
purse							

Lowering of high and midhigh vowels preceding nasals

/i/	Rz	/ɪ/	Rz	/ei/	Rz	/ou/	Rz	/ɔ/	Rz
ice-cream		chin		chain		cone		room	
cream		Jim		stain		comb			
green		pin		rain		stone			
beans		Lynne		train		phone			
team		robin		plane		Joan			
stream		basin				bone			
clean		tin							
dream		chimney							
queen		king							
		skin							

/u/

/u/	
spoon	
baboon	
balloon	
June	

179

References

Bates, S. A. R. (1995). Towards a definition of schwa: An acoustic investigation of vowel reduction in English. Ph.D. thesis, University of Edinburgh.

Bates, S. A. R., Hewlett, N. F. R., Kaighin, S., et al. (1992). Distortion and possible neutralisation within the vowel systems used by some Edinburgh children presenting with phonological disorder. Supplement to the Proceeding of the Second International Conference on Spoken Language Processing. Banff, Alberta, Canada.

Bates, S., and Watson, J. (1995). Consonant-vowel interactions in developmental phonological disorder. In Caring to Communicate: Proceedings of the Golden Jubilee Conference of the Royal College of Speech and Language Therapists, York, October, 1995. London: Royal College of Speech and Language Therapists, 274–279.

Bernhardt, B. H., and Stemberger, J. P. (1998). Handbook of phonological development from the perspective of constraint-based nonlinear phonology. San Diego: Academic.

Bradford, A., and Dodd, B. (1996). The motor-planning abilities of phonologically disordered children. European Journal of Disorders of Communication, 29, 349–370.

Braine, M. D. S. (1974). On what constitutes a learnable phonology. Language, 50, 270–300.

Browman, C. P., and Goldstein, L. (1986). Towards an articulatory phonology. Phonology Yearbook, 3, 219–252.

Browman, C. P., and Goldstein, L. (1989). Gestural structures and phonological patterns. Status Report on Speech Research, SR-97/80, Haskins Laboratories.

Camerata, S., and Gandour, J. (1984). On describing idiosyncratic phonological systems. Journal of Speech and Hearing Research, 49, 262–266.

Catts, H. W., and Kamhi, A. G. (1984). Simplification of /s/+stop consonant clusters: A developmental perspective. Journal of Speech and Hearing Research, 27, 556–561.

Chomsky, N., and Halle, M. (1968). The sound pattern of English. New York: Harper.

Davis, B. L., and MacNeilage, P. F. (1990). Acquisition of correct vowel production: A quantitative case study. Journal of Speech and Hearing Research, 33, 16–27.

Davis, B. L., and MacNeilage, P. F. (1995). The articulatory basis of babbling. Journal of Speech and Hearing Research, 38, 199–211.

Davis, B. L., MacNeilage, P. F., Gildersleeve-Neumann, C., and Teixeira, E. (1999). Cross-language studies of consonant-vowel co-occurrence constraints in infants and adults: Ambient language effects in first words. Oral presentation at the Twentieth Annual Child Phonology Conference, July 7-10, 1999. Bangor: University of Wales.

Davis, B. L., and Matyear, C. L. (1997). Babbling and first words: Phonetic similarities and differences. Speech Communication, 22, 269–277.

de Boysson-Bardies, B., Sagart, J., Halle, P., and Durand, C. (1986). Acoustic investigation of cross linguistic variability in babbling. In B. Lindblom and R. Zetterstrom (Eds.), Precursors of early speech (pp. 113–127). Basingstoke, England: Macmillan.

de Boysson-Bardies, B., and Vihman, M. M. (1991). Adaptation to language: Evidence from babbling and early words in four languages. Language, 61, 297–319.

de Boysson-Bardies, B., Vihman, M. M., Roug-Hellichius, L., et al. (1992). Material evidence of infant selection from target language: A cross linguistic study. In C. A. Ferguson, L. Menn, and C. Stoel-Gammon (Eds.), Phonological development: Models, research, implications (pp. 369–391). Timonium, Md.: York Press.

Ferguson, C., and Farwell, C. (1975). Words and sounds in early language acquisition: English initial consonants in the first 50 words. Language, 51, 419–439.

Fudge, E. C. (1969). Syllables. Journal of Linguistics, 5, 253–286.

Gay, T. (1977). Articulatory movements in VCV sequences. Journal of the Acoustical Society of America, 62, 183-193.

Gibbon, F. E. (1998). Lingual articulation in children with developmental speech disorders. Ph.D. thesis. Luton, England: University of Luton.

Gibbon, F. E. (1999). Undifferentiated lingual gestures in children with articulation/phonological disorders. Journal of Speech, Language, and Hearing Research, 42, 382–397.

Gibbon, F., Shockey, L., and Reid, J. (1992). Description and treatment of abnormal vowels. Child Language Teaching and Therapy, 8(1), 30–59.

Gierut, J. A. (1990). Differential learning of phonological oppositions. Journal of Speech and Hearing Research, 33, 540–549.

Goodell, E. W., and Studdert-Kennedy, M. (1993). Acoustic evidence for the development of gestural coordination in the speech of 2-year-olds: A longitudinal study. Journal of Speech and Hearing Research, 36, 707–727.

Grundy, K., and Harding, A. (1995). Developmental speech disorders. In K. Grundy (Ed.), Linguistics in clinical practice (2nd ed.) (pp. 329–357). London: Whurr.

Grunwell, P. (1981). The nature of phonological disability in children. New York: Academic.

Grunwell, P. (1985). Phonological assessment of child speech (PACS). Windsor: NFER-Nelson.

Harris, J., Watson, J. M. M., and Bates, S. A. R. (1999). Prosody and melody in vowel disorder. Journal of Linguistics, 35, 489–525.

Hewlett, N. (1985). Phonological versus phonetic disorders: Some suggested modifications to the current use of the distinction. British Journal of Disorders of Communication, 20, 155–164.

Hezelwood, B. (1998). A phonetically-based feature geometry for the analysis and classification of disordered pronunciation. In W. Ziegler and K. Deger (Eds.), Clinical phonetics and linguistics (pp. 115–123). London: Whurr.

Hodge, M. (1989). A comparison on spectral-temporal measures across speaker age: Implications for an acoustic characterization of speech maturation. Ph.D. thesis. Madison: University of Wisconsin.

Jakobson, R., and Halle, M. (1971). Fundamentals of language (2nd ed.). The Hague: Mouton.

Johnson, K. (1997). Acoustic and auditory phonetics. Oxford: Blackwell.

Jusczyk, P. (1997). The discovery of spoken language. London: MIT Press.

Kent, R. D. (1983). The segmental organization of speech. In P. MacNeilage (Ed.), The production of speech (pp. 57–89). New York: Springer-Verlag.

Kent, R. D. (1984). Psychobiology of speech development: Co-emergence of language and a movement system. American Journal of Physiobiology, 246, 888–894.

Kent, R. D. (1992). The biology of phonological development. In C. A. Ferguson, L. Menn, and C. Stoel-Gammon (Eds.), Phonological development: Models, research, implications (pp. 65–90). Timonium, Md.: York Press.

Kent, R. D., and Bauer, H. R. (1985). Vocalizations of one-year olds. Journal of Child Language, 13, 491–526.

Kent, R. D., and Murray, A. D. (1982). Acoustic features of infant vocalic utterances at 3, 6 and 9 months. Journal of the Acoustical Society of America, 72, 353–365.

Kühnert, B., and Nolan, F. (1999). The origin of coarticulation. In W. J. Hardcastle and N. Hewlett (Eds.), Coarticulation: Theory, data and techniques (pp. 7–30). Cambridge, England: Cambridge University Press.

Lancaster, G., and Pope, L. (1989). Working with children's phonology. Bicester, England: Winslow Press.

Leonard, B. D., Devescovi, A., and Ossella, T. (1987). Context-sensitive phonological patterns in children with poor intelligibility. Child Language Teaching and Therapy, 3(2), 125–132.

Leonard, L., Newhoff, M., and Mesalam, L. (1980). Individual differences in early child phonology. Applied Psycholinguistics, 1, 7–31.

Levelt, C. C. (1994). On the acquisition of place. HIL dissertations in linguistics 8. Leiden, The Netherlands: Holland Institute of Linguistics.

Levelt, C. C. (1996). Consonant vowel interactions in early child speech. In B. Bernhardt, J. Gilbert, and D. Ingram (Eds.), Proceedings of the UBC

International Conference on Phonological Acquisition (pp. 229–239). Somerville Mass.: Cascadilla Press.

Lindsey, G., and Harris, J. (1995). The elements of phonological representation. In J. Durand and F. Katamba (Eds.), Frontiers of phonology: Atoms, structures, derivations (pp. 34–79). Harlow, England: Longman.

Macken, M. A. (1979). Developmental reorganization of phonology: A hierarchy of basic units of acquisition. Lingua, 49, 11–49.

MacNeilage, P. F. (1998). Acquisition of speech. In W. J. Hardcastle and J. Laver (Eds.), The handbook of phonetic sciences (pp. 300–332). London: Blackwell.

MacNeilage, P. F., and Davis, B. L. (1990a). Acquisition of speech production: The achievement of segmental independence. In W. J. Hardcastle and A. Marchal (Eds.), Speech production and speech modelling (pp. 55–68). Dordrecht, The Netherlands: Kluwer.

MacNeilage, P. F., and Davis, B. L. (1990b). Acquisition of speech production: Frames then content. In M. Jeannerod (Ed.), Attention and performance XIII: Motor representation and contol (pp. 453–476). Hillsdale, N.J.: Lawrence Erlbaum.

McCune, L., and Vihman, M. M. (1987). Vocal motor schemes. Papers and Reports in Child Language Development, 26, 72–79.

Menn, L. (1983). Development of articulatory, phonetic and phonological capabilities. In M. Butterworth (Ed.), Language production (pp. 3–50). London: Academic.

Nittrouer, S. (1983). The emergence of mature gestural patterns is not uniform: Evidence from an acoustic study. Journal of Speech and Hearing Research, 30, 319–329.

Nittrouer, S. (1992). Age-related differences in perceptual effects of formant transitions within syllables and across syllable boundaries. Journal of Phonetics, 20, 351–382.

Nittrouer, S. (1993). The emergence of mature gestural patterns is not uniform: Evidence from an acoustic study. Journal of Speech and Hearing Research, 36(5), 959-972.

Nittrouer, S., and Studdert-Kennedy, M. (1987). The role of coarticulatory effects in the perception of fricatives by children and adults. Journal of Speech and Hearing Research, 30, 319–329.

Nittrouer, S., Studdert-Kennedy, M., and McGowan, R. S. (1989). The emergence of phonetic segments: Evidence from the spectral structure of fricative-vowel syllables spoken by children and adults. Journal of Speech and Hearing Research, 32, 120–132.

Nittrouer, S., Studdert-Kennedy, M., and Neely, S. T. (1996). How children learn to organise their speech gestures: Further evidence from fricative-vowel syllables. Journal of Speech and Hearing Research, 39, 379–389.

Piske, T. (1995). Articulatory patterns in early speech production. In Proceedings of the Thirteenth International Congress of Phonetic Sciences 2, 698–702. Stockholm, Sweden: Royal Institute of Technology (KTH, Kungl Tekniska Högskolan).

Piske, T. (1997). Phonological organization in early speech production: Evidence for the importance of articulatory patterns. Speech Communication, 22, 279–295.

Pollock, K. E., and Keiser, N. J. (1990). An examination of vowel errors in phonologically disordered children. Clinical Linguistics and Phonetics, 4(2), 161–178.

Recasens, D. (1984). V-to-C coarticulation in Catalan VCV sequences: An articulatory and acoustic study. Journal of Phonetics, 12, 61–73.

Recasens, D. (1991). An electropalatographic and acoustic study of consonant-to-vowel coarticulation. Journal of Phonetics, 19, 177–192.

Repp, B. H. (1986). Some observations in the development of anticipatory coarticulation. Journal of the Acoustical Society of America, 79, 1616–1619.

Reynolds, J. (1990). Abnormal vowel patterns. The British Journal of Disorders of Communication, 25(2), 115–148.

Scobbie, J. M., Gibbon, F., Hardcastle, W. J., and Fletcher, P. (1997). Longitudinal phonological and phonetic analyses of two cases of disordered /s/+stop cluster acquisition. In A. Sorace, C. Heycock, and R. Shillcock (Eds.), Proceedings of the GALA '97 Conference on Language Acquisition (pp. 278–283). Edinburgh, Scotland: University of Edinburgh.

Scobbie, J. M., Gibbon, F., Hardcastle, W. J., and Fletcher, P. (1998). Covert contrast and the acquisition of phonetics and phonology. In W. Ziegler and K. Deger (Eds.), Clinical phonetics and linguistics (pp. 147–156). London: Whurr.

Scobbie, J. M., Gibbon, F., Hardcastle, W. J., and Fletcher, P. (2000). Covert contrast as a stage in the acquisition of phonetics and phonology. In M. Broe and J. Pierrehumbert (Eds.), Papers in laboratory phonology 5: Language acquisition and the lexicon (pp. 194–207). Cambridge, England: Cambridge University Press.

Stevens, K. N., and House, A. S. (1963). Perturbation of vowel articulations by consonantal context: An acoustical study. Journal of Speech and Hearing Research, 6, 111–128.

Stoel-Gammon, C. (1983). Constraints on consonant-vowel sequences in early words. Journal of Child Language, 10, 455–457.

Stoel-Gammon, C., and Herrington, P. B. (1990). Vowel systems of normally developing and phonologically disordered children. Clinical Linguistics and Phonetics, 4(2), 145–160.

Studdert-Kennedy, M. (1987). The phoneme as a perceptuomotor structure. In A. Allport, D. MacKay, W. Prinz, and E. Scheerer (Eds.), Language perception and production (pp. 67–84). London: Academic.

Studdert-Kennedy, M. (1991a). Comment: The emergent gesture. In I. G. Mattingly and M. Studdert-Kennedy (Eds.), Modularity and the motor theory of speech perception: Proceedings of a conference to honour Alvin M. Liberman (pp. 85–90). Hillsdale, N.J.: Lawrence Erlbaum.

Studdert-Kennedy, M. (1991b). Language development from an evolutionary perspective. In N. A. Krasnegor, D. M. Rumbaugh, R. L. Schiefelbusch, and M. Studdert-Kennedy (Eds.), Biological and behavioural determinants of language development (pp. 5–28). Hillsdale, N.J.: Lawrence Erlbaum.

Studdert-Kennedy, M., and Goodell, E. W. (1995). Gestures, features and segments in early child speech. In B. De Gelder and J. Morais (Eds.), Speech and reading (pp. 65–88). London: Erlbaum, Taylor, and Francis.

Tyler, A. A., and Langsdale, T. E. (1996). Consonant-vowel interaction. First Language, 16, 159–191.

Vihman, M. M. (1996). Phonological development: The origins of language in the child. Oxford: Blackwell.

Vihman, M. M., Ferguson, C. A., and Elbert, M. (1986). Phonological development from babbling to speech: Common tendencies and individual differences. Applied Psycholinguistics, 7, 3–40.

Vihman, M., and Velleman, S. (2000). Phonetics and the origins of phonology. In N. Burton-Roberts, P. Carr, and G. Docherty (Eds.), Phonological knowledge: Conceptual and empirical issues (pp. 305–339). Oxford: Oxford University Press.

Waters, D. (1995). Speech motor control in children with phonological acquisition difficulties. In Caring to Communicate: Proceedings of the Golden Jubilee, Conference of the Royal College of Speech and Language Therapists, York, October, 1995 (pp. 296–301). London: Royal College of Speech and Language Therapists.

Waterson, N. (1971). Child phonology: A prosodic view. Journal of Linguistics, 7, 179–211.

Watson, J. M. M. (1997). Sibilant-vowel coarticulation in the perception of speech of children with phonological disorder. Ph.D. thesis. Edinburgh, Scotland: Queen Margaret College.

Williams, A. L., and Dinnsen, D. A. (1987). A problem of allophonic variation in a speech disordered child. Innovations in Linguistics Education, 5, 85–90.

Wolfe, V. I., and Blocker, S. D. (1990). Consonant-vowel interaction in an unusual phonological system. Journal of Speech and Hearing Disorders, 25(2), 115–148.

6

Clinical Phonology of Vowel Disorders

Martin J. Ball

A wide range of phonological approaches have been applied to disordered speech data for the dual purpose of helping plan remediation and aiming to understand the underlying deficit (Ball and Kent, 1997; Grunwell, 1987). Disordered data have also been used as a way of testing the phonological theory itself. However diverse the theories themselves, they fall into the following broad categories regarding the methods used to account for the surface patterns of the disordered data:

1. Rule-based approaches. These normally take the target form as input, and provide the surface output through a series of rewrite rules (normally based on primarily binary feature systems). Such an approach, of course, explicitly claims that the disordered speaker has access to the target system, and that the disorder lies in the correct combination of different feature values.

2. Process-based approaches. Processes were originally envisaged as a set of natural constraints imposing motorically easier sounds as replacements for more difficult ones (such as stops for fricatives). Whereas in Stampe's original (1973) formulation, processes were seen as psycholinguistically real entities, they have generally been used in speech pathology approaches as atheoretical descriptive devices which can be added to at will with little underpinning of phonetic naturalness.

3. Constraint-based approaches. These have become very popular in recent times, and have begun to be applied to disordered speech (Bernhardt and Stemberger, 1998). This type of phonology avoids rewrite rules (and the implications that flow from them), preferring to posit sets of constraints on the output phonology. The ordering of the constraints, and how easy or otherwise it is to break them, vary from language to language. For example, languages that do not allow closed

syllables will have a *no coda* constraint; languages, such as English, that do allow a coda consonant, will not rank no coda highly. To describe disordered speech, constraints can be changed in rank, or new constraints can be devised.

4. Element-based approaches. Elements, in approaches such as government phonology (Ball, 1997), are the equivalent of features. However, instead of being binary, they are unary (either present or not). Flexibility is introduced through the ability of unary elements to enter into governing relations that distinguish basic sound types (where the element is by itself), or complex types (where elements in varying relationships coexist). Disordered speech can be accounted for by restrictions to the number and type of governing relationships entered into by the elements.

5. Gestural-based approaches. In articulatory phonology, the basic unit of analysis is the gesture, which can be divided into constriction location and degree. Temporal aspects can also be described, so that the final *gestural score* (that is, arrangement of gestures in time, location, and degree) is particularly suited for describing coarticulatory effects in speech.

In this chapter, I will take just one part of the phonology (vowels), and examine how the different approaches deal with typical disordered vowel systems reported in the literature. I will demonstrate that rule-based approaches are limited in their explanatory adequacy by the need to operate with binary feature systems often offering counterintuitively complex solutions to seemingly straightforward substitution patterns.

Further, processes, unless based on cross-linguistic, developmental, and disordered data together with some metric of motoric simplicity, seem to be little more than handy labels. Constraint-based approaches have an advantage in that they do not claim explicitly that the disordered phonology has to be derived directly from the target. However, like processes, constraints sometimes appear to be ad hoc devices thought up solely for a specific problem, and might well use the binary feature systems already noted as problematic. Researchers in articulatory phonology have concentrated much of their work on coarticulation, and their schema allows for four basic vowel constrictions. It is, therefore, difficult to see an easy way of describing the three-vowel system found in the examples discussed in this chapter.

An element-based description of disordered vowel systems is shown to be one that restricts the appearance of certain vowels within the phonological system itself (by restricting governing relationships between elements). In this way, the specific sounds are not available to the phonology, and so do not need to be rewritten away, or constrained in their appearance by later devices. It is argued that this approach best accounts for the data, and, further, provides a potential route into remediation by explicitly showing some sounds as inherently more complex than others.

Of course, data reported in the literature (Gibbon, Shockey, and Reid, 1992; Penney, Fee, and Dowdle, 1994; Pollock and Hall, 1991; Pollock and Keiser, 1990; Reynolds, 1990; Stoel-Gammon and Herrington, 1990; Walton and Pollock, 1993; Watson, Martineau, and Hughes, 1994), and that reported elsewhere in this volume, illustrate a wide range of vowel disorder patterns. It is beyond the scope of this kind of chapter to cover all of them. For the purpose of exemplifying different phonological approaches, therefore, I will restrict the disordered data to a type commonly reported: simplification of the vowel system to the *corner* vowels (that is, /i, a, u/), though on occasion we might also look at slightly less simplified systems. The following sections illustrate the five approaches described above, and then these are compared and contrasted. This evaluation will not only be in terms of which approach seems the most elegant and insightful, but also for its clinical applicability in therapeutic intervention for speakers with disordered vowel systems.

Rule-Based Approaches

What I am terming *rule-based approaches* are those ultimately deriving from Chomsky and Halle's (1968) *Sound Pattern of English* (SPE). While recognizing, of course, that many developments and refinements have taken place since SPE first described generative phonology, as in Ingram (1997), there remains the basic concept of rules linking different levels of description in rule-based approaches. We illustrate this by a commonly cited example. At the *systematic phonemic* level of description, vowel segments preceding nasal consonant segments retain their status as oral sounds (thus allowing simpler descriptions at this level). At the *systematic phonetic* level, however, these vowels preceding nasal consonants are described as nasal (thus reflecting the phonetic reality). These two levels are linked by rewrite rules: The systematic phonemic level serves as the input (the *structural description* or SD), while the systematic phonetic level is the output (the *structural change* or SC). These rules can change phonological features, and also add, delete, or reorder entire segments. This type of phonology, therefore, is derivational in that the surface form is derived through a set of rules from a simpler underlying form. We will return to rules, and how we might apply them to disordered vowel systems; but first we must consider phonological features in more detail.

Features

As Ohala (1992,166) states, "the segmental or articulated character of speech has been one of the cornerstones of phonology since its beginnings some two-and-a-half millennia ago." Durand (1990,12–13) also discussed this issue. However, as phonologists have long realized, units smaller than the segment can be posited, and, indeed, are needed if we want to make statements about natural classes of segments, and the phonological processes affecting them. The answer to this problem has normally been some kind of feature, or component, that might be thought of as making up a segment in conjunction with others.[1] Such a feature can then be isolated, and serve as the input to a phonological process, or as a method of grouping segments together into natural classes, and so on.

The notion of the phonological feature as commonly found in modern phonological approaches derives largely from the work of the Prague School of linguistics. However, while Trubetzkoy (1969 [original 1939]) considered a range of feature types, later work by Chomsky and Halle (1968); Jakobson, Fant, and Halle (1952); and Jakobson and Halle (1956) drew on only a subset of these feature types. In particular, they proposed systems of phonological distinctive features that were binary, while alternative unary and scalar features, considered in earlier work, were not included. Scalar features later re-emerged in work by Ladefoged (1971) and Durand (1990), amongst others, and unary features are found in several recent theoretical approaches discussed later in the text.

Another area of debate concerns equipollent and privative oppositions in feature theory, as found in Durand (1990, 72) and Harris (1994, 92). An equipollent opposition is one in which both the plus and minus values of a binary feature specify a particular property (the minus value does not imply mere absence of the feature, but a different specification of it). For example, as noted by Durand (1990) the [+voice] feature refers to a particular glottal configuration; [-voice] should not be read as simply the lack of that glottal configuration, but should be understood as referring to a different glottal configuration: that needed to produce voicelessness.

On the other hand, a feature such as that proposed by Chomsky and Halle's (1968) SPE for tongue height—[± high]—is arguably not equipollent, but privative. A privative opposition is one in which the minus value of the feature is interpreted as mere absence of the plus, rather than as some configuration in its own right. If we consider vowel systems, the SPE feature [+high] refers to an oral configuration in which the tongue is raised above a midpoint, and groups together as a natural class vowels such as /i, y, u/. On the other hand, [-high] is not to be understood as a specific tongue position (for example, lowered below a midpoint), but rather as simply not raised above that midpoint. The minus value of this feature, therefore, can group both mid and low vowels together. The [±low] feature works in the same way, and by using these two, we can isolate three different vowel heights: high [+high, –low], mid [–high, –low], and low [–high, +low]. The combination [+high, +low] is ruled out as being physically impossible.

That last point is worth further consideration. Clearly, features whose very names appear to demonstrate how unlike they are, are not expected to operate together in defining a class of sounds. The fact that the minus values can operate this way demonstrates that the opposition for both these features is privative, not equipollent. An equipollent opposition might have allowed [−high] to represent a mid vowel tongue configuration, but not a low vowel one as well. As Harris (1994) points out, the position adopted in SPE specified that features were uniformly expressed in terms of equipollent oppositions. Nevertheless, as our example has shown, this was not always realized. As Durand (1990, 77) notes, "the possible defect of two interpretations of binary distinctive features . . . was discarded in the interests of formal unity."

Relationships between Features

Another problem area concerned the relationships between features. For example, the feature [+sonorant] is much more likely to co-occur with the feature [+voice], than with [−voice]; the feature [+strident] has to co-occur with the feature [−sonorant]; the feature [+del rel] has to co-occur with [+consonantal], and so on. Classical SPE-type generative phonology attempted to deal with these relationships through markedness theory (again adapted from Prague School ideas). We do not have the space to go into this in any detail, as can be found in Durand's (1990) and Harris' (1994) discussion, but basically, markedness is an attempt to show which feature values and which feature combinations are more *natural* than others.[2] Natural, of course, might be interpreted as a universal characteristic of phonologies of all languages, or it might be natural in terms of the language under investigation. Markedness conventions, moreover, are external to the basic notation of generative phonology: They operate as a kind of mathematical table referred to in order to convert from u, and m values (unmarked and marked) to + and − ones. As Harris (1994, 93) points out, "a more radical solution is to build markedness relations directly into phonological representations"; and goes on to suggest that this is best done through a framework in which phonological oppositions are uniformly privative.

Attempts to express relationships between features in generative phonology have been termed *feature geometry*. In SPE, features were viewed as independent, but in more recent phonological work, it has been recognized that dependency relations exist between features, as we have just noted. If features (whether of the SPE binary type, or other privative types) are given some kind of dependency structure in terms of each other, then it will become easier to specify more from less natural phonological process. Roca (1994, 98) notes that if all place features are gathered together into one node, then assimilation process, such as found in many languages between nasals and following obstruents, can be ex-

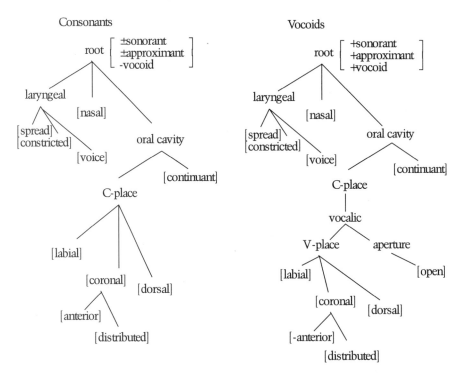

Figure 6-1   An example of a feature tree proposed for consonants and for vocoids.

pressed very simply, and in such a way as to rule out only partial assimilation of place.

Those working within this area have constructed feature trees to express dependency relations between the wide range of features in SPE and post-SPE phonology. Roca (1994), for example, discussed some of the adaptations to features since SPE. An example of a feature tree proposed for consonants and for vocoids by Clements and Hume (1995) is shown in Figure 6-1.

Feature geometry has proved a valuable tool in constraining the generative power of SPE-type rules, but there is no reason why such formalism should be restricted to binary features of the type traditionally found in generative phonology.[3]

Rules

We noted previously that rules use features to link the SD with the SC. We now return to the example given regarding the nasalization of vowels before nasal consonants. The rule schema normally note those features needed to distinguish the segments concerned from any others. We note that the feature value [–nasal] has changed to [+nasal], and that this happens with vowels only, occurring when they precede consonants that are also [+nasal]. Using a fairly basic SPE-type approach, this rule is shown as follows

$$[\text{--nasal}] \;\rightarrow\; [\text{+nasal}] \;/\; \begin{bmatrix} \text{--cons} \\ \text{+voc} \end{bmatrix} \qquad \begin{bmatrix} \text{+cons} \\ \text{--voc} \\ \text{+nasal} \end{bmatrix}$$

SD   SC   context

and read as: "the feature minus nasal changes to plus nasal in vowels which are followed by consonants that are plus nasal."

How has this approach been applied to clinical phonology? As described in Grunwell (1987), generative phonology has been adapted with disordered data such that the two levels of description are reinterpreted to stand for the target pronunciation, and the disordered realization. The speaker is assumed to be aiming for the SD pronunciation, but the SC pronunciation is what actually occurs. This usage explicitly links the target with the realization. This is fine if the researcher believes that all disordered speakers have full knowledge of the target phonology, but it is a problem if the researcher wishes to claim otherwise, or treat the disordered speech patterns as a phonology in their own right.

Disordered Vowels

In this subsection I will illustrate how a generative rule approach, as described previously, can be applied to the simplified vowel system we noted in the introduction. The language of exemplification will be English, and assuming a traditional SPE set of vowel features, the following features are needed to cover the monophthongs of English (we exclude the diphthongs in this account to avoid bringing in extra formalism):

- [+high] vowels with the tongue raised above the midpoint
- [–high] vowels with the tongue not raised above the midpoint
- [+low] vowels with the tongue lowered below the midpoint
- [–low] vowels with the tongue not lowered below the midpoint
- [+back] vowels with the tongue retracted behind the central point
- [–back] vowels with the tongue not retracted behind the central point
- [+round] vowels with a rounded lip shape
- [–round] vowels with a spread or neutral lip shape
- [+tense] vowels uttered with high muscular tension (normally peripheral to the vowel area)
- [–tense] vowels uttered with low muscular tension (normally central to the vowel area)

As shown in Carr (1993), I have also included a feature [long] as a means of distinguishing long schwa from /eː/: [+long] are vowels with a long duration, [–long] are vowels with a short duration.

The following is a list of the monophthongs of a representative accent of English (Southern British Standard): /i, ɪ, e, æ, ʌ, ɑ, ɒ, ɔ , ʊ, u, ə, ɜ/. These vowels can be displayed in a feature matrix, as shown in Table 6-1.

We assume the following patterns of substitutions to a reduced three corner vowel system:

1. /i, ɪ, e, ə, ɜ/ → [i]
2. /æ, ʌ, ɑ, ɒ/ → [a]
3. /ɔ, ʊ, u/ → [u][4]

We now need a rule that will describe these substitutions. It appears difficult, however, to find a single rule that accounts for this simplification using the features noted earlier in the text, so the following three rules are listed: The first substitution pattern would need this first rule:

$$\begin{bmatrix} -\text{high} \\ -\text{tense} \end{bmatrix} \rightarrow \begin{bmatrix} +\text{high} \\ +\text{tense} \end{bmatrix} / \begin{bmatrix} +\text{voc} \\ -\text{cons} \\ -\text{low} \\ -\text{round} \end{bmatrix}$$

To meet the second substitution pattern, we need this second rule:

$$\begin{bmatrix} +\text{back} \\ +\text{round} \\ -\text{tense} \end{bmatrix} \rightarrow \begin{bmatrix} -\text{back} \\ -\text{round} \\ +\text{tense} \end{bmatrix} / \begin{bmatrix} +\text{voc} \\ -\text{cons} \\ +\text{low} \end{bmatrix}$$

Finally, this third rule describes the third substitution pattern:

$$\begin{bmatrix} -\text{high} \\ -\text{tense} \end{bmatrix} \rightarrow \begin{bmatrix} +\text{high} \\ +\text{tense} \end{bmatrix} / \begin{bmatrix} +\text{voc} \\ -\text{cons} \\ -\text{low} \\ +\text{round} \end{bmatrix}$$

We now need to see whether these three rules can be collapsed to show the unity of the simplification of vowels into the three corner units. Clearly, the first rule and the third rule can be collapsed, using the *alpha* notation convention so that the input can take either + or – [round] causing this feature to remain unchanged in the output, as shown in the end result of this final rule.

$$\begin{bmatrix} -\text{high} \\ -\text{tense} \end{bmatrix} \rightarrow \begin{bmatrix} +\text{high} \\ +\text{tense} \end{bmatrix} / \begin{bmatrix} +\text{voc} \\ -\text{cons} \\ -\text{low} \\ \alpha\text{round} \end{bmatrix}$$

Table 6-1   Distinctive Feature Matrix for English Monophthongs

	i	ɪ	e	æ	ʌ	ɑ	ɒ	ɔ	ʊ	u	ə	ɜ
high	+	+	–	–	–	–	–	–	+	+	–	–
low	–	–	–	+	+	+	+	–	–	–	–	–
back	–	–	–	–	–	+	+	+	+	+	–	–
round	–	–	–	–	–	–	+	+	+	+	–	–
tense	+	–	+	+	–	+	–	+	–	+	–	+
long	+	–	–	–	–	+	–	+	–	+	–	+

However, the second rule noted previously cannot be joined to the final rule for two reasons. First, the [+low] feature in the context clashes with [–low] requirement in the context for the last rule. Second, the change from [+round] to [–round] in the second rule clashes with the [αround] (that is, unchanged value to round) requirement in the final rule's context.

We have couched this discussion in very traditional SPE formalism. However, even using more recent developments in generative phonology, it is difficult to see how a rule-based approach can unify the vowel simplification we are considering.

Process-Based Approaches

Stampe (1969, 443) defines a phonological process as follows: "A phonological process merges a potential phonological opposition into that member of the opposition which least tries the restrictions of the human speech capacity," and further (1970, 1): "A phonological process is a mental operation that applies in speech to substitute, for a class of sounds or sound sequences presenting a common difficulty to the speech capacity of the individual, an alternative class identical but lacking the difficult property."

However, it was not intended that processes would be ad hoc devices; rather, they should be grounded in naturally occurring patterns. These patterns can be found through investigating phonological acquisition across languages, and by looking at systemic and structural constraints across languages. In other words, if, in phonological acquisition cross-linguistically, children replace fricatives with plosives, this can be considered a natural process. Also, if adult phonologies cross-linguistically display a preference for final voiceless obstruents over voiced, that, too, can be considered a natural process. It is worth noting that Stampe believed that processes were not just helpful descriptive labels, but were linguistically innate.

However, in his description of natural phonology, Stampe did not restrict himself to natural processes as descriptive devices. He also believed that phonological rules were needed to describe language-specific (morpho)phonological changes that could not be grounded in natural, phonetic explanations. For example, Stampe notes that changes such as palatalization in fast speech in English (/t/+/j/ → /tʃ/ in "what you . . .") is a natural process, whereas /k/ → /s/ in "electric, electricity" is not natural and so must be accounted for through a rule. Generally, Stampe and adherents of natural phonology eschew the formalism of other approaches to phonology. Therefore, we do not encounter rule or process formalisms in their expositions; rather, phonological changes tend to be written out as descriptions (such as fricative stopping: all fricatives are realized as stops). This does not mean, however, that natural phonology operates at the level of the segment. As noted previously, Stampe sees processes as replacing the *difficult property* of a class of sounds with an easier property. We can only interpret this to mean some kind of phonological (or maybe phonetic) feature.

What is difficult to ascertain, however, is whether natural phonology is derivational in the sense explored in the previous section, "Rule-Based Approaches." In describing phonological acquisition, natural phonologists claim that the child has access to the full adult system, but that different sets of natural phonological processes operate at different stages to simplify this target phonology. Indeed, phonological acquisition can be seen as a process whereby natural processes are eliminated one by one, until the only ones left are those still operating on the adult target phonology. In this sense, then, acquisition can be thought of as derivational in that the adult phonology is realized by the child through a filtering layer of natural processes.

But what about the target system itself? I feel that, as far as natural processes are concerned (that is the set of processes that still apply, are supposed to apply, for that particular language, and these will differ from language to language), natural phonology is nonderivational. The processes act as constraints on the set of phonological units available to the language (the phonological system) and on the combination of these units at the syllable/word level, (the phonological structure). These processes can be seen as derivational only in the sense of the link between all possible units and all possible combinations. On the other hand, the phonological rules (as far as these have been described) are presumably derivational, as seen in the "electric, electricity" example given earlier. Such a hybrid approach to phonology might be viewed as a drawback to a coherent theory of speech organization, although polysystemic approaches to linguistics have always been supported by some, so different theories for different aspects might be a strength.

Processes

Processes can be broadly divided into those that effect systemic simplification (simplifying the set of units available to the phonology), and those that effect structural simplification (simplifying the possible combinations of units allowed at the syllable/word level). We illustrate this distinction with some typical natural processes found both in language acquisition, and in adult natural language phonologies.

Systemic simplification can be seen in the following processes:

Fricative stopping. All fricatives are realized as stops: found cross-linguistically in phonological acquisition, and presumably in the 6.6% of languages in the UCLA Phonological Segment Inventory Database that lack fricatives (Maddieson, 1984). In the acquisition data, fricatives are normally replaced by stops at the nearest place of articulation (such as /f/ by /p/, /s/ by /t/), so that it is the fricative property that is being simplified. In binary feature systems of the SPE type, we would need rules specifying that both [+continuant] and, where appropriate, [+strident] were changed to negative values, as well as rules adjusting for place differences (such as /ʃ/ to /t/). The process is much simpler, though the lack of formalism does not make explicit within the theory how the simplification works, or its phonetic motivation, or how classes of sounds may be grouped together.

Velar fronting. All velar consonants realized further forward (usually as alveolars/dentals). This is widely found in acquisition data. There are also many languages that do not utilize the velar place of articulation for all, or some of their consonant types. English, for example, now lacks velar fricatives (though a velar fricative phoneme did exist in Old English). Historically, some kind of fronting of English velar fricatives appears to have happened, in that the spelling "gh" (a sign that originally a velar fricative was present) can be realized as /f/ in some cases (*rough, cough*). However, a total deletion process also appears to have occurred, as in *though, through.* Velar to alveolar changes in SPE phonology requires changes to the three features: [anterior], [coronal], and [back].

Structural simplification can be seen in the following processes:

Final consonant deletion. This is common in acquisition, and there are also languages, such as Italian, in which no (or very few) words end with a consonant.

Final devoicing. It is also common in acquisition to encounter only voiceless obstruents in word-final position. This is illustrated in many of the Germanic languages in which only voiceless obstruents may occur word-finally.

Cluster reduction. This process covers a variety of subprocesses whereby clusters of consonants are simplified at different positions in the word. Children acquiring English display cluster reduction in word-initial position in the following two ways: /s/ plus consonant clusters will simplify by deleting the /s/ (such as *stop* [tɒp], *snow* [noʊ]), while consonant plus approximant clusters will delete the approximant (such as *blue* [bu], *quick* [kɪk]). At first, these two sub-processes might co-occur, but later the first might be retained while the second is discarded. In natural language, too, we may find a range of constraints on consonant clusters, both in terms of the number and type of consonants allowed. For example, Arabic only allows two consonants in word-final clusters (English can have up to four), while Hawaiian has severe limitations on consonant clusters of any kind.

Processes and Disordered Vowels

The application of natural phonology to disordered speech (as discussed by Grunwell, 1997) has a long history. It has been seen as a relatively formalism-free (and so unthreatening) approach to the description of disordered speech. Many of the processes used to describe disordered speech are the same as those used in language acquisition and natural language description. They are thus grounded in cross-linguistic data as well as in phonetic simplicity effects.

However, not all disordered speech is of a simple delay type: What do we do when we encounter unusual or idiosyncratic patterns, or patterns that do not immediately appear to have a phonetic simplification motivation? Stampe's discussion leads me to assume that we should call these phonological rules, but, as noted previously, it is not easy to determine from published work in natural phonology precisely how these differ from processes in their formalism or their ordering. Usually, work on natural phonology and disordered speech have coined new processes as needed to cover whatever unusual patterns are encountered.

If processes are being used as simple shorthand devices to remind a speech-language therapist what a pattern looks like, and if all pretensions to the innateness of processes as opposed to rules are abandoned, then coining new processes as required does not cause any problems. If, however, we are attempting to use natural phonology as a theory of the structure and control of sound systems, then such an approach negates any theoretical integrity, and we cannot claim to provide any coherent insights on phonology or therapy.

This becomes problematic when we consider disordered vowel systems. In both acquisition studies, and those of disordered speech, vowels have been neglected until somewhat recently. It is difficult, therefore, to find published data describing natural processes in vowel acquisition. Grunwell (1997) lists the vowel processes described in Reynolds (1990):

1. Lowering of (midfront) vowels to /a/
2. Fronting (of lowback vowels) to /a/
3. Diphthong reduction (or monophthongization)

On the other hand, the type of reduction to the corner vowels noted previously could be described by three processes as follows:

1. Front vowel raising
2. Back vowel raising
3. Open vowel lowering

I argued in the previous section that these three processes (found in the "Rule-Based Approaches" section) are manifestations of a single substitution pattern, which could be termed *vowel cornering.*

Clearly, the problem we are encountering in this instance is that clinical natural phonologists have fallen into a trap of inventing a process to deal with their data without grounding this process in the way Stampe outlined. Currently, we are not able to say that a vowel-cornering process is as well motivated as velar fronting or final consonant deletion. Such ad hoc labeling may supply us with a handy descriptive label for what is going on, but it has no theoretical value, and, further, cannot inform the clinician's intervention strategy. The work reported in the contributions to this volume by Donegan, Reynolds, and Pollock provides us with a firmer idea regarding patterns of vowel acquisition. Still, due to the range of patterns, drafting a list of commonly occurring natural processes remains difficult.

Constraint-Based Approaches

Recent developments in theoretical phonology have centered on constraint-based approaches to the description of sound systems (Archangeli and Langendoen, 1997; Bernhardt and Stemberger, 1998; Prince and Smolensky, 1993; Stemberger and Bernhardt, 1997). To some extent, these developments hark back to the natural phonology framework just described. In natural phonology processes (based on naturally occurring cross-linguistic patterns) constrain what speakers can produce phonologically. If a language has the process of final devoicing, then speakers of that language are constrained to produce only final voiceless obstruents.

However, as we pointed out, natural phonology allows rules as well, and, in that respect at least, is derivational. We also noted that the process part of the phonology could be deemed nonderivational. Constraint-based phonology, (as found within the overall framework of optimality theory [OT] described in Archangeli and Langendoen, 1997), on the other hand, has constraints only, and is overtly nonderivational. By this last point, we mean that phonological descriptions do not set out to derive a surface realization from an underlying general phonological description through a set of rules. The relation between the input and the output of the phonology is mediated by the ranking of a set of constraints. This point is described in Roca (1997). Nevertheless, the constraints themselves, like natural processes, need to be grounded somehow, instead of being ad hoc mechanisms.

This grounding need not, though, be linked to innateness as claimed by Stampe (1973). The constraints can be grounded in considerations of phonetic complexity and perceptual clarity (Bernhardt and Stemberger, 1998). Indeed, one of the criticisms of innate processes is that it appears to be counterintuitive to suggest that learning how to produce a target phonology should involve unlearning a set of restrictions. This would imply that the child starts off with a more complex phonology than the adult. In constraint-based phonology, however, it would be argued that children simply acquire the correct ranking of the set of constraints, and that immature patterns demonstrate that this ranking has yet to be mastered. We can best illustrate this approach by looking at some examples of phonological constraints and how they are ranked.

Constraints

Archangeli and Langendoen (1997) describe the operation of OT as containing three basic components: the generator (GEN), the evaluator (EVAL), and the universal set of constraints (CON). The universal set of constraints, which might be phonological, morphological, or syntactic, are ranked differently for different languages. What might be inviolable in one language (such as restrictions on consonant clusters) might be violable in another.

However, constraints are not present or absent (such as rules), but because they are all potentially violable, they need to be ranked. The generator is the device for linking inputs with potential outputs. It can add, delete, and rearrange items similar to the approach used by generative phonological rules. Its potential outputs are judged by the EVAL. The evaluator compares all the outputs produced by GEN to the language-specific ranking of CON. The evaluator then selects as the optimal output the one that best satisfies the ranked constraints. In this regard, it should be noted that violation of a lower-ranking constraint is tolerated if it satisfies a higher-ranking constraint. On the other hand, if various candidates all satisfy (or indeed violate) higher-ranking constraints, then the optimal candidate will be the one that satisfies more lower-ranking constraints.

Let us see how this might work with one of the processes we noted earlier: final consonant deletion. To do this, we will consider a range of possible syllable structures produced by GEN (we are being illustrative here, rather than comprehensive): V, CV, CVC, VC, CCV, VCC, and so on (where C stands for consonant, and V stands for vowel). Many languages, of course, allow only a subset of these possible syllable types, while others (such as English) allow all of them. In constraint-based approaches to phonology, the CON component contains a set of constraints on syllable structure grounded in cross-linguistic evidence (for example, of commonly and less commonly occurring types), and in consideration of phonetic simplicity and perceptual clarity. We list some of these as follows:[5]

PEAK	syllables have one peak
ONSET	syllables begin with a consonant
*COMPLEX	syllables have at most one consonant at an edge
NOCODA	syllables end with a vowel

Now, in any particular language, these constraints might be ranked differently; further, some constraints might be violable, others not. In OT, this is shown by listing the constraints, with higher constraints separated from lower by a double arrow, and equally ranked constraints separated by commas. In the following examples, it is assumed that constraints to the left of the double arrow are inviolable. A language that must have a vocalic peak and that does not allow any consonant clusters would rank PEAK and *COMPLEX to the left of the other constraints: PEAK, *COMPLEX >> ONSET, NOCODA. On the other hand, a language which allows initial clusters, but not vowel initials or final consonants, might have the following ranking: PEAK, ONSET, NOCODA >> *COMPLEX. In order to see how the EVAL component evaluates competing structures, we display a tableau of possible forms, as is often done in OT. The tableaux in Table 6-2 and Table 6-3 display the two rankings just noted.

In Table 6-2, violated constraints are marked by *, while *! marks those violated constraints that are inviolable for the particular language. The ☞ sign marks the syllable structures (or, of course, any output) that break no inviolable constraint. We can see from this table that CV is the most basic syllable type (breaking none of the constraints), but that VC and CVC are also possible. Our other language type is shown in Table 6-3.

Table 6-3 demonstrates the difference between OT and natural phonology: The latter posits an innate process that deletes final consonants, while the former proposes a high ranking to a universal constraint on allowing final consonants.

Table 6-2 PEAK, *COMPLEX >> ONSET, NOCODA

	PEAK	*COMPLEX	ONSET	NOCODA
CC	*!	*!		
CCV		*!		
☞ CV				
☞ VC			*	*
☞ CVC				*

Table 6-3   PEAK, ONSET, NOCODA >> *COMPLEX

	PEAK	ONSET	NOCODA	*COMPLEX
CC	*!			*
VC		*!		
CVC			*!	
☞ CV				
☞ CCV				*

Constraints and Disordered Vowels

Optimality theory has recently been applied to normal and disordered phonological acquisition in a series of studies (Barlow, 2001; Bernhardt and Stemberger, 1998; Dinnsen, 2001; Gierut, 2001; Gilbers, 2001; O'Connor, 2001; Stemberger and Bernhardt, 1997; Ueda and Davis, 2001). It is clear that the idea of ranking constraints is very useful in describing how disordered speech differs from target pronunciations. If constraints are reranked, and if inviolable constraints become violable or vice versa, then disordered patterns can be justified. To return to final consonant deletion, NOCODA is violable in target, adult English, but might be ranked as inviolable by speakers exhibiting this variety of restricted syllable type. Further, if *COMPLEX were classified as inviolable, this could account for patterns of cluster reduction.

However, we also need to consider how problems with specific sounds (such as velar fronting, or voicing problems) can be dealt with in OT. At this level of detail, we need to appeal to constraints that act on features: specifically, the co-occurrence of features. For example, to account for velars fronting to alveolars, Stemberger and Bernhardt (1997) propose the following ranking:

1. NOT(DORSAL) >> SURVIVED(DORSAL) >> NOT(LABIAL) >> NOT(CORONAL)[6]

This schema means that the constraint forbidding dorsal place (such as velars) outranks the one allowing dorsal inputs to survive as dorsal outputs. Further, the ranking of the last two constraints predicts that coronals (such as alveolars) rather than labials will be the most favored place, so velars will front to alveolars. To account for final consonant devoicing, we need to access co-occurrence constraints. One way of achieving this would be with a constraint such as:

2. NOTCOOCCURRING ([–sonorant] [+voice])

However, this just bans any voiced obstruent. We want to ban only those at the end of words. We could rephrase the previous constraint to add in context in the manner that traditional generative rules do, as in the following constraint.

a. NOTCOOCCURRING ([−sonorant] [+voice] / __ #)

Alternatively, we can make use of the syllable level terminology of onset, rime, and coda that (as we have seen in the NOCODA constraint) is often used in OT, to give us the following constraint:

b. NOTCOOCCURRING (Coda[−sonorant] [+voice])

Finally, we can also consider that these types of restrictions might better be portrayed as positive rather than negative constraints, reflecting natural tendencies for certain segment types to be voiced or voiceless. We can recast the final devoicing pattern, therefore, in terms of what voicing type must co-occur with which segment type:

3. COOCCUR (Coda[−sonorant] → [−voice])

Turning to vowels, we see again that little attention has been paid to this group by OT researchers so far. The exception to this is Bernhardt and Stemberger (1998) who examine a range of acquisition patterns, and propose a number of constraints to account for them. These include co-occurrence and nonco-occurrence constraints, some *not* constraints linked to specific features, and *survived* constraints, again linked to specific features. Of course, an approach like OT does not need to use any specific set of features, but those working within the framework have tended to use the current set of binary (and sometimes unary) features such as those portrayed in Figure 6-1 shown previously in the text. As we noted in the "Rule-Based Approaches" section, the rules to give us vowel cornering require several features to be included. This suggests that a constraint-based approach will need to use co-occurrence constraints. I propose that to account for our vowel substitution patterns, we would need the following inviolable constraints:

4. No([−tense]), NOTCOOCCUR([−high] [−low]), NOTCOOCCUR([+back] [+low] Labial)

No([−tense]) will remove the [−tense] feature from the nonperipheral vowels, and normally their other place features will ensure their correct realization as [i], [a], or [u]. The NOTCOOCCUR([−high] [−low]) constraint prohibits the mid vowels (such as /e/, /ɔ/). By manipulating the ranking of other violable constraints, we can ensure that these either raise (to [i] and [u]) or lower (to [a]). The NOTCOOCCUR ([+back] [+low] Labial) is required to deal with the realization of lowback rounded /ɒ/ as [a]; as this vowel is not found in some accents of English (such as General American). This constraint would not be required for those varieties. We can see how this system might work in the simplified tableau in Table 6-4 (simplified because I have omitted most of the violable constraints).

Looking at Table 6-4 it could be argued that the constraint NOTCO-OCCUR([+back] [+low] Labial) is not actually required, as the vowel /ɒ/ is prohibited by the No([−tense]) constraint. However, while No([−tense]) bans [−tense]

Table 6-4   No([−tense]), NotCooccur([−high] [−low]), NotCooccur([+back] [+low] Labial) >> No([+back])

	No([−tense])	NotCooccur ([−high] [−low])	NotCooccur ([+back] [+low] Labial)	No([+back])
/ɪ/	*!			
/ʊ/	*!			*
/e/		*!		
/ɔ/		*!		*
/ɒ/	*!		*!	*
/ə/	*!	*!		
☞/i/, /a/				
☞/u/				*

vowels, it would not deal with the fact that /ɒ/ is labial ([+round] in earlier feature systems). This could result in the realization of some kind of tense low rounded vowel, which we clearly do not want.[7] This problem arises partly due to the reliance on the mostly binary feature system adopted, and an alternative system might well provide a better answer as shown in the "Element-Based Approaches" section.

Constraints, therefore, provide an alternative route to rules and to processes to account for the original pattern. However, we are still left with a minimum of three inviolable constraints providing us with the cornering pattern of vowel realization. Arguably, we could construct a constraint that prohibited all non-corner vowels. In order to achieve this, we need a feature system that can account for corner vowels in a parsimonious and elegant manner.

Element-Based Approaches

In some comparatively recent work within phonology, the emphasis has shifted away from the use of equipollent, binary features to privative unary elements.[8] This can be seen within work in dependency phonology (Anderson and Durand, 1986; 1987; Anderson and Ewen, 1987; Durand, 1990; Lass, 1984), but also in other frameworks derived from dependency phonology. Ewen (1995), Harris (1994), Schane (1995), and van der Hulst (1989) refer to other work on this subject. Privative phonological elements are either present, in which case the value of the unit is realized, or absent, in which case no alternative value is realized. There is only one possible value associated with the unit, which is shown to be unary as opposed to the binary possibilities of equipollent features.

Van der Hulst (1989) comments that the central motivation for a unary approach is that it constrains the phonology. Binary distinctive feature approaches allow a large number of natural classes (both + and − a feature), phonological systems, and processes. On the other hand, a unary system only allows classes of segments that share a component, not classes that do not share a component. Harris (1994) sees unary accounts as ways of reducing the range of processes available to those that are observed in natural language data, thus avoiding theoretical add-ons (such as markedness conventions).

There is a further claim made about unary components by many who work with them: that they have phonetic interpretability, or at least that some of the components do (Harris, 1994, 94; van der Hulst, 1989, 261). In any theory of phonological units below the level of the segment we might validly ask whether the units have independent phonetic interpretation. In the case of traditional binary distinctive features, the answer is clearly negative. They might have phonetic content of some kind (for example, [+voice] can be linked to an articulatory configuration), but this content can only manifest itself when joined with other feature values filling the feature matrix of a specific segment. Therefore, these binary phonological features (at a late stage in the derivation) have to be mapped onto phonetic features (often viewed as multivalued) for the string concerned to be interpreted phonetically.

Harris (1994) notes that a system of unary components (where the components are phonetically interpretable primes) signifies that, at all levels of phonological derivation, segments are phonetically interpretable. This is clearly not possible with underspecification approaches adopted in other theoretical stances. Harris (1994, 94–95) outlines detailed psycholinguistic critique of underspecification. That this is desirable becomes clear when we consider the roles of the phonology and phonetics in such an approach:

> Since phonological representation uniformly adheres to the principle of full phonetic interpretability, there is no motivation for recognizing an autonomous level of systematic phonetic representation. Any phonological representation at any level of derivation can be directly submitted to articulatory or perceptual interpretation. Derivation is thus not an operation by means of which abstract phonological objects are transformed into increasingly concrete physical objects. Rather it is a strictly generative function, which defines the grammaticality of phonological strings. (Harris, 1994, 96)

Such a view of phonology differs from that held in traditional SPE-like accounts, but is similar to that of OT discussed in the previous section. As Harris claims, this structure, together with phonetically interpretable phonological elements, might well be psycholinguistically more plausible. So, what we are tentatively claiming is that, in this instance, unary privative components, of the type described in this section, are psycholinguistically more plausible than binary distinctive features. We now should consider how such an approach operates. For the purposes of this chapter, we will use the formalism of government phonology (GvP).

Government Phonology

Government phonology (Harris, 1990; 1994; Harris and Lindsey, 1995; Kaye, Lowenstamm, and Vergnaud, 1985; 1990) can be viewed to some extent as an offshoot of dependency phonology. This was prompted, at least in part, by a desire to constrain the overgenerative power of the former approach. Dependency phonology allows four different dependency relations (nongoverning, mutual governing, a governing b, and b governing a), and a relatively high number of phonological units. Therefore, a large number of phonological relations can be generated by the theory. This can be seen as a disadvantage, as it is likely to produce more combinations than are needed to characterize natural language. (However, we must bear in mind that this might, to some extent, be useful in the description of atypical speech.) Successor theories to dependency phonology, therefore, were concerned, to some extent, with reducing both the number of relationships allowed to hold between units and the number of units themselves. This is still an area of controversy, which will be discussed later, but we briefly outline a version of GvP that has been featured in the recent literature.

John Harris, in several recent publications (such as in Harris, 1994; Harris and Lindsey, 1995), develops a version of government phonology in which the atoms of phonological structure clearly owe a lot to dependency phonology, but also to other developments in phonological theory, notably feature geometry (such as Clements, 1985; Sagey, 1986). In his 1994 publication, Harris promoted the use of unary phonological primes, as opposed to the traditional binary distinctive features of most approaches to phonology since Chomsky and Halle (1968).

Brockhaus (1995) clearly describes the concerns of GvP, both at the level of the word and above. There are also broader phonological concerns, such as the status of derivation and interfaces between phonology and the lexicon and phonology and phonetics. These are discussed in Harris and Lindsey (1995) and Kaye (1995). We concentrate in this section, however, on the elements of phonological structure (sometimes termed the *melodic primes*), as this will be of particular use to our attempts at characterizing vowel cornering. Originally, Kaye, Lowenstamm, and Vergnaud (1985; 1990) proposed ten active elements used in defining segmental expressions:

A	nonhigh	R	coronal
U	labial/round	ʔ	occluded
I	front/palatal	h	aperiodic energy (noise)
Ɨ	ATR	H	stiff vocal cords
N	nasal	L	slack vocal cords

Since those publications by Kaye and colleagues, there has been considerable debate within the GvP literature as to the desirability of reducing the number of elements in order to constrain the generative power of the theory. Following Harris (1994), therefore, we can present an element geometry tree of the elements found in that approach to GvP in Figure 6-2.

To see how these elements are used to describe particular segments, we will examine a selection of both vowels and consonants. Harris (1994) assumes a prime @ that represented centrality in vowels and dorsal (but nonpalatal) in consonants, that is to say velar.[9]

Vowels represented by the simple three vowel elements are:

A	[a][10]
I	[i]
U	[u]

Combinations of elements will provide a wider vowel set, of course. However, in combinations, one element is normally deemed to be the *head* (or *governor*), and others are dependent on the head. In GvP formalism, the head element is underlined; if no element is underlined, then the elements are in nongoverning relationship. If we examine some English vowels, we can see this process in operation:

[I, @]	/ɪ/
[A, I, @]	/ɛ/
[I, A]	/æ/
[U, A]	/ɒ/
[U, @]	/ʊ/
[@]	/ʌ/
[A, @]	[ɐ]

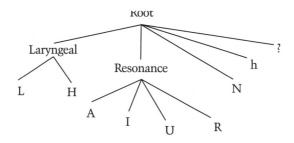

Figure 6-2   Geometry tree of the elements found in approach to GvP

As can be seen, those short vowels of English that are generally considered to be lax vowels as well, are governed by the neutral element @. Looking at long vowels, it should be noted that in GvP these are considered to occupy two segment slots (like diphthongs), and can be characterized as follows:[11]

Turning now to consonants, we will give (as with vowels) the phonetic interpretation of the elements most frequently used to characterize them. It should be noted that the slightly different exponence of the **I** and the **U** elements derives from their no longer being dominated by a nucleus node in word structure.

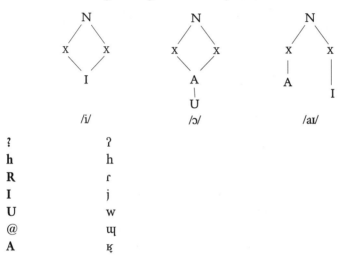

The following will serve as illustrations of the use of both place and manner features in a range of consonants (these examples are all voiceless to avoid the inclusion of the laryngeal node elements that control the voicing distinction among other aspects):

[h, U, ʔ]	p
[h, R, ʔ]	t
[h, @, ʔ]	k
[**h̲**, U]	f
[**h̲**, R]	s
[h, **R̲**]	θ
[**h̲**, R, I]	ʃ (alternatively [**h̲**, I])
[**h̲**, @]	x
[**h̲**, A]	χ
[h, **A̲**]	ħ
[R, ʔ]	l

Other consonants found in English are included above as the exponence of the simple elements, although consonants such as nasals can be characterized through the inclusion of the element **N**. Ritter (1996) provides an alternative to avoid the use of this element.

Government Phonology and Disordered Vowels

Government phonology has not yet been used to any extent in the description of disordered speech. For more discussion, see Harris, Watson, and Bates (1999). However, it has been used to describe phonological acquisition (Ball, 1996; Harrison, 1996), so we could easily extend those kinds of analyses to processes in disordered speech.

Lenition and fortition processes of consonants are both found in disordered speech: fortition in such processes as fricative stopping, and lenition in the weakening found in some dysarthric speech. In GvP, both fortition and lenition can be characterized as the progressive adding or deleting of elements, or the alteration of dependency relations between elements. The lenition of /t/ is shown in the following illustration (the fortition would, of course, require the reversal of the steps shown), with x standing for the consonantal place in structure:

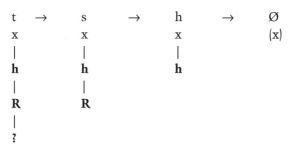

This process is seen as the gradual elimination of melodic material until an empty slot is obtained. In terms of processes such as fricative stopping, we are assuming that an element such as **?** is attached to all consonantal nodes, and the removal of such an element is accomplished at a later stage of phonological development. In the case of disordered phonology, this might not be accomplished. This differs from traditional SPE-type feature approaches, where it is assumed an extra feature such as [continuant] has to be learned, and has echoes, perhaps, of approaches such as natural phonology.

A pattern such as velar fronting requires a simple substitution of **R** for **@**, unlike the complex of features that need to be changed in a feature approach. Voicing changes, too, can be dealt with for English through manipulating the element **H** (for voiceless aspirated) at the laryngeal level with the neutral element (zero; representing the generally devoiced characteristics of English voiced consonants).

Finally, the vowel errors considered in this chapter show patterns of mid vowel raising to close positions with both front and back vowels, and for lower mid vowels there is a process of vowel lowering to an open position, again affecting front and back vowels. In a GvP account of such processes, we see a simplification of the segmental description, with vowels becoming progressively more like I, U, or A, as shown below. Harris, Watson, and Bates (1999) provide a detailed GvP account of a variety of disordered vowel systems.

$$[A, I, @] \rightarrow [I, @] \rightarrow [\underline{I}]$$
$$/\epsilon / \rightarrow /\mathrm{I}/ \rightarrow /\mathrm{i}/$$

$$[A, \underline{U}] \rightarrow [\underline{A}, U] \rightarrow [\underline{A}]$$
$$/ɔ/ \rightarrow /ɒ/ \rightarrow /ɑ/$$

The various patterns we have considered have only required manipulation of elements. This might be in the form of changing governing relations between elements, deleting or adding elements, or changing one element for another. In most cases, we have seen patterns accounted for through the manipulation of a single element, unlike the multiple feature rules we encountered in rule-based approaches, or the multiple constraints we found in OT.

Gestural or Articulatory Phonology

We have not yet considered in this chapter another influential approach to phonological analysis: gestural or articulatory phonology (Browman and Goldstein, 1986; 1989; 1992; Kent, 1997). In articulatory phonology, the main units of analysis consist of, among others, articulator shapes, sometimes termed *tract variables* (such as lip protrusion, and tongue body constriction location and degree). For the description of vowels, tongue body constriction location is used, with four different places noted: palatal, velar, uvular, and pharyngeal (this is similar, in many respects, to Catford's suggestion [1977], although he uses six locations). These constrictions can occur with different degrees of tongue body constriction degree, namely wide or narrow (or, as Browman and Goldstein, 1989, note, with as many extra intermediate degrees as needed for a particular vowel system).

While the literature on gestural phonology does not describe clearly all possible vowel types using this approach, we list the main vowels with their locations and degrees in Table 6-5.

If we examine Table 6-5, we can see that the simplified three-vowel system considered in this chapter consists of narrow vowels at the palatal, velar, and pharyngeal constriction locations.[12] We could envisage, therefore, a constraint on tongue body constriction degree allowing only narrow passages of air. This, however, would have to be augmented by some constraint allowing three tongue body constriction locations (palatal, velar, and pharyngeal), but ruling out one (uvular). There does not appear to be any device within the theory, or anything

Table 6-5   Characterization of Vowels in Gestural Phonology

Location	Degree	Vowel
Palatal	Narrow	[i]
	Mid	[e]
	Wide	[ɛ]
Velar	Narrow	[u]
	Wide	[ʊ]
Uvular	Narrow	[o]
	Mid	[ɔ]
	Wide	[ʌ]
Pharyngeal	Narrow	[ɑ]
	Mid	[ä]
	Wide	[a]

obvious extra-theoretically,[13] to justify what appears to be an ad hoc exclusion. We do not, therefore, feel that this approach to phonological analysis is of help in the case described in this chapter.

Conclusion

The survey of phonological approaches we have undertaken in this chapter has pointed out strengths and weaknesses in terms of how economical a description is, and how well grounded the different mechanisms are. In this conclusion, however, I return to the *clinical* part of the title of the chapter. In other words, how clinically useful are the different approaches. In order to do this, I consider where in the phonology the various devices used to account for our vowel cornering pattern are situated. This enables us to see where the theory predicts intervention should take place. Our knowledge of remediation strategies helps us determine how successful therapy would be. Table 6-6 displays this information, together with a recapitulation of the bases of the different approaches.

We see that both rule-based accounts and process-based accounts require vowel cornering to be located at the level of the derivation of the disordered form from the target form. This requires that we assume a model of disordered phonology in which the target form is known, but the speaker has difficulties realizing it (this might, indeed, be so, but this debate is not crucial to our discussion). This signifies that intervention must be targeted at reversing rules or eliminating processes that are already in the phonology. Constraint-based approaches posit that the EVAL component is the area in which reranked universal constraints are dealt with, and the component that would, therefore, pro-

Table 6-6   Comparison of Phonological Approaches to Vowel Cornering

	Basic units	Number of operations for vowel cornering	Location of vowel cornering
Rule-based	features; mostly binary	2 rules	derivational level
Process-based	? features	3 processes (or 1?)	derivational level
Constraint-based	features; mostly binary	3 constraints	evaluator level
Element-based	unary elements	1 restriction on element combinations	segmental level
Gesture-based	gestures	1 constraint on degree, 1 constraint on location	gestural scoring

hibit noncorner vowels. Intervention, then, must be targeted at EVAL, in order to change constraint ranking, and so allow segments that would otherwise be prohibited.

Gestural or articulatory phonology requires us to posit constraints at the point in which gestures are combined to produce a gestural score. This can be viewed as a similar process to traditional derivation. Only element-based phonology provides us with a location of the disorder at the segmental level (and with a single operation, using phonetically realizable elements). I contend that this fits well with therapists' intuitions: If a child cannot produce a sound, then the problem is at the segmental level; if a group of sounds are similarly affected, then it is a single problem. To remediate this problem, we need (where possible) to work on a single characteristic that will help produce improvement in a group of sounds.

This does not mean, of course, that only one approach to phonological disorder is correct or useful. Clearly, we might consider using a constraint-based model of description, but combined, not with binary features, but with unary ones such as described in GvP. Furthermore, until we have seen whether recent approaches such as OT and GvP are useful therapeutic tools (Harris, Watson, and Bates 1999; Stemberger and Bernhardt, 1997, provide preliminary work), the jury must remain out.

Endnotes

1. By this, we mean phonologically.
2. Underspecification theory can be thought of as having developed out of markedness approaches, but we do not have the space to follow those developments here. Roca (1994) provides a fuller account of the development of underspecification.

3. We have not discussed at all developments in nonlinear, or tiered phonology, as they do not bear directly on the concerns of this chapter.
4. Of course, slightly different patterns may be involved in a reduction to corner vowels. Reynolds (1990), for example, reports /e/ lowering to /a/.
5. A variety of names and abbreviations are used in optimality theory for constraints. We adopt those of Archangeli and Langendoen (1997).
6. I have retained the authors' constraint names, which often differ from those of other researchers, but have reinstated the convention of using small capital letters in constraint names.
7. An alternative of ranking No(Labial) highly among the violable constraints would cause problems with raising to [u].
8. This section is based, to some extent, on Ball (1997).
9. @ was omitted from the tree because it represents a default value or *blank canvas*.
10. This vowel is presumed to be somewhere between Cardinal Vowel 4 and 5. In this, and other lists of symbols, International Phonetic Alphabet values are followed.
11. N in the following diagrams stands for nucleus, not the nasal element.
12. It is, of course, debatable whether the low vowel of the reduced vowel systems discussed earlier is best described as a lowback vowel, a lowfront vowel, or simply a low vowel with a range of possible realizations. This point does not affect our discussion on gestural or articulatory phonology.
13. This is assuming that one accepts the four locations for vowels.

References

Anderson, J., and Durand, J. (1986). Dependency phonology. In J. Durand, (Ed.), Dependency and non-linear phonology (pp. 1–54). London: Croom Helm.

Anderson, J., and Durand, J. (Eds.) (1987). Explorations in dependency phonology. Dordrecht, The Netherlands: Foris.

Anderson, J., and Ewen, C. (1987). Principles of dependency phonology. Cambridge, England: Cambridge University Press.

Archangeli, D., and Langendoen, T. (1997). Optimality theory. An overview. Oxford: Blackwell.

Ball, M. J. (1996). An examination of the nature of the minimal phonological unit in language acquisition. In B. Bernhardt, J. Gilbert, and D. Ingram (Eds.), Proceedings of the UBC International Conference on Phonological Acquisition (pp. 240–253). Somerville, Mass.: Cascadilla Press.

Ball, M. J. (1997). Monovalent phonologies: Dependency phonology and an introduction to government phonology. In M. J. Ball and R. D. Kent, (Eds.), The new phonologies (pp. 127–161). San Diego: Singular.

Ball, M. J., and Kent, R. D. (Eds.) (1997). The new phonologies. San Diego: Singular.

Barlow, J. (2001). A preliminary typology of initial clusters in acquisition. Clinical Linguistics and Phonetics, 15, 9–13.

Bernhardt, B., and Stemberger, P. (1998). Handbook of phonological development. San Diego: Academic.

Browman, C., and Goldstein, L. (1986). Towards an articulatory phonology. Phonology Yearbook, 3, 219–252.

Browman, C., and Goldstein, L. (1989). Articulatory gestures as phonological units. Phonology, 6, 201–251.

Browman, C., and Goldstein, L. (1992). Articulatory phonology: An overview. Phonetica, 49, 155–180.

Carr, P. (1993). Phonology. London: Macmillan.

Catford, J. (1977). Fundamental problems in phonetics. Edinburgh, Scotland: Edinburgh University Press.

Chomsky, N., and Halle, M. (1968). The sound pattern of English. Cambridge, Mass.: MIT Press.

Clements, G. (1985). The geometry of phonological features. Phonology Yearbook, 2, 225–252.

Clements, G., and Hume, E. (1995). The internal organization of speech sounds. In J. Goldsmith (Ed.), The handbook of phonological theory (pp. 245–306). Oxford: Blackwell.

Dinnsen, D. (2001). New insights from optimality theory for acquisition. Clinical Linguistics and Phonetics, 15, 15–18.

Durand, J. (1990). Generative and non-linear phonology. London: Longman.

Ewen, C. (1995). Dependency relations in phonology. In J. Goldsmith (Ed.), The handbook of phonological theory (pp. 570–585). Oxford: Blackwell.

Gibbon, F., Shockey, L., and Reid, J. (1992). Description and treatment of abnormal vowels in a phonologically disordered child. Child Language Teaching and Therapy, 8, 30–59.

Gierut, J. (2001). A model of lexical diffusion in acquisition. Clinical Linguistics and Phonetics, 15, 19–22.

Gilbers, D. (2001). Conflicting phonologically based and phonetically based constraints in the analysis of liquid-nasal substitutions. Clinical Linguistics and Phonetics, 15, 23–28.

Grunwell, P. (1987). Clinical phonology (2nd ed.). London: Croom Helm.

Grunwell, P. (1997). Natural phonology. In M. J. Ball and R. D. Kent, (Eds.), The new phonologies (pp. 35–75). San Diego: Singular.

Harris, J. (1990). Segmental complexity and phonological government. Phonology, 7, 255–300.

Harris, J. (1994). English sound structure. Oxford: Blackwell.

Harris, J., and Lindsey, G. (1995). The elements of phonological representation. In J. Durand and F. Katamba (Eds.), Frontiers of phonology (pp. 34–79). London: Longman.

Harris, J., Watson, J., and Bates, S. (1999). Prosody and melody in vowel disorder. Journal of Linguistics, 35, 489–525.

Harrison, P. (1996). The acquisition of melodic primes in infancy. Paper presented at the 4th Phonology Meeting, University of Manchester, England.

Ingram, D. (1997). Generative phonology. In M. J. Ball and R. D. Kent, (Eds.), The new phonologies (pp. 7–33). San Diego: Singular.

Jakobson, R., Fant, G., and Halle, M. (1952). Preliminaries to speech analysis. Cambridge, Mass.: MIT Press.

Jakobson, R., and Halle, M. (1956). Fundamentals of language. The Hague: Mouton.

Kaye, J. (1995). Derivations and interfaces. In J. Durand and F. Katamba (Eds.), Frontiers of phonology (pp. 289–332). London: Longman.

Kaye, J., Lowenstamm, J., and Vergnaud, J.-R. (1985). The internal structure of phonological elements: A theory of charm and government. Phonology Yearbook, 2, 305–328.

Kaye, J., Lowenstamm, J., and Vergnaud, J.-R. (1990). Constituent structure and government in phonology. Phonology, 7, 193–232.

Kent, R. D. (1997). Gestural phonology: Basic concepts and applications in speech-language pathology. In M. J. Ball and R. D. Kent (Eds.), The new phonologies (pp. 247–268). San Diego: Singular.

Ladefoged, P. (1971). Preliminaries to linguistic phonetics. Chicago: University of Chicago Press.

Lass, R. (1984). Phonology. Cambridge, England: Cambridge University Press.

Maddieson, I. (1984). Patterns of sound. Cambridge, England: Cambridge University Press.

O'Connor, K. (2001). When is a cluster not a cluster? Clinical Linguistics and Phonetics, 15, 53–56.

Ohala, J. J. (1992). The segment: Primitive or derived? In G. Docherty and R. Ladd (Eds.), Papers in laboratory phonology II. Gesture, segment, prosody (pp. 166–183). Cambridge, England: Cambridge University Press.

Penney, G., Fee, E. J., and Dowdle, C. (1994). Vowel assessment and remediation: A case study. Child Language Teaching and Therapy, 10, 47–66.

Pollock, K. E., and Hall, P. K. (1991). An analysis of the vowel misarticulations of five children with developmental apraxia of speech. Clinical Linguistics and Phonetics, 5, 207–224.

Pollock, K. E., and Keiser, N. (1990). An examination of vowel errors in phonologically disordered children. Clinical Linguistics and Phonetics, 4, 161–178.

Prince, A., and Smolensky, P. (1993). Optimality theory: Constraint interaction in generative grammar. RuCCs Technical Report No. 2. Piscataway, N.J.: Rutgers University Center for Cognitive Science.

Reynolds, J. (1990). Abnormal vowel patterns in phonological disorder: Some data and a hypothesis. British Journal of Disorders of Communication, 25, 115–148.

Roca, I. (1994). Generative phonology. London: Routledge.

Roca, I. (Ed.) (1997). Derivations and constraints in phonology. Oxford: Clarendon Press.

Ritter, N. (1996). An alternative means of expressing manner. Paper presented at the 4th Phonology Meeting, University of Manchester, England.

Sagey, E. (1986). The representation of features and relations in non-linear phonology. Ph.D. dissertation. Cambridge, Mass.: MIT.

Schane, S. (1995). Diphthongization in particle phonology. In J. Goldsmith (Ed.), The handbook of phonological theory (pp. 586–608). Oxford: Blackwell.

Stoel-Gammon, C., and Herrington, P. (1990). Vowel systems of normally developing and phonologically disordered children. Clinical Linguistics and Phonetics, 4, 145–60.

Stampe, D. (1969). The acquisition of phonetic representation. In Papers from the Fifth Regional Meeting, Chicago Linguistics Society (pp. 443–454).

Stampe, D. (1973). A dissertation on natural phonology. Doctoral dissertation, University of Chicago. New York: Garland Press.

Stemberger, J., and Bernhardt, B. (1997). Optimality theory. In M. J. Ball and R. D. Kent, (Eds.), The new phonologies (pp. 211–245). San Diego: Singular.

Trubetzkoy, N. ([1939] 1969) Principles of phonology. Berkeley: University of California Press.

Ueda, I., and Davis, S. (2001). Promotion and demotion of phonological constraints in the acquisition of the Japanese liquid. Clinical Linguistics and Phonetics, 15, 29–33.

van der Hulst, H. (1989). Atoms of segmental structure: Components, gestures and dependency. Phonology, 6, 253–284.

Walton, J. H., and Pollock, K. E. (1993). Acoustic validation of vowel error patterns in developmental apraxia of speech. Clinical Linguistics and Phonetics, 7, 95–111.

Watson, M., Martineau, D., and Hughes, D. (1994). Vowel use of phonologically disordered identical twin boys: A case study. Perceptual and Motor Skills, 79, 1587–1597.

7

Therapy for Abnormal Vowels in Children with Phonological Impairment

Fiona E. Gibbon
Janet Mackenzie Beck

Therapy for vowel errors has received scant attention in the extensive literature on phonological impairment. As a result, speech clinicians currently have little evidence on which to base clinical decisions about therapy for children whose speech contains vowel errors. The beginning of this chapter is devoted to a review of the few studies that have reported therapy for abnormal vowels systems in children with phonological impairment. The tentative conclusion that emerges from the limited evidence is that direct therapy for vowel errors has a positive effect, with improvements in vowel production occurring over and above that expected from spontaneous development.

The latter part of this chapter discusses a range of therapy approaches that are of potential, although as yet unproven, value for increasing vowel production accuracy. Included in this section are approaches designed originally for consonant errors, along with examples illustrating how approaches can be adapted for vowel errors. Also included are approaches involving computer-assisted techniques. Some computer techniques aim to develop children's auditory receptive skills in vowel identification and discrimination, others aim to improve vowel production skills through the provision of real-time visual feedback of speech features.

The information contained in this chapter is intended to be of interest and relevance to speech clinicians responsible for the management of children with phonological impairment. These clinicians are likely to have on their caseloads at least some children whose speech contains mild-to-moderate, if not severe, vowel errors. It is hoped that the issues raised throughout the chapter will stimulate future research into vowel errors and factors that influence therapy outcome.

Phonological Impairment and Vowel Errors

Children with phonological impairment have developmental speech disorders that cannot be attributed to identifiable organic pathology, such as hearing impairment, neurological deficit, or structural abnormality of the vocal tract (Leonard, 1995). Research concerning effective therapy for these children is particularly relevant to clinicians because phonological impairment is one of the most frequently encountered communication disorders affecting children in the preschool years. It is estimated that approximately 10% of preschool children fail to develop intelligible speech in the absence of identifiable etiology. Furthermore, 80% of this group require speech and language therapy services, with the result that children with phonological impairment make up a large proportion of many speech clinicians' pediatric caseloads (Weiss, Gordon, and Lillywhite, 1987).

The literature on phonological impairment focuses almost entirely on abnormal consonant production. The percentage of children with abnormal vowel systems is not known for certain, although it is clear that vowel errors are less frequent than consonant errors (Eisenson and Ogilvie, 1963; Stoel-Gammon and Herrington, 1990). Pollock and Keiser (1990) studied vowel errors in 15 children with moderate-to-severe phonological impairment. They found that one child had severe difficulty with vowels, while eight more children (53%) displayed mild or moderate difficulties. Although less frequent than consonantal difficulties, vowel errors may occur in as many as 50% of children with phonological impairment, if Pollock and Keiser's estimate is accurate. In addition, the likelihood of vowel errors occurring increases as the severity of the children's consonantal difficulty increases (see preliminary results from the Memphis Vowel Project in Chapter 3).

Although mild-to-moderate vowel problems might be common, speech clinicians often do not detect vowel errors in routine examinations of children's speech based on perceptual analysis (Pollock and Keiser, 1990). There are several possible explanations for vowel errors remaining undetected in clinical assessments. First, many standard speech assessment procedures do not allow for a full range of vowels to be elicited, so vowel errors are not always recorded. Second, clinicians might not be aware of the types of errors that can affect vowels, and, as a result, fail to identify vowel error patterns. Third, Stoel-Gammon (1990) suggests that listeners find vowels difficult to transcribe reliably, and that normal dialectal differences in vowel systems make listeners more tolerant of abnormal variations in vowel productions. A final difficulty is that we still have a rather incomplete understanding of normal patterns of vowel development. This was also discussed earlier in Chapter 1. Recent research into vowel production in the spontaneous speech of typically developing Scottish toddlers (aged 18 to 36 months) found a high level of variability in patterns of vowel acquisition (Matthews, 2001). Matthews' study also found that errors involving target /u/ were frequent in the children investigated, casting some doubt on the view that corner vowels are always the first to be produced in a consistently accurate way (Stoel-Gammon and Herrington, 1990).

Some researchers have suggested that children with vowel errors form a subgroup of phonological impairment. Adler, Rees, Serwer, and Stocker (1968) studied a group of 42 children (aged 3 to 12 years) with vowel errors associated with functional articulation disorders. The children presented with a number of distinct clinical features. For instance, boys with vowel errors outnumbered girls by a ratio of 6:1 (2:1 is a typical ratio in phonological impairment). Many children had additional prosodic abnormalities affecting speech rate, rhythm, stress, and intonation. The combination of vowel errors and abnormal prosody gave the "impression that these children had foreign accents" (Adler, Rees, Serwer, and Stocker, 1968, 52). Another feature was that a high proportion of the children showed signs of social/behavioral immaturity. These clinical features led Adler and colleagues to conclude that children with vowel errors formed a subgroup distinct from other developmental speech disorders. Although it is possible that such a subgroup exists, the evidence is weak because no studies have compared the clinical characteristics of children with and without vowel errors.

The overwhelming majority of therapy procedures have been developed for improving consonant error patterns, providing a wide range of approaches in routine clinical use. The various approaches are based on diverse assumptions about underlying speech processing deficits in phonological impairment. As a result, approaches emphasize different therapy goals and employ a range of therapy strategies. Clinicians select a therapy approach based on their judgement about the most complementary matching between the assumed underlying deficit/s and the orientation and strategies employed in that particular therapy approach.

Many diverse therapy approaches are reported as having positive effects on children's consonant systems (Bernthal and Bankson, 1998; Gierut, 1998). Positive effects include greater accuracy in production of speech sounds, increased phonetic repertoires, more adultlike use of phonological contrasts, more complex syllable structures, and overall improved intelligibility. The benefits of therapy for improving speech in children with phonological impairment have been documented in numerous descriptive case studies, and experimental studies involving single cases and groups.

Although there is a large body of evidence showing the benefits of therapy for phonological impairment, treatment efficacy studies focus almost exclusively on improvements in the consonant system. In contrast to the extensive literature on therapy for consonant error patterns, relatively few approaches mention their application to vowel error patterns, and few studies investigate the effects of therapy for vowel errors in phonological impairment. Gierut's (1998) wide-ranging review of the literature on treatment efficacy specifically highlights the need for research into therapy programs for improving abnormal vowel systems in children with phonological impairment.

Why Target Vowels in Therapy?

There are several reasons why it is desirable for clinicians to resolve children's vowel errors as part of a therapy program. A successful therapy program could

- *Improve intelligibility.* Vowel errors often have a significant and detrimental effect on intelligibility (Metz, Schiavetti, Samar, and Sitler, 1990), and improving accuracy of vowels is likely to improve speech intelligibility.
- *Increase speech acceptability.* In mild-to-moderate vowel errors, the issue of acceptability of speech quality might arise. Even quite minor residual vowel errors having little impact on intelligibility, might cause distress by making children's overall speech quality inappropriate for their accent group. Some children with vowel errors also have unusual prosodic patterns, further reducing speech acceptability. Therapy that improves abnormal vowels is likely to increase speech acceptability.
- *Restore a normal developmental pattern.* Children with typically developing speech master the vowel system earlier than the consonant system (Stoel-Gammon, 1990). A developmental perspective suggests, therefore, that vowel errors should be targeted before consonant errors to restore a normal developmental pattern.

Although these are good reasons for focusing therapy directly on vowel errors, one contraindication is where vowel errors are systematically conditioned by adjacent consonant errors (as discussed in Chapter 5). In these cases, it is logical to target the consonant error in therapy, and observe whether the vowel error improves spontaneously.

Studies Reporting Therapy for Vowel Errors

This section reviews studies of direct therapy for vowel errors in children with phonological impairment. Direct therapy includes goals and activities designed specifically for children's vowel errors. Despite an early study concluding that vowel errors "tend to be highly resistant to speech therapy" (Adler, Ross, Serwer, and Stocker, 1968, 55), the review presents an optimistic picture of the benefits of direct therapy for vowel errors. Also discussed are reports of vowel errors resolving either spontaneously or as a result of indirect therapy (that is, therapy for consonant errors).

Direct Therapy for Vowel Errors

Four studies of direct therapy for vowel error patterns in children with phonological impairment are examined. These studies were conducted by Gibbon, Shockey, and Reid (1992); Hargrove, Dauer, and Montelibano (1989); Penney, Fee, and Dowdle (1994); and Pollock (1994). These four studies report therapy targeting a range of error patterns and employing a variety of therapy approaches.

Hargrove and colleagues (1989) described therapy for atypical vowels in 4-year-old identical twin boys with highly unintelligible speech. In addition to vowel difficulties, the twins had abnormal syntax and prosody. The boys produced over a quarter of vowel targets as errors of distortion (such as prolongation affecting long and short vowel targets) and inconsistent vowel substitutions. Hargrove and colleagues discussed a therapy program conducted over 8 months to decrease the duration of the twins' prolonged vowels. Therapy strategies included contingent reinforcement, verbal feedback, auditory/visual cues, imitation, and modeling, and involved a series of 11 objectives in which vowel targets occurred in increasingly demanding contexts. At Stage 1, the clinician elicited isolated vowels in imitation of a model, while at Stage 11, the twins produced vowels spontaneously in connected speech. The twins responded positively to therapy as targeted vowels became shorter and more similar to those of an age-matched comparison child. The authors noted that there were carryover problems, however, as vowel errors occurred in connected speech even when the twins demonstrated vowel production accuracy in clinic-based activities.

Gibbon and colleagues (1992) described therapy for abnormal vowels in the speech of a 4-year-old boy (D) with a phonological impairment. Child D had highly unintelligible speech, with both consonant and vowel systems affected. Data was gathered at three stages (prevowel therapy, 4 months postvowel therapy, and 8 months postvowel therapy) from naturalistic conversation and spontaneous picture-naming activities. Analysis of Child D's vowel errors showed diphthong reduction affecting /eɪ/, /aɪ/, /ɒɪ/, /əʊ/ targets. Child D also lacked differentiation between vowels in the mid to high region of the vowel space, effectively neutralizing the /i/, /ɪ/ contrast, and /ʊ/, /ɜ/, /u/ contrasts. A stimulability task involving isolated vowel targets showed that Child D could produce some vowel targets (such as /ɒɪ/), but not other vowels (such as /u/, /eɪ/, /aɪ/, /əʊ/).

The therapy program described by Gibbon and colleagues focused on the development of diphthongs in six weekly sessions. Therapy included the development of a suitable vocabulary to discuss distinguishing features of monophthongs and diphthongs. A sliding analogy was used for the notion of articulatory movement from one component of the diphthong to the other. Therapy developed awareness of the difference between monophthongs and diphthongs, and Child D was encouraged to produce a diphthong/monophthong contrast elicited from pictures of minimal pair words. Following the six sessions that focused on vowels, therapy continued, but the focus shifted from vowel to consonant targets. Data recorded 4 months after the vowel therapy sessions showed that the highfront and highback vowels and diphthongs, which had all previously shown errors, had improved to the extent that all contrasts were now differentiated, and fewer errors affected vowel targets. Data gathered 8 months after the vowel sessions showed further improvement, with all vowels except one produced with 100% accuracy.

Penney and colleagues (1994) described intervention strategies for abnormal /u/, /æ/ targets produced by a 4-year-old girl (CG) with a phonological impairment. Child CG's speech was highly unintelligible and contained multiple articulation errors in both consonant and vowel systems. A vowel assessment of Child CG's speech revealed a reduced vowel inventory, and a low overall percentage of correct vowels. Assessment showed that back vowels contained the lowest correct rate (35%), followed by front vowels (85% correct), with central vowels being the most accurate (100% correct). Improving the accuracy of vowels /u/, /æ/ was a therapy goal because these targets had the lowest percentage correct scores, and also because the vowels have a high frequency of occurrence in English. Intervention was constructed in the form of a hierarchy involving perception (auditory detection and discrimination), and production (imitation and elicitation) of target vowels from isolated vowels to spontaneous speech. Therapy strategies included auditory bombardment, detection of target vowels, vowel discrimination, and phonetic placement of vowels. Child CG's vowels responded positively. As an example, /u/, /æ/ were highly stimulable after therapy, and Child CG attained 80% accuracy for /u/ at all levels of the hierarchy apart from spontaneous speech.

Pollock (1994) described therapy for vowel errors in a 4-year-old boy (P) with a phonological impairment. Child P's vowel inventory was reduced, and vowel errors showed patterns of lowering, backing, centralization, and diphthong reduction. Child P showed a severe difficulty with vowels, with only 33% correctly produced. More specifically, 41% of nonrhotic monophthongs were correct, 11% of nonrhotic diphthongs were correct, and rhotic monophthongs were 0% correct. Only /i/, /ɑ/, were produced with 100% accuracy prior to therapy. Four vowels (/aɪ/, /aʊ/, /e/, /o/) showing zero correct production on baseline probes were selected as therapy goals.

Child P attended for three 50-minute therapy sessions per week for two semesters. Approximately half of the sessions focused on vowels, with the remaining sessions focused on consonant targets. Therapy approaches included drill and drill-play activities with small sets of words containing the target vowels. The clinician provided auditory and visual cues as needed. Minimal pairs activities were used to facilitate the concept of contrast. Child P made rapid progress with diphthong target /aɪ/, (targeted in the first semester), and by the end of this period, Child P had reached 100% accuracy on untrained probe words. The second semester focused on /aʊ/, with similar success to /aɪ/, with 40% accuracy of untrained probe words at the end of this period.

As in the case described by Gibbon and colleagues, therapy for diphthongs described by Pollock also was successful. Child P's progress with midvowels /e/, /o/ was less successful, however. Child P was not stimulable for /e/, even with multiple auditory, visual, tactile, and verbal cues, and production of /e/ remained at 0% correct throughout both semesters. Some progress with /o/ occurred, as Child P could manage a close approximation with multiple cues, although production remained variable on untrained words. Pollock concluded that therapy had been successful in bringing about improvement in three out of four vowel targets. Since vowel errors did not change during baseline probes, and only began to improve when therapy was initiated, this evidence suggested that therapy, and not spontaneous development, was responsible for improved vowel production in Child P's case.

Spontaneous Resolution of Vowel Errors

Some research suggests that vowel errors resolve spontaneously during the school years due to maturational factors (Adler, Rees, Serwer, and Stocker, 1968), whereas other research indicates that vowel errors can resolve without direct therapy during the preschool years (Watson, Martineau, and Hughes, 1994). Watson and colleagues studied 3-year-old identical twin boys with phonological impairment over a 16-month period. Despite the presence of phonological disorder, the parents of the twins decided not to enroll them in therapy, and the changes that were documented occurred in the absence of any formal therapy input. The twins initially presented with expressive syntax delays, using phonological processes affecting speech intelligibility. The boys had reduced vowel inventories, with neither twin producing vowels /ɔ/, /ʊ/, /ɚ/, /ɝ/. Although the boys differed somewhat in their vowel errors, and in their development over time, as the boys' phonological systems developed spontaneously, so did their correct use of vowels. Their improvement in vowel use reflected normal vowel development, as described by Stoel-Gammon and Herrington (1990). In other words, the first vowels to develop were the corner vowels /i/, /a/, /u/, and the last were the rhotic vowels /ɚ/, /ɝ/. This evidence suggests that some children's vowel errors can improve spontaneously in the absence of formal intervention.

Counterevidence of spontaneous or maturational resolution of vowel errors comes from a rare study of seven siblings aged 6 to 14 years, all having moderate-to-severe phonological impairment (Radford and Gentry, 1997). These children were unusual because none had attended school, and none had received speech therapy prior to the data collection reported in the study. Although this study contains few details of the children's vowel or consonant systems, the speech samples from the children show evidence of vowel errors. Given that all the children presented with significant speech disorders, irrespective of their ages, the authors concluded that phonological impairment does not resolve spontaneously in all children in the absence of direct intervention.

Therapy for Consonants Indirectly Benefiting Vowel Errors

Another clinically relevant issue is whether maximum benefits are gained from targeting vowels directly, or whether therapy focusing on improving the consonant system has an indirect, but equally beneficial, effect of improving the vowel system. The view that targeting consonants can have an indirect and beneficial impact on vowel production is supported by a study conducted by Robb, Bleile, and Yee (1999). They adopted an indirect approach to treating vowels in a 4-year-old girl (J) with a phonological impairment affecting both consonants and vowels. The study employed transcription data and acoustic analysis to evaluate changes in Child J's vowel productions over a 10-week period. Treatment consisted of 20 sessions focusing on developing consonant production, in this case postvocalic obstruent voicing. This program involved a minimal pair approach contrasting the phonemes /z/ and /g/ with their voiceless counterparts /s/ and /k/. No emphasis was placed on accurate vowel production during the course of therapy. At the conclusion of therapy, the size of this child's vowel inventory and overall vowel accuracy had improved.

Robb and colleagues (1999) commented that, although therapy did not directly focus on vowel accuracy, it was possible that the activities undertaken in their therapy program facilitated correct vowel production. Specifically, the variations in place and manner of articulation of the consonants targeted in therapy could have resulted in a general improvement in speech motor control abilities resulting in more accurate vowel production.

Preliminary findings from eight children studied longitundinally in the Memphis Vowel Project, described by Pollock in Chapter 3, partially support the view that vowel errors resolve with indirect therapy. Pollock found that most of the children improved in vowel accuracy over time with intervention for consonant errors. Several children, however, continued to exhibit vowel errors 18 months after initial testing, suggesting that indirect therapy benefits some, but not all, children.

Vowel Therapy: Principles and Approaches

The previous section shows that relatively few studies have specifically investigated vowel therapy in children with phonological impairment. Nonetheless, we can draw on knowledge from research in other areas when formulating general principles for vowel therapy. An assumption made throughout the ensuing discussions about therapy is that children with vowel errors do not form a subgroup separate from those with consonant errors. This view allows us to apply to vowel errors the same general principles and therapy approaches that apply to consonant errors in children with phonological impairment. A proviso is that any approach requiring children to focus on their own articulatory activity might be somewhat more difficult with vowels than it is with consonants. The high degree of vocal tract constriction involved in consonant production generally results in a high level of tactile feedback, enhancing awareness of articulatory placement. With the exception of close vowels, such as /i/, /ɪ/, this tactile feedback is greatly decreased during vowel production.

The discussion regarding principles is followed by descriptions of therapies that clinicians can adapt for use with vowel errors. These diverse approaches are not intended to be mutually exclusive. Rather, it is assumed that effective management of phonological impairment involves the clinician selecting and sequencing different approaches to meet children's needs, as therapy progresses (Dodd and Bradford, 2000).

General Principles

A prerequisite for effective identification and treatment of vowel errors is that clinicians should have good perceptual skills to analyze vowels, and be able to relate the findings to expected vowel productions in the child's sociolinguistic group. Clinicians need to formulate therapy goals in the light of a clear description of the adult target vowel system (that is, if and how the target system differs from standard systems). Clinicians' vowel production skills are also important, because clinicians might need to model a full range of vowel qualities during therapy activities. The need for vowel analysis and production skills is especially great when the clinician and child have different target accents. The issue of developing clinicians' phonetic perceptual and production skills in relation to vowels is revisited at the end of this chapter.

A second general principle is that clinicians need to select appropriate therapy goals and intervention approaches based on detailed phonetic and phonological analyses of the child's speech, an assessment of speech and language processing skills (Stackhouse and Wells, 1997), as well as relevant information gathered as part of routine clinical assessment. The phonetic and phonological analyses provide a descriptive account of speech error patterns, which the clinician can use to formulate therapy goals. Although an essential part of the assessment process, phonological analyses provide a descriptive, rather than an explanatory, account of children's speech difficulties.

A psycholinguistic profile will, however, suggest which aspect or aspects of speech processing to focus on in intervention, and which approach is most likely to facilitate improved speech intelligibility. For instance, some children have auditory perceptual deficits, whereas others have cognitive/linguistic deficits associated with the phonological structure of the language (Dinnsen, 1984; Elbert and Gierut, 1986; Ingram, 1976). A third possibility is that motoric/artic-ulatory deficits affect the movements and coordination necessary for normal speech production. These different levels of speech processing form the ration-ale for the structure of the second part of this chapter, which describes a range of therapy approaches that develop processing skills at these levels.

It is worth noting that there is some controversy in the literature about whether therapy is most effective when it targets processing deficits directly. One view is that, "intervention targeting the primary area of deficit for children is likely to be more effective than other treatment techniques" (Dodd and Bradford, 2000, 191). Dodd and Bradford would presumably argue that, in cases in which assessment reveals auditory discrimination deficits, the most effective therapy approach is one that focuses directly on improving auditory discrimi-nation skills. An alternate view is that the most effective therapy approach is one that bypasses children's specific area of difficulty. Waters (2001) adopted this alternate view in a therapy program capitalizing on input and cognitive process-ing strengths to overcome a motor/articulatory difficulty in a 5-year-old boy with a severe developmental speech disorder.

A third view is that certain therapy approaches are effective irrespective of children's underlying processing deficits. For instance, Shuster, Ruscello, and Toth (1995) view visual feedback as effective, because feedback improves pro-duction directly regardless of deficits at auditory perceptual, cognitive/linguistic, or motor/articulatory levels.

Approaches to Vowel Therapy

Some therapy approaches described in the following text were developed primarily for consonant errors in children with phonological impair-ment. Other approaches were developed for vowel errors occurring in speech pathologies other than phonological impairment, such as developmental apraxia of speech and hearing impairment. Altogether, six approaches are considered. The first three approaches focus on children's auditory/perceptual skills, linguistic/ phonological abilities, and motor/articulatory skills. The final three approaches involve the use of computer-based instrumentation to develop children's perceptual skills, provide children with visual feedback of acoustic information, and provide visual feedback of direct articulatory information. Examples illustrate how approaches could be adapted to target a range of vowel error patterns.

Auditory/Perceptual Approaches

Vowel errors in children with phonological impairment might be associated with auditory perceptual deficits. Examples of auditory perceptual approaches to therapy are auditory input therapy (Flynn and Lancaster, 1996), and auditory bombardment (Hodson and Paden, 1983). Auditory input therapy "aims to enhance the auditory salience of target speech sounds and structures in a natural context" (Flynn and Lancaster, 1996, 51). This approach is also called structured listening and does not require children to produce target sounds. Flynn and Lancaster feel that it is not necessary to include production practice, because the increased opportunities to hear target speech sounds are sufficient to induce positive changes in output in many children.

Auditory input therapy aims to enhance the auditory salience of target speech sounds through children experiencing increased opportunities to hear well-formed adult productions during naturalistic contexts (such as structured stories and games). The approach maximizes auditory salience of target speech sounds by placing them in contexts involving maximally clear productions. For example, target speech sounds are placed in syllables that have primary stress, and placed in nouns occurring at the ends of phrases. If the target sound is /aɪ/, for instance, activities might involve structured stories or games including multiple opportunities for the adult to produce, and for the child to hear, words such as *tie, pie, dye, pipe*. Because children are not put under pressure to correct their errored productions, auditory input therapy is considered an ideal intervention for parents to carry out as home-based programs.

Auditory bombardment is a component of the cycles approach to phonological therapy (Hodson and Paden, 1983; 1991). In auditory bombardment, children listen for a few minutes to a small set (12–15) of selected words containing the target sound using minimal amplification. Bombardment takes place at the beginning and end of therapy sessions, and once a day at home. Like auditory input therapy, children are not required to produce target sounds during auditory bombardment activities. Although Hodson and Paden view amplification as an integral part of auditory bombardment, Flynn and Lancaster (1996) point out that no empirical research has compared the effects of amplification versus no amplification during bombardment activities. Flynn and Lancaster view structured auditory input without amplification as effective.

Monsen and Shaughnessy (1978) described a vowel therapy program based on structured listening drills emphasizing articulatory relations between vowel sounds. The procedure consisted of comparison drills, which involved the client listening to vowel sequences produced by the clinician. The front vowel sequence was /i/, /ɪ/, /ɛ/, /æ/, and its purpose was to demonstrate how vowels are related in degree of mouth opening and tongue height. In the sequence /i/ to /æ/, there is gradual mouth opening, and, at the same time, tongue lowering. Although the drills described by Monsen and Shaughnessy were used with individuals with hearing impairment, increasing awareness of articulatory relationships between vowels might be valuable, at least for older children with phonological impairment.

Following are examples of therapy activities to develop auditory perceptual skills (see also minimal pair discrimination later in the text). The activities use real and nonwords, with success in these activities requiring phonetic level auditory processing skills. The demands involved in the three activities need to be matched carefully to the processing abilities of individual children. These activities provide multiple opportunities for children to hear target vowels, as does auditory input therapy, but they also involve children in various types of decision making, so placing additional demands on their processing skills.

1. Same/different judgements (real words). These activities involve children listening to and judging whether two real words produced by the clinician are the same or different. The words are selected according to the speech errors made by the child. Word pairs for a child who neutralized the /ɛ/, /æ/ vowel contrast might include: *bad, bad* (same); *bad, bed* (different). If a child found minimal distinctions difficult, vowels involving maximal distinctions, such as *bad, bad* (same); *bad, bead* (different) could be used.

2. Same/different judgements (nonwords). In these activities, the child judges whether two nonwords produced by the clinician are the same or different. Judgements about nonwords require a different level of perceptual processing from real words, because nonwords have no phonological representations. Therefore, semantic or other higher level language processes do not assist in this task. Words are again selected according to the speech errors made by the child. Nonword pairs for a child who neutralized the /ɛ/, /æ/ vowel contrast might include: /bæm/, /bæm/ (same); /bæm/, /bɛm/ (different). Once again, if minimal distinctions were difficult, maximal distinctions such as /bæm/, /bæm/ (same); /bæm/, /bɒɪm/ (different) could be used.

3. Right/wrong judgements. Activities involving the child identifying the clinician's correct and incorrect vowel productions could help to develop processing skills. Initially, errors could be gross, with a move towards subtle errors, and, more importantly, errors that the child makes. If the target vowel was /ɒɪ/, for instance, the clinician could devise an activity involving the child in making yes/no decisions about the accuracy of the clinician's productions of the word

toy. In this case the clinician could ask the child, "is this a [tɪ]?" (correct answer: no); "is this a [tɒ]?" (correct answer: no); "is this a [tɒɪ]?" (correct answer: yes).

Several studies reviewed in the beginning of this chapter incorporated auditory perceptual approaches as part of their therapy programs. Penney, Fee, and Dowdle (1994) employed auditory bombardment, auditory detection of target vowels, and same/different vowel discrimination. Gibbon, Shockey, and Reid (1992) developed auditory awareness of the monophthong/diphthong contrast in Child D's therapy program.

Linguistic/Phonological Approaches

Linguistic/phonological approaches emphasize the importance of contrasts and communicating meaning as integral components of the therapy process. In addition, therapy is typically directed towards targeting whole sound classes, rather than individual segments. Examples of phonological approaches are minimal pair contrast therapy (Blache, Parsons, and Humphreys, 1981; Elbert, Rockman, and Saltzman, 1980; Weiner 1981), maximal oppositions (Elbert and Gierut, 1986), and Metaphon (Dean and Howell, 1986; Howell and Dean, 1994). A phonological approach focuses on "awareness and discrimination of minimal differences and on the child's attempts to produce a difference of some kind in a case where they usually neutralized a distinctive opposition" (Reynolds, 1990, 145). Reynolds views phonological approaches as appropriate, particularly for younger children with vowel errors in their speech.

Minimal pair therapy, also referred to as minimal pair contrast therapy, is probably the best known and most researched phonological therapy. Therapy typically involves a game format presenting pairs of words that the child produces as identical (that is, homophonous). For instance, children with vowel errors often neutralize the /ɛ/, /æ/ distinction, producing the minimal pair bed, *bad* as homophonous [bæd]. In relation to vowels, minimal pairs can vary along the dimensions high/low, front/back, long/short, and so on.

The use of minimal pairs encourages children to produce the word pairs distinctly in order to communicate a message to the listener. The clinician engineers situations in which communication breaks down if children produce homophonous word pairs. Breakdown occurs when the listener (the clinician) cannot distinguish between children's identical forms. In order to repair the breakdown, children attempt to change their habitual errored productions in some way in order to get the message across. Through confrontation of minimal pairs, children learn the communicative importance of producing contrasts that are sufficiently distinct for listeners to detect.

Minimal pairs can be used in a variety of game formats during therapy. One application is barrier game formats (Bunce, 1989). Like other phonological approaches, barrier games emphasize contrast and communicating meaning to the listener. The activities involve the child and clinician giving and following directions, and subsequently evaluating the success of their communication. A barrier or screen of some type separates the child from the clinician. A typical activity using minimal pairs might involve child and clinician having identical sets of pictures (or objects). The child arranges the pictures in a particular sequence on one side of the barrier, and then describes the sequence to the clinician who is on the other side of the barrier and cannot see the child's picture sequence. At this point, the clinician has to listen to the child's instructions and follow them, thus attempting to replicate exactly the child's picture sequence. If the child's productions are ambiguous, the clinician can query the child's intention by saying "did you say *bed* or *bad*?" and there is an opportunity for repair.

When the sequences are complete, the barrier is removed, and the child and clinician discuss the success of their communications (that is, whether the two sequences on either side of the barrier matched). The child and clinician then switch roles, so the clinician is the speaker and the child the listener. Switching roles not only preserves the normal turn-taking of games. When the clinician is the speaker, the situation is ideal for the clinician to model the correct production of the minimal pair words. When the child is the listener, there is an opportunity for the clinician to check the child's auditory discrimination of minimally distinct words. Barrier game formats do not require a clinician to participate, and interesting communications can occur when there is a child on each side of the barrier.

Although clinicians can use minimal pairs in creative and flexible ways during therapy, one limitation is that success requires that the child has adequate motor/articulatory ability to produce the target sound in the minimal pair words. Articulatory ability to produce target sounds is not present in all children who neutralize phonological contrasts in their speech. For example, the child with a phonological impairment and vowel errors described by Pollock (1994) was unable to produce /e/, even with multiple auditory, visual, tactile, and verbal cues. Production of /e/ remained at 0% correct throughout the therapy period. Minimal pairs involving the target sound /e/ would probably have proved both frustrating and unsuccessful in this case. An additional practical difficulty can be finding sufficient minimal pairs involving appropriate vocabulary for preschool children, although Baker (1981) provides a useful resource of pictures and vocabulary for a range of vowel targets, including minimal pairs.

The previous description of minimal pair therapy focuses on eliciting production. Minimal pairs can also be used to check and develop the children's perception of minimally distinct words. In minimal pair discrimination activities, word pairs are presented to the child in the form of pictures/objects, and the child points to or selects in some way the word spoken by the clinician. Minimal pairs embedded in sentences and paragraphs can follow discrimination at a single word level. Minimal pair discrimination tasks involve high level cognitive/linguistic processing skills, because success depends on the child having accurate stored phonological representations of the minimal word pairs. Difficulties with this type of task often reflect high-level processing difficulties such as with establishing phoneme category boundaries or with words that have underspecified phonological representations.

The maximal opposition approach (Elbert and Gierut, 1986; Gierut 1989), like the minimal pair approach, presents a conceptual approach to phonological therapy. In minimal pairs, phonological oppositions typically vary in one feature, whereas in maximal opposition, the phonological oppositions vary along multiple dimensions of voice, manner, and place of articulation. In relation to vowels, target vowels are selected on the basis that they also vary on a number of dimensions. For example, the vowels /i/, /ɑ/ are maximally opposed (on the height and front/back dimension), as are /æ/, /u/.

Gierut (1989) suggests that the maximal opposition approach is suitable for children with significant gaps in their phonological systems, or for those who find making the subtle distinctions in minimal pairs difficult. For these children, grosser distinctions might be easier for them to produce, thus avoiding frustration, particularly in the early stages of therapy. Furthermore, a practical advantage of this approach is that clinicians have a wider choice of vocabulary from which to select words to use in therapy activities. A final important point is that Gierut (1990) has found maximal opposition therapy to be more effective than minimal pair therapy. All of these advantages suggest that the maximal opposition approach is potentially effective, and it is, therefore, surprising that studies have not reported its use with vowel errors.

Another phonological approach is Metaphon developed by Dean and Howell (1986). Metaphon aims to increase children's ability to use phonological contrasts by building metaphonological and metacommunicative awareness, and, at the same time, developing children's ability to use repair strategies.

Metaphon has two phases. The first phase aims to build a shared vocabulary that the child and clinician can use to explore the phonetic properties of speech sound contrasts. Phase one capitalizes on children's naturally occurring interest in sounds. In phase one, children become increasingly aware of their own and the adult target system, and are given opportunities to experiment with new articulatory gestures. Although there are few accounts of using Metaphon for vowel errors, the approach could be adapted easily for this purpose. Therapy could develop appropriate vocabulary and visual referents for short and long vowels, lip rounding versus spreading, movement for diphthongs (Gibbon, Shockey, and Reid, 1992, used a sliding analogy for the movement for diphthongs) and perhaps high/low and back/front tongue position.

Phase two of therapy builds on the awareness of sounds that children have developed in phase one. Phase two encourages children to use newfound sound knowledge to make distinctions between minimal pairs, and to repair errors when communication breaks down.

Several therapy studies reviewed in the beginning of this chapter incorporated linguistic/phonological approaches. Most studies targeted vowel error patterns, using different vowels and diphthongs as examples of the targeted sound classes. In addition, most emphasized the importance of phonological contrasts by using approaches such as minimal pairs and Metaphon in their therapy programs (Gibbon, Shockey, and Reid, 1992; Pollock, 1994).

Motor/Articulatory Approaches

Therapy to develop motor/articulatory skills follows general principles of motor learning, emphasizing the importance of providing repetitive, intensive, and systematic practice drills. These drills are used to establish accuracy in articulation and reduce variable performance. Motor approaches emphasize the importance of knowledge of results in the form of verbal, visual, tactile, and kinesthetic feedback on performance. Articulatory approaches include the traditional method (Van Riper, 1947), contextual facilitation (Kent, 1982), phonetic placement (Scripture and Jackson, 1925), and the use of tactile and gestural cues (Chumpelik, 1984; Passy, 1990).

Van Riper's traditional method (Van Riper, 1947; Van Riper and Emerick, 1984) proceeds in four stages:

1. Sensory/perceptual training (ear training). This stage focuses on identifying the target sound and discriminating it from error productions.

2. Production training. This stage aims to change production of the error sound. The approach introduces different syllable positions throughout therapy, gradually increasing the motor complexity of tasks. If the vowel target were /æ/, words containing the target vowel would be introduced in increasingly complex consonant/vowel (CV) sequences such as: *am* (VC); *ham* (CVC); *ant* (VCC); *pram* (CCVC); *stamp* (CCVCC).

3. Stabilization. This stage strengthens the correct production, helping children to produce newly acquired sound quickly and easily, with what has been termed *articulatory ease*. Methods used to establish articulatory ease include prolonging/whispering the target sound, and alternating between the correct/ error sound, or between the correct/another sound.

4. Transfer. This stage ensures carryover of the newly acquired sound into syllables, words, and, ultimately, into everyday communicative situations.

Most therapies, including the traditional method, grade the motor complexity of tasks in some way, and this principle is incorporated in motor-based approaches to therapy. Another example of an approach that grades motor complexity, and which specifically includes vowels, is the Nuffield Dyspraxia Programme (Connery, 1994). In this program, each vowel target has an associated visual referent. The diphthong /ɒɪ/ is associated with a picture of a parrot, for instance, and the vowel /i/ with a mouse. The program provides numerous drill/play exercises, building from sounds in isolation to simple alternating sequences, and gradually to phrases. The program has been used with children aged 3 years and older who have been diagnosed with developmental apraxia of speech.

Some articulatory approaches emphasize the role of phonetic context surrounding target vowels in facilitating correct sound production (such as contextual facilitation, Kent, 1982). In children with variable productions of vowels, some phonetic environments or linguistic conditions may be more likely to facilitate correct vowel production than others. An awareness of the impact of context on production accuracy is useful. Clinicians will want to proceed through a hierarchy, from maximally facilitative contexts to less-facilitative or nonfacilitative contexts, as therapy progresses.

Kent identified stress as a factor that could influence accuracy of sound production. For example, syllable stress helps to "assure distinctive and well-formed (nonreduced) articulations" (Kent, 1982, 67). In addition, vowel durations are longer in stressed syllables, and more extreme in their articulatory placement than in unstressed syllables. Consequently, the increased acoustic information available in stressed syllables results in vowels being more perceptually distinct to the listener, and might supply children with enhanced motor and auditory feedback. These are good reasons for selecting words that have target vowels in stressed syllables, at least at stages in therapy requiring the vowel to occur in maximally facilitative contexts.

Physiological factors can act to either facilitate or hinder correct sound production. By way of illustration, it might be expected that a bilabial such as /b/ would be a facilitating context for correct production of the diphthong /ɒɪ/. The reason is that production of /ɒɪ/ involves the tongue, whereas /b/ does not. Therefore, /b/ production does not directly interfere or compete with tongue movements involved in /ɒɪ/ production. In other words, the word *boy* would be more facilitative for correct /ɒɪ/ than the words *toy* or *coy*.

Phonetic similarity between adjacent sounds might also have a facilitative effect. Gallagher and Shriner (1975, 631) stated that, "large articulatory adjustments seem to place more constraints on the speech production mechanism, and correspondingly, the chance of error for segments within the motoric unit is increased." The relevance of phonetic similarity to vowel therapy is that facilitative contexts involve relatively small articulatory adjustments, so for high-front vowels /i/, /ɪ/, facilitative contexts are alveolar consonants (such as /t/, /d/,

/n/), whereas facilitative contexts for highback vowels /u/, /ʊ/ are velar consonants (such as /k/, /g/, /ŋ/). Similarly, facilitative contexts for rising diphthongs /aɪ/, /eɪ/ are sequences such as /eɪt/ or /eɪn/ in which the raising movement of the tongue for the diphthong offglide is compatible with the following alveolar sound, which also involves tongue tip/blade raising.

In addition to inherently facilitative phonetic contexts for vowels, correct vowel production will be further assisted by considering the child's consonant system, and the constraints operating on it. Crystal (1985, 5) reminds clinicians to "teach one thing at a time." When applied to vowel therapy, the implication is that correct vowel production is facilitated in contexts involving well-established, correctly produced consonants and syllable structures. The application of this principle will, in almost all cases, limit the choice of words available for use in therapy, because most children with vowel errors also have reduced consonant inventories and syllable shapes.

Phonetic placement (Scripture and Jackson, 1925) is a motor-based technique used when children are unable to produce a particular sound in any phonetic context. In these cases, the clinician provides instructions to children regarding how to produce that sound. Placement methods include manipulating or holding articulators in place with a tongue depressor or the clinician's fingers (these procedures require strict adherence to health and safety guidelines). The use of mirrors to illustrate and provide feedback of lip and jaw position provides additional visual clues about lip position for vowels such as /i/, /a/, /u/. Clinicians can use a variety of illustrative material, including vocal tract and mouth posture diagrams, as a basis for discussions with children regarding how vowel targets are articulated. Details of vowel elicitation techniques can be found in Secord (1981) and Shriberg (1975).

Although phonetic placement techniques might elicit targets in some cases, Pollock's (1994) experience is that techniques such as phonetic placement are not always successful. Pollock goes further, suggesting that nonstimulable vowel targets are less likely than stimulable ones to improve as a result of therapy. It might be that some vowel features are more amenable to a phonetic placement approach than others. Without some form of computer-based visual feedback device, it is difficult to describe tongue position in the vocal tract in a way that is meaningful to young children (Reynolds, 1990). Lip posture, on the other hand, might be more amenable to phonetic placement because the lips are visually accessible.

Some articulatory-based therapy approaches for speech disorders use tactile and gestural cues for vowel errors. Prompts for restructuring oral muscular phonetic targets, developed by Chumpelik (1984), is an approach that involves applying a system of external tactile cues (using the clinician's hands) to the external regions of the child's vocal tract. The application of these tactile cues, or *prompts*, are altered in terms of degree of pressure and tension applied to specific muscle groups, and also in terms of the duration and speed of application. These tactile cues are applied to the vocal tract structures associated with voicing, nasality, and jaw opening. There is a different prompt for each phoneme, including vowels.

Cued vowels (Passy, 1990) are gestural cues involving hand signs representing tongue position for vowels. The hand signs also indicate whether there is lip rounding or not, and whether vowels are long, or short monophthongs, or diphthongs.

Motor/articulatory approaches were incorporated in several of the studies of therapy for vowel error patterns described in the beginning of this chapter. Pollock's (1994) therapy included drill and drill-play activities, and Hargrove, Dauer, and Montelibano (1989) used feedback, visual cues, and modeling. The hierarchy of difficulty from imitation to conversational speech used by Penney, Fee, and Dowdle (1994) and Hargrove and colleagues is typical of motor/articulatory approaches. Although some aspects of Hargrove and colleagues' approach resembled the traditional method, the program they described omitted traditional carryover phases. This could explain the poor generalization of accurate vowel production to connected speech occurring in this case.

Computer-Based Systems to Develop Perceptual Skills

Computer technology offers new possibilities for engaging children in auditory discrimination and identification tasks by the use of a variety of material, including synthetic speech material, which allows for selective cue manipulation (Hazan, Wilson, Howells, et al., 1995; Watson and Hewlett, 1998). Rvachew (1994) described a procedure known as speech assessment and interactive learning system for presenting receptive contrast activities. This procedure is a computer game (developed for children aged 3 to 9 years) used for the assessment and treatment of phonemic perception and phoneme identification, and for establishing appropriate phonemic boundaries. The basis for the program is a series of auditory stimuli representing correct and incorrect productions of words. The child identifies whether a production they hear is correct or incorrect. Rvachew found that children who received this auditory/perceptual program in combination with therapy focusing directly on production, made better progress than children who received therapy for production only.

Hazan and colleagues (1995) described a speech pattern audiometer, which is a computer-based speech perception assessment and therapy system. The system tests children's perceptual abilities to detect changes in temporal patterns, steady and transient formants, fundamental frequency, aperiodic versus periodic patterns, and nasality. A series of minimal pairs presented on a screen tests children's ability to categorize phonemic contrasts. Meaningful words, represented by pictures, are produced by high quality computer-generated syntheses. Elements of the words are individually manipulated, thereby producing a continuum of six stimuli in which the speech patterns under investigation are varied in small equal steps between the values appropriate for the original words. The system includes tests for vowel contrasts such as /u/,/i/; /o/,/u/; /i/,/ɪ/; /ɛ/,/æ/. Hazan and colleagues suggested that the system is applicable to treat impaired vowel perception in children who do not produce normal vowel contrasts.

Visual Feedback of Vowel Production

Visual feedback systems for vowel production can utilize either physiological or acoustic information and convert this into meaningful displays. The use of visual feedback in therapy derives its effectiveness from making ambiguous internal cues explicit, and enabling conscious control of such cues to develop. In relation to therapy for speech disorders, Shuster, Ruscello, and Smith (1992) suggested that biofeedback is particularly effective if details of target sound production are difficult to describe to clients. This applies especially to movement of the visually inaccessible articulators, such as the tongue during production of vowels. Thus, subconscious cues are made explicit and brought to conscious attention, and through interaction and practice, children can develop control over tongue position and movement. For example, in relation to consonant production, under normal circumstances, children are not aware that their anterior tongue should be positioned precisely on the alveolar ridge with a delicate groove formed through which the air is channeled during production of sibilant /s/. When undergoing visual feedback therapy with electropalatography, however, tongue positioning and grooving can be visualized, bringing these features to children's conscious attention (Hardcastle and Gibbon, 1997).

In terms of vowels, children might not be consciously aware of the height of the tongue during vowel production; however, F2 formant location on spectrographic displays reflects tongue height. Visual feedback of F2 can be used to make speakers aware of this feature. Increased awareness assists children's subsequent interactions with the feedback displays. At the same time as visualizing their speech, children can hear their own productions, thus allowing access to simultaneous visual and auditory information regarding their own correct and errored productions.

There are several clinical systems available that provide visual feedback of vowel production, based on acoustic analysis, although there has been little research on what type of visual feedback is of most value to children at particular ages. One issue concerns the timing of the feedback. For feedback to be effective, it must follow speech output as quickly as possible, but real-time displays might be too transitory to allow children to interpret the feedback.

Moreover, the delayed nature of the clinician's feedback might not allow children to recognize tactile and kinesthetic cues and associate them with correct tongue placement and posture as they occur. Many feedback systems, therefore, involve some mechanism for *freezing* the visual image. Another issue concerns the nature of the visual display. Some feedback displays attempt a visual representation of the articulators, which can support a direct articulatory approach to therapy. Others use abstract displays or games in which the visual display is unrelated to the mechanism of speech production, and the aim is to maintain children's attention and reward success.

Carter (1998) studied children's responses to types of visual feedback included in the autonomous speech rehabilitation system for hearing impaired people (Rooney, Carraro, Dempsey, et al., 1994). Carter found that this system evoked high levels of cooperation and positive evaluations from children with speech and language disorders aged 3 to 6 years, some of whom had phonological impairment. The types of visual feedback varied from abstract game activities (such as changing the height of an airplane by altering pitch) to explicit articulatory diagrams (such as a dynamic vocal tract diagram showing the tongue moving between alveolar and postalveolar placement, depending on the acoustic characteristics of the fricative produced).

Although Carter's (1998) findings must be treated with caution, as the speech tasks involved in each module were not directly comparable, it is interesting that children appeared more engaged and more able to modify their speech output when shown an abstract representation of vowels as *clouds* than when shown a vocal tract diagram. This study did not evaluate ongoing therapy and it might be that articulatory diagrams would be more effective in the context of an explicitly articulatory approach to therapy, or with older clients.

A game-playing approach is used by the IBM SpeechViewer II, which offers the vowel accuracy module to improve production accuracy of vowels. The screen in the vowel accuracy module shows two monkeys and a coconut tree. If the child produces a vowel that matches a preset threshold of acceptability, the lower monkey climbs the tree and pushes the upper monkey to release a coconut. The distance between the lower and upper monkeys is intended to represent the closeness of the match between the acoustic properties of the child's production and a template for the vowel target. The software has the facility to create different vowel target models, making it possible to customize the module for individual children.

The efficacy of the vowel accuracy module has been investigated in children with hearing impairment (Pratt, Heintzelman, and Deming, 1993; Ryalls, Michallet, and Le Dorze, 1994). Pratt and colleagues described the use of the vowel accuracy module with six preschool children. The vowels /ɑ/, /i/, /u/ were targeted over a 4-month therapy period. Positive effects of therapy for these vowels occurred in most children, although one child did not comply with therapy using the system. Out of the group, four children showed improvements in production of /u/, two for /ɑ/, and one for /i/, and these children demonstrated some generalization to untreated vowel targets.

Although positive treatment effects were observed in the study by Pratt and colleagues, there were some practical difficulties associated with the vowel accuracy module. These included inaccuracies in the feedback on low intensity, hypernasal, and high-pitched utterances, and an inability to sustain the attention of preschoolers over multiple sessions. Masterson and Rvachew (1999) reported difficulties similar to those identified by Pratt and colleagues with SpeechViewer. At present, it seems that although the SpeechViewer has potential to provide visual feedback for vowel errors in children with phonological impairment, there are some practical difficulties with its use.

Anecdotal reports from clinicians (Jocelynne Watson, personal communication) suggest that several modules available in the IBM SpeechViewer 3 program are valuable adjuncts to therapy for vowel errors. Useful modules include phoneme accuracy, multiphoneme chains, and two- and four-phoneme contrast modules. The phoneme accuracy module involves a game format requiring children to produce a single sustained phoneme, such as vowels /ɛ/ or /æ/. Accurate productions move a mobile character (such as a snail) up an incline, and the closer the children can match their productions to the target, the more progress the character makes up the incline. The multiphoneme chains module aims to improve accuracy of up to four phonemes produced in a sequence. The module is, therefore, useful for developing diphthongs from monophthong sequences (such as monophthongs /a/ and /ɪ/, which can be combined in a multiphoneme chain to produce diphthong /aɪ/).

The two- and four-phoneme contrast modules in SpeechViewer 3 are particularly useful as they provide children with not only multiple opportunities to produce contrasting monophthongs, but also powerful demonstrations of the consequences of homophony in their speech. The two phoneme contrast module involves driving a mobile (such as a jeep) around an obstacle course (such as wild animals in a safari park). The game could be set up so that the jeep moves right following production of /ɛ/, and moves left following production of /æ/. This arrangement would be appropriate if a child neutralized the /ɛ/, /æ/ contrast, thus producing both vowel targets as homophonous /æ/. The dramatic result of homophony, in this case, is that the child can only make the jeep move to the left; therefore, little progress is made through the safari park.

Confronting children with the consequences of their vowel neutralizations in this way prompts them to change their productions. Children often experiment at this stage by making interesting phonetic alterations to their vowel productions (such as lip spreading, vowel lengthening, volume changes) as they attempt to separate vowel contrasts. At this point, children are often receptive to phonetic placement or other cues that will enable them to produce more accurate vowels, and, consequently, succeed in controlling the jeep's movements.

The four-phoneme contrast module is similar to the two-phoneme contrast module, but involves a more complex activity. In this module, the production of four different phonemes steers a mobile square left, right, up, or down around mazes of varying difficulty. The four-phoneme contrast module is a useful way of contrasting a target phoneme with adjacent vowels in the vowel space. If the target vowel is /ɛ/, for instance, the four contrasting vowels could be front vowels /i/, /ɪ/, /ɛ/, /æ/. Although anecdotal reports suggest that SpeechViewer 3 is useful in helping children with phonological impairment to establish new vowel contrasts and to improve accuracy of productions, its use in therapy has not been investigated in controlled studies.

The use of spectrographic displays for improving vowel production in children with phonological impairment has received limited research attention, although there are reports of positive responses with vowel errors associated with other speech pathologies. Spectrograms provide cues for important speech features associated with vowels, with the location and shape of formant bands being the most visually salient cues for vowel identification (see Chapter 2). Ertmer, Stark, and Karlan (1996) used spectrographic displays to improve vowel production in two 9-year-old children with hearing impairment. The vowel production therapy involved four stages:

1. Presentation of spectrographic models helps learners recognize the visually displayed acoustic characteristics of a vowel target and discriminate acceptable from unacceptable vowel productions.
2. Instruction in articulator placement (such as tongue posture) focuses the learners' attention on the articulatory events needed to produce a target vowel.
3. Self-evaluation of spectrographic feedback helps learners recognize the spectrographic features of their vowel productions and to associate correct productions with orosensory cues.
4. Orosensory cues enable maintenance of correct productions as visual cues are phased out.

Ertmer and colleagues (1996) found that both children improved in at least some of the vowels targeted, and there was some evidence of carryover of practiced vowel targets to untrained words. The authors viewed one child's rapid progress as due to a sudden insight into the relationship between spectrographic patterns and positioning of the articulators for vowels. The authors stated that the relatively concrete, consistent, and immediate feedback provided by the displays allowed the children to be active learners through interaction with the visual displays.

Shuster, Ruscello, and Toth (1995) used visual feedback with a 10-year-old boy and a 14-year-old girl (with functional articulation disorders) who had failed to attain correct production of /r/ or /ɜ/, despite years of treatment. Intervention used a real-time spectrograph to display a correct /ɜ-/, produced by the investigator, located beside an incorrect /ɜ-/, produced by the child, on a computer screen. The two versions displayed side by side made visual inspection of differences possible, and allowed discussions about these differences to take place. Acoustic measures of the clients' productions, before and after treatment, indicated that older children and adolescents are able to use this type of visual feedback to attain correct production when other methods have failed.

Povel and Wansink (1986) used a vowel corrector with profoundly hearing-impaired people. The technique depicts vowels spoken in isolation, or in monosyllables, as small light spots on a screen, with different vowel sounds appearing in different areas of the screen. The system provides information about whether a speaker has produced a vowel correctly, or as an error. If the vowel is an error, the system indicates to what extent, and in what direction, the error deviates from the intended vowel. Although this system has potential for exploring the vowel space and for learning gross vowel differentiation, the authors stated that it has limited ability to detect subtle vowel differences. This probably restricts its usefulness as a therapy tool for children with phonological impairment.

Although there are obvious potential benefits for children to be gained from the use of computer-based visual feedback systems, and the systems might offer valuable support to clinicians' perceptual monitoring of vowel quality, the feedback provided needs to be treated with some caution (van Doorn, Shakeshaft, Winkworth, et al., 1998). Analysis and feedback relating to durational features should be quite robust in most systems. The signal processing problems associated with acoustic analysis of vowels in very young speakers with high F0, low intensity, nasality, or unstable F0 might set some insurmountable limitations on their use for precisely monitoring vowel quality in children with phonological impairment.

Visual Feedback of Vowel Production Using Physiological Techniques

Visual feedback about tongue position can be achieved using techniques such as glossometry (Fletcher, 1983; Fletcher, Dagenais, and Critz-Crosby, 1991), electropalatography (Dagenais, Critz-Crosby, Fletcher, and McCutcheon, 1994; Hardcastle and Gibbon, 1997), and ultrasound (Shawker and Sonies, 1985; Stone, 1997). Physiological techniques can provide feedback about articulatory features, such as tongue height and its relative position in the front/back dimension. An important advantage of these techniques over indirect acoustic information is that the visual feedback provided is both evaluation and informative, with direct articulatory information given regarding why mismatches occur and how to correct errors.

Glossometry has been used to provide visual models and feedback of tongue posture during vowel production in children with hearing impairment (Fletcher,

Dagenais, and Critz-Crosby, 1991). Glossometry is a technique involving light-emitting diodes and photosensor pairs mounted on an artificial plate molded to fit against the hard palate. The pairs are located in the midline of the plate. Light emitted from the diodes is scattered by the tongue, with the light reflected back to the photosensors being detected. The distance between the sensor and the tongue is computed and displayed on a computer screen. During therapy, model tongue positions are outlined on the computer screen, and a dynamic display provides real-time feedback of the vertical location of the tongue's position in the oral cavity.

Fletcher and colleagues used glossometry to teach the four corner vowels /i/, /æ/, /u/, /ɑ/ to six children aged 4 to 16 years with profound hearing impairment. Prior to glossometry therapy, the children had centralized tongue positions during vowel productions. After 15 to 20 therapy sessions, all the children showed greater diversification of tongue postures for the vowels, especially for tongue height. Fletcher and colleagues' study showed that glossometry enabled some children to produce more intelligible vowels and to use an expanded vowel space. These authors reported that several children showed increased tongue arching after therapy, suggesting that motor control for lingual postures became more independent from the jaw following therapy.

Electropalatography is a technique for recording, visually observing, and analyzing the tongue's contact with the hard palate during continuous speech (Hardcastle and Gibbon, 1997). Electropalatography has a facility for providing direct visual feedback of tongue-palate contact patterns. An essential component of electropalatography is a thin custom-made, artificial plate molded to fit the speaker's hard palate. A number of sensors embedded in the artificial plate detect the presence of contact between the tongue and the hard palate. Electropalatography is used primarily to provide visual feedback for lingual consonants. The technique can also be used for vowel errors involving the relatively close front vowels /i/, /ɪ/, /ɛ/, /u/ and diphthongs with a close front vowel component, such as /eɪ/, /aɪ/, /ɔɪ/ (Hardcastle and Gibbon, 1997). For further discussion of this technique, see Chapter 2.

Ultrasound is a noninvasive procedure used to display tongue position during normal and abnormal vowel production (Stone, 1997). Ultrasound uses the reflective properties of sound waves, with a piezoelectric crystal emitting an ultra high frequency sound wave and receiving the reflected echo. When the sound reaches the air at the surface of the tongue, it reflects back, thereby creating an image of the tongue consisting of a bright white line. It is possible to gain an image of the tongue by placing a transducer below the chin.

Although we do not know of any studies of ultrasound in vowel therapy, the technique has been used in a therapy program to establish consonants that are phonetically vowel-like. Shawker and Sonies (1985) employed real-time ultrasound biofeedback with a 9-year-old girl with a persisting speech disorder affecting target /r/, which she produced as [w]. Visual feedback was provided during speech exercises, enabling a comparison to be made between the child's tongue position and an ultrasound image showing the correct tongue placement prerecorded onto videotape by a speech clinician. Ultrasound feedback resulted in 100% accuracy of /r/, both during, and immediately after, therapy. Although accuracy fell somewhat after a 3-month nontreatment interval, some improvements in production of /r/ were maintained. Shawker and Sonies noted that success in therapy using ultrasound depends on the speaker's ability to interpret the tongue's image presented on the screen.

Although glossometry and electropalatography are potentially useful for vowel errors, their widespread use in therapy for children with phonological impairment is unlikely in the near future. There are several reasons for this. First, the financial cost of manufacturing custom-made plates for individuals undergoing therapy usually is warranted only if the speech difficulty is particularly severe, or has proved unresponsive to previous therapeutic efforts. Second, the procedural demands of these techniques make them unsuitable for use with young children, thus excluding many children with phonological impairment. Third, these techniques are not widely available in pediatric speech therapy clinics. Ultrasound is a promising technique for imaging the tongue during vowel production, and has practical advantages over glossometry and electropalatography because it does not require the manufacture of artificial plates.

Conclusion

The conclusion that emerges from the studies reviewed in the beginning of this chapter is that direct therapy for vowel errors had a positive outcome in the cases described. The view that progress was made in response to a variety of approaches is supported by Gierut's (1998) review. She reached a similar conclusion regarding therapies for consonant errors. Despite this optimistic picture of the effects of therapy, at present we do not know whether all children with vowel errors respond positively to direct therapy.

Although the studies examined contribute to our understanding of therapy for vowel errors, they are nevertheless limited in certain respects. The studies report small numbers of cases, so it is not possible to generalize the findings to other children with phonological impairment. Another limitation is that some studies did not report adequate baseline data, so it is unclear whether the progress reported was a result of therapy, or due to some other factor, such as spontaneous development.

The approaches discussed in the latter part of this chapter illustrate the wide range of options available to clinicians when devising therapy programs for vowel errors. Speech clinicians are familiar with many approaches (auditory/-perceptual, cognitive/linguistic, and motor/articulatory) because they are routinely used in clinical contexts for consonant errors. These approaches can be adapted with relative ease in order to target vowel errors. It is likely that the application of some instrumental approaches to vowel errors will be limited in clinical contexts at present, however, because some clinicians do not have access to computer-based technology and instrumentation. Despite the problem of limited access, new technologies offer exciting new opportunities for using visual feedback as a component of a therapy program for vowel errors.

Although a wide range of therapy options for vowel errors exists, clinicians still have limited empirical evidence on which to base decisions regarding which therapy approach is best suited to an individual child. Pollock (1994) stated that clinicians should not be discouraged by the current lack of clinical and research evidence, and urged clinicians to develop and implement therapy programs targeting vowel errors, and to document the results. Future research also needs to investigate factors influencing therapy outcome. Children's linguistic capability, and their degree of motivational effort during therapy, for instance, might influence outcome as much as the clinician's choice and implementation of a particular therapy approach (Kwiatkowski and Shriberg, 1993). Finally, there is a need to investigate the relative efficacy of different approaches so that clinicians know which are the most effective for vowel errors.

The Future: Developing Clinicians' Skills for Working with Vowels

One way to encourage further clinical research into vowel errors is to develop clinicians' confidence and skills in working with vowels. Experience suggests that vowel analysis is an aspect of phonetics that clinicians and students find particularly difficult. This is probably due to a combination of factors, including the fact that we accept a wide range of accent-related variations in vowels as normal, as Pollock and Keiser (1990) pointed out. In addition, vowels seem to be intrinsically more difficult to analyze in any categorical manner, because of the free variation between duration, anterior-posterior and close-open dimensions of tongue position and lip position.

A further compounding factor might be the lack of attention to vowels on phonetics curricula. A survey of curricular content of phonetics courses within speech and language therapy education programs in the United Kingdom (House, 1996) suggested that analysis of vowels was not given high priority on some courses. Many students are given practice in broad transcription only of Received Pronunciation, or of a limited set of accent types.

The increasing awareness of the importance of vowel disorders (evidenced in this book) highlights the necessity of teaching students to develop a high level of skill in vowel analysis and production. It is important that students develop their ability to analyze vowels in a way that integrates perceptual quality with articulatory parameters, taking into account factors such as duration and vowel movement. Curricula could develop skills in vowel mapping, by using a system such as the Cardinal Vowel system (Jones, 1917), provide familiarity with a wide range of normal and disordered vowel systems, and encourage confidence in using appropriate diacritics to modify vowel symbols of the international phonetic alphabet.

References

Adler, B., Rees, N. S., Serwer, B. L., and Stocker, B. (1968). Implications of vowel diphthong distortions. Exceptional Children, 35, 51–55.

Baker, A. (1981). Ship or sheep? An intermediate pronunciation course. Cambridge, England: Cambridge University Press.

Bernthal, J. E., and Bankson, N. W. (1998). Articulation and phonological disorders (4th ed.). Boston: Allyn and Bacon.

Blache, S. E., Parsons, C. L., and Humphreys, J. M. (1981). A minimal-word-pair model for teaching the linguistic significance of distinctive feature properties. Journal of Speech and Hearing Disorders, 46, 291–296.

Bunce, B. (1989). Using a barrier game format to improve children's referential communication skills. Journal of Speech and Hearing Disorders, 54, 33–43.

Carter, G. (1998). An evaluation of a visual feedback system (HARP) and its use with phonologically and pragmatically impaired children. Unpublished honours project. Edinburgh, Scotland: Queen Margaret University College.

Chumpelik, D. (1984). The PROMPT system of therapy: Theoretical framework and applications for developmental apraxia of speech. Seminars in Speech and Language, 5, 139–156.

Connery, V. (1994). The Nuffield Dyspraxia Programme: Working on the motor programming of speech. In J. C. Law (Ed.), Before school: A handbook of approaches to intervention with preschool language impaired children (pp. 125–141). London: Association for All Speech Impaired Children.

Crystal, D. (1985). Putting profiles into practice. Speech Therapy in Practice, 1, 4–5.

Dagenais, P. A., Critz-Crosby, P., Fletcher, S. G., and McCutcheon, M. J. (1994). Comparing abilities of children with profound hearing impairments to learn consonants using electropalatography or traditional aural-oral techniques. Journal of Speech and Hearing Research, 37, 687–699.

Dean, E., and Howell, J. (1986). Developing linguistic awareness: A theoretically based approach to phonological disorders. British Journal of Disorders of Communication, 21, 223–238.

Dinnsen, D. A. (1984). Methods and empirical issues in analyzing functional misarticulation. In M. Elbert, D. A. Dinnsen, and G. Weismer (Eds.),

Phonological theory and the misarticulating child (pp. 5–17). ASHA monographs No. 22. Rockville, Md.: American Speech Hearing Association.

Dodd, B., and Bradford, A. (2000). A comparison of three therapy methods for children with different types of developmental phonological disorder. International Journal of Language and Communication Disorders, 35, 189–209.

Eisenson, J., and Ogilvie, M. (1963). Speech correction in the schools. New York: Macmillan.

Elbert, M., and Gierut, J. (1986). Handbook of clinical phonology: Approaches to assessment and treatment. San Diego: College Hill Press.

Elbert, M., Rockman, B., and Saltzman, D. (1980). Contrasts: The use of minimal pairs in articulation training: Clinicians' manual. Austin, Tex.: Exceptional Resources, Inc.

Ertmer, D. J., Stark, R. E., and Karlan, G. R. (1996). Real-time spectrographic displays in vowel production training with children who have profound hearing loss. American Journal of Speech-Language Pathology, 5, 4–16.

Fletcher, S. G. (1983). New prospects for speech by the hearing impaired. In N. Lass (Ed.), Speech and language: Advances in basic research and practice (pp. 1–42). New York: Academic.

Fletcher, S. G., Dagenais, P. A., and Critz-Crosby, P. (1991). Teaching vowels to profoundly hearing-impaired speakers using glossometry. Journal of Speech and Hearing Research, 34, 943–956.

Flynn, L., and Lancaster, G. (1996). Children's phonology sourcebook. Bicester, England: Winslow.

Gallagher, T. M., and Shriner, T. H. (1975). Contextual variables related to inconsistent /s/ and /z/ production in the spontaneous speech of children. Journal of Speech and Hearing Research, 18, 623–633.

Gibbon, F., Shockey, L., and Reid, J. (1992). Description and treatment of abnormal vowels in a phonologically disordered child. Child Language Teaching and Therapy, 8, 30–59.

Gierut, J. A. (1989). Maximal opposition approach to phonological treatment. Journal of Speech and Hearing Disorders, 54, 9–19.

Gierut, J. A. (1990). Differential learning of phonological oppositions. Journal of Speech and Hearing Research, 33, 540–549.

Gierut, J. A. (1998). Treatment efficacy: Functional phonological disorders in children. Journal of Speech, Language, and Hearing Research, 41, 85–100.

Hardcastle, W. J., and Gibbon, F. (1997). Electropalatography and its clinical applications. In M. J. Ball and C. Code (Eds.), Instrumental clinical phonetics (pp. 149–193). London: Whurr.

Hargrove, P. M., Dauer, K. E., and Montelibano, M. (1989). Reducing vowel and final consonant prolongations in twin brothers. Child Language Teaching and Therapy, 5, 49–63.

Hazan, V., Wilson, G., Howells, D., et al. (1995). Speech pattern audiometry for clinical use. European Journal of Disorders of Communication, 30, 116–123.

Hodson, B., and Paden, E. (1983). Targeting intelligible speech: A phonological approach to remediation. San Diego: College Hill Press.

Hodson, B., and Paden, E. (1991). Targeting intelligible speech: A phonological approach to remediation (2nd ed.). Austin, Tex.: PRO-ED.

House, J. (1996). NetPHON: Network for education and training in phonetics. Final report to Department of Education and Employment. London: University College.

Howell, J., and Dean, E. (1994). Treating phonological disorders in children: Metaphon—theory to practice (2nd ed.). London: Whurr.

Ingram, D. (1976). Phonological disability in children. London: Edward Arnold.

Jones, D. (1917). An English pronouncing dictionary (1st ed.). London: Dent.

Kent, R. D. (1982). Contextual facilitation of correct sound production. Language, Speech, and Hearing Services in Schools, 13, 66–76.

Kwiatkowski, J., and Shriberg, L. D. (1993). Speech normalization in developmental phonological disorders: A retrospective study of capability focus theory. Language, Speech, and Hearing Services in Schools, 24, 10–18.

Leonard, L. B. (1995). Phonological impairment. In P. Fletcher and B. MacWhinney (Eds.), The handbook of child language (pp. 573–602). Oxford: Blackwell.

Masterson, J. J., and Rvachew, S. (1999). Use of technology in phonological intervention. Seminars in Speech and Language, 20, 233–249.

Matthews, B. (2001). On variability of vowels in normally developing Scottish children (18–36 months). Ph.D. dissertation. Edinburgh, Scotland: Queen Margaret University College.

Metz, D. E., Schiavetti, N., Samar, V. J., and Sitler, R. W. (1990). Acoustic dimensions of hearing-impaired speakers' intelligibility: Segmental and suprasegmental characteristics. Journal of Speech and Hearing Research, 33, 476–487.

Monsen, R. B., and Shaughnessy, D. H. (1978). Improvement in vowel articulation of deaf children. Journal of Communication Disorders, 11, 417–424.

Passy, J. (1990). Cued vowels. Ponteland, United Kingdom: STASS Publications.

Penney, G., Fee, E. J., and Dowdle, C. (1994). Vowel assessment and remediation: A case study. Child Language Teaching and Therapy, 10, 47–66.

Pollock, K. E. (1994). Assessment and remediation of vowel misarticulations. Clinics in Communication Disorders, 4, 23–37.

Pollock, K. E., and Keiser, N. J. (1990). An examination of vowel errors in phonologically disordered children. Clinical Linguistics and Phonetics, 4, 161–178.

Povel, D. J., and Wansink, M. (1986). A computer-controlled vowel corrector for the hearing impaired. Journal of Speech and Hearing Research, 29, 99–105.

Pratt, S. R., Heintzelman, A. T., and Deming, S. E. (1993). The efficacy of using the IBM SpeechViewer vowel accuracy module to treat young children with hearing impairment. Journal of Speech and Hearing Research, 36, 1063–1074.

Radford, N. T., and Gentry, B. (1997). Speech delay in seven siblings with unusual sound preferences. Perceptual and Motor Skills, 85, 1067–1072.

Reynolds, J. (1990). Abnormal vowel patterns in phonological disorder: Some data and a hypothesis. British Journal of Disorders of Communication, 25, 115–148.

Robb, M. P., Bleile, K. M., and Yee, S. S. L. (1999). A phonetic analysis of vowel errors during the course of treatment. Clinical Linguistics and Phonetics, 13, 309–321.

Rooney, E., Carraro, F., Dempsey, W., et al. (1994). HARP: An autonomous speech rehabilitation system for hearing impaired people. Institute of Acoustics 1994 Autumn Conference: Speech and Hearing. Windermere Hydro Hotel, 24–27 November 1994.

Rvachew, S. (1994). Speech perception training can facilitate sound production learning. Journal of Speech and Hearing Research, 37, 347–357.

Ryalls, J., Michallet, B., and Le Dorze, G. (1994). A preliminary evaluation of the clinical effectiveness of vowel training for hearing-impaired children on IBM's SpeechViewer. Volta Review, 96, 19–30.

Scripture, M. K., and Jackson, E. (1925). A manual of exercises for the correction of speech disorders. Philadelphia: F.A. Davis.

Secord, W. (1981). Eliciting sounds: Techniques for clinicians. San Antonio: Texas Psychological Corporation.

Shawker, T. H., and Sonies, B. C. (1985). Ultrasound biofeedback for speech training: Instrumentation and preliminary results. Investigative Radiology, 20, 90–3.

Shriberg, L. D. (1975). A response evocation program for /ɝ/. Journal of Speech and Hearing Disorders, 40, 92–105.

Shuster, L. I., Ruscello, D. M., and Smith, K. D. (1992). Evoking [r] using visual feedback. American Journal of Speech-Language Pathology, 1, 29–34.

Shuster, L. I., Ruscello, D. M., and Toth, A. R. (1995). The use of visual feedback to elicit correct /r/. American Journal of Speech-Language Pathology, 4, 37–44.

Stackhouse, J., and Wells, B. (1997). Children's speech and literacy difficulties: A psycholinguistic framework. London: Whurr.

Stoel-Gammon, C. (1990). Issues in phonological development and disorders. In J. F. Miller (Ed.), Research on child language disorders: A decade of progress (pp. 255–265). Austin, Tex.: PRO-ED.

Stoel-Gammon, C., and Herrington, P. (1990). Vowel systems of normally developing and phonologically disordered children. Clinical Linguistics and Phonetics, 4, 145–160.

Stone, M. (1997). Laboratory techniques for investigating speech articulation. In W. J. Hardcastle and J. Laver (Eds.), Handbook of phonetic sciences (pp. 11–32). Oxford, England: Blackwell.

van Doorn, J., Shakeshaft, J., Winkworth, A., et al. (1998). Models of Australian English vowels for commercial visual feedback systems. Proceedings of European Speech Communication Association Workshop of Speech Technology in Language Learning (STiLL 98) (pp. 53–56). Stockholm: Department of Speech, Music and Hearing, Royal Institute of Technology (KTH, Kungl Tekniska Hogskolan).

Van Riper, C. (1947). Speech correction: Principles and methods (2nd ed.). New York: Prentice Hall.

Van Riper, C., and Emerick, L. (1984). Speech correction: An introduction to speech pathology and audiology. Englewood Cliffs, N.J.: Prentice Hall.

Waters, D. (2001). Using input processing strengths to overcome speech output difficulties. In J. Stackhouse and B. Wells (Eds.), Children's speech and literacy difficulties 2: Identification and intervention (pp. 164–203). London: Whurr.

Watson, J., and Hewlett, N. (1998). Perceptual strategies in phonological disorder: Assessment, remediation and evaluation. International Journal of Language and Communication Disorders, 33 (supplement), 475–480.

Watson, M. M., Martineau, D., and Hughes, D. (1994). Vowel use of phonologically disordered identical twin boys: A case study. Perceptual and Motor Skills, 79, 1587–1597.

Weiner, F. (1981). Treatment of phonological disability using the method of meaningful minimal contrast: Two case studies. Journal of Speech and Hearing Disorders, 46, 97–103.

Weiss, C. E., Gordon, M. E. and Lillywhite, H. S. (1987). Clinical management of articulatory and phonologic disorders. Baltimore: Williams and Wilkins.

Index